PRAISE FOR *THE JOURNEY THROUGH CANCER*

"A timely addition to the medical bookshelf. . . . Dr. Geffen lauds the benefits of complementary practices in treating the person as a whole. But he does not advocate swallowing these notions and potions instead of proven treatments. [He tries] . . . to address the emotional and spiritual needs of his patients and provide traditional care. These efforts will sound refreshing for cancer patients, many of whom feel they are simply cases being run through a treatment mill."

—*New York Times*

"When a sixty-nine-year-old friend was recently diagnosed [with cancer] . . . his family and friends wondered how he would manage his late-stage disease. Dr. Geffen's *The Journey Through Cancer* will be my gift to him to help him on his journey. . . . Dr. Geffen's calm, balanced voice of experience convinced me that he is on to something."

—*Journal of the National Cancer Institute*

"Oncologist Jeremy R. Geffen, MD, has done medicine—physicians, nurses, allied health providers, patients, and their families—an extraordinary service in giving us this sensitive, thoughtful, beautifully written book."

—*The Integrative Medicine Consult*

"Dr. Jeremy Geffen is an oncologist of the future, one who integrates the best of traditional and nontraditional approaches. He addresses the physical as well as the psychosocial, emotional, and spiritual dimensions of health and healing. It is unfortunate that all people who are concerned with cancer can't have Dr. Geffen as their doctor; this book is the next best thing."

—Dean Ornish, MD, president of the Preventive Medicine Research Institute and author of *Dr. Dean Ornish's Program for Reversing Heart Disease* and *Love and Survival*

D1016215

"I finished *The Journey Through Cancer* and immediately thought, 'The world is a better place because Jeremy Geffen is in it.' To find an oncologist who combines the latest medical knowledge with the wisdom of the heart is a miracle. Step-by-step he leads the reader through every dimension of cancer and healing, from the nitty-gritty of the physical to the importance of the spiritual. This is the single best book ever written for those with cancer and those who love them."

—Joan Borysenko, PhD,
author of *Minding the Body, Mending the Mind*

"*The Journey Through Cancer* is a priceless gift. With love and grace, Dr. Jeremy Geffen creates a practical guide that stepwise builds enduring, complete healing of the body, mind, heart, spirit, and community. It can transform your *very next day* in the clinic to one of wholeness, joy, and endless possibility, and will in time reclaim for cancer medicine its fullest potential."

—John W. Rieke, MD, FACP,
Medical Director, Multicare Regional Cancer Center, Tacoma, Washington

"Dr. Geffen's vast knowledge, experience, insight, and compassion in the treatment of cancer patients shine radiantly through in *The Journey Through Cancer*. This is a useful book for anyone facing this serious challenge."

—Deepak Chopra, MD,
author of *Quantum Healing* and *Ageless Body, Timeless Mind*

"*The Journey Through Cancer* is an extraordinary book—a must-read for anyone facing cancer. Dr. Geffen's understanding of oncology and healing, combined with his compassion and caring, raise the bar for oncology care."

—Congressman Dan Burton

"This is a superb contribution to the literature on integrating the best of conventional and alternative cancer therapies."

—Michael Lerner, president of Commonweal and
author of *Choices in Healing*

"Dr. Jeremy Geffen offers all of us a wise, warm, and deeply informed vision of the kind of care that everyone with cancer should have. If you have cancer, buy this book."

—James S. Gordon, MD, director of the Center for Mind-Body Medicine and author of *Comprehensive Cancer Care: Integrating Alternative, Complementary, and Conventional Therapies*

"*The Journey Through Cancer* is an invaluable contribution for patients, families, physicians, nurses, and others involved in living with, treating, and caring for cancer patients. In this wonderfully engaging book, Dr. Jeremy Geffen provides both a practical guide and a range of choices through his seven-level program that will greatly enhance the lives of persons with cancer."

—Philip R. Lee, MD, professor of social medicine, emeritus, senior staff, Institute of Health Policy Studies, UCSF School of Medicine

"*The Journey Through Cancer* is written by a compassionate physician from the depths of his heart. The book captures, in a wonderful way, the importance of 'body, mind, heart, and spirit' as dimensions of ourselves and illuminates their roles in the healing process. It is a brilliant piece of work that undoubtedly will have an enormously positive impact on the lives of people with cancer and their families."

—Fawzy I. Fawzy, MD, professor of psychiatry, UCLA School of Medicine

"*The Journey Through Cancer* is a profound and deeply inspired guide for anyone dealing with cancer. Dr. Geffen skillfully leads you through every aspect of healing and transformation in a completely unique and practical way. His vision of multidimensional medicine is remarkable, real, and urgently needed. Don't miss this important book."

—Shirley Watson, DC, CCN, VoiceAmerica Network

THE

JOURNEY

THROUGH

CANCER

Healing and Transforming the Whole Person
NEWLY REVISED AND UPDATED

A Comprehensive Guide by
a Leading Pioneer in Integrative Medicine and Oncology

JEREMY R. GEFFEN, MD

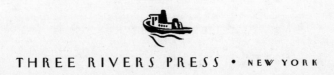

THREE RIVERS PRESS • NEW YORK

Originally published in slightly different form in the United States in hardcover by
Crown Publishers, an imprint of the Crown Publishing Group,
a division of Random House, Inc., New York, in 2000.

Library of Congress Cataloging-in-Publication Data
Geffen, Jeremy R.
The journey through cancer : healing and transforming the whole person /
Jeremy R. Geffen.— [2nd ed.]
"Newly Revised and Updated."
Includes bibliographical references and index.
1. Cancer—Popular works. 2. Cancer—Alternative treatment.
3. Integrative medicine. I. Title.
RC263.G426 2006
616.99'4—dc 22   2006002463

ISBN-13: 978-0-307-34181-5
ISBN-10: 0-307-34181-X

Printed in the United States of America

Design by Maria Elias

10 9 8 7 6 5 4 3 2 1

Revised Edition

*Dedicated to the spirit of freedom
and love
in the heart of all beings*

IF THE HEALING ART IS MOST DIVINE, IT MUST OCCUPY ITSELF
WITH THE SOUL AS WELL AS WITH THE BODY.

—APOLLONIUS OF TYANA,
FIRST CENTURY A.D.

AUTHOR'S NOTE

This book is not intended as a substitute for the medical advice of physicians. The reader should regularly consult his or her doctor in matters relating to health, symptoms that may require diagnosis or medical attention, and treatments. Every person is unique, and diagnosis and treatment must be individualized for the reader by his or her doctor.

CONTENTS

PREFACE

Six years have passed since the first printing of *The Journey Through Cancer*, a book written from my heart as well as from my experience as a Western-trained, board-certified medical oncologist. *The Journey Through Cancer* also drew on my background in Eastern philosophy and medicine, and complementary and alternative therapies. Then, as now, my intention was to guide and assist people dealing with cancer to find comfort, healing, and a greater sense of possibility and hope at every step along their journey. My intention has also been to provide an inspiring and practical model of how every dimension of human beings can be honored and cared for with equal skill and integrity on the cancer journey, and to demonstrate how this can be accomplished within the context of modern medicine and modern life.

Though the greatest truths about wellness and healing are timeless and remain unchanged, in recent years remarkable technological advances in science and medicine have made treatments for cancer and other serious illnesses possible that were unimagined even a decade ago. Many were not available when *The Journey Through Cancer* was first published, and many more are on the horizon. Despite these advances, millions of people are still seeking an approach to medicine and healing that is more holistic, compassionate, and sensitive to their needs as a whole person. This is particularly true for those facing the extraordinary challenges encountered with a diagnosis of cancer. In light of this, when I was asked to prepare an update to *The Journey Through Cancer*, I felt it was something that had to be done. Thus, this revised and updated edition was born.

In one way or another, cancer impacts virtually all of our lives. On an individual level, it is a life-transforming experience that often challenges the mind, heart, and spirit of patients and family members as deeply—if not *more deeply*—than it challenges the physical body. More than ever before, patients, family members, and health professionals must grapple with a dizzying array of conventional as well as nonconventional treatment options, which are ever-changing and often openly in conflict with each other. Those dealing with cancer must make decisions in the midst of what, for many, is the greatest health crisis of their lives. They must do so while searching simultaneously for meaningful ways of embracing the mental, emotional, and spiritual dimensions of healing. This process has never been more complex or challenging.

In this context, a number of very important questions arise: What is the most conscious, empowered, and comprehensive response to a diagnosis of cancer? How can we honor and care for the *whole person* along the way? What constitutes a truly integrative or multidimensional approach to health and healing? What are the essential elements of a comprehensive healing program? And how can all of this be accomplished within the context of modern medicine and modern life?

The Journey Through Cancer addresses these questions and more. Offering practical guidance, it describes seven essential areas of inquiry and exploration that are necessary for healing and transforming the whole person—the Seven Levels of Healing. This approach embraces the best of conventional medicine as well as complementary and alternative therapies. It also embraces every dimension of who we all are as human beings, and serves patients, practitioners, and caregivers alike.

While writing the first edition of *The Journey Through Cancer* I was directing the Geffen Cancer Center and Research Institute, in Vero Beach, Florida. I had established the Center explicitly to provide answers and solutions for cancer patients and family members seeking a genuinely holistic approach to understanding and treating their illness and themselves—in addition to receiving meticulous, conventional cancer care. It demonstrated, in a real-life, clinical setting, a new and inspiring paradigm of medicine: one that promotes awareness, healing, and transformation at the deepest levels of the body, mind, heart, and spirit.

For more than a decade, I was privileged to serve as physician, guide, mentor, and coach for thousands of patients and their family members on their personal journeys through cancer. During this time, I discovered the principles of the Seven Levels of Healing, and directly saw their power to positively impact the experience of everyone involved. Through this compelling process—working with individuals from all walks of life, facing illness of all types and stages—I became increasingly convinced of the universal nature and applicability of the Seven Levels.

In 2003 I closed the Center to focus full-time on sharing the ideas and principles of the Seven Levels of Healing with a much wider audience, through writing, speaking, and working with individuals and organizations. The experience I gained from my years of research and clinical work with the Seven Levels, as well as my understanding of cancer as a *journey,* has deepened my conviction in the power of this whole-person approach.

Since *The Journey Through Cancer* was first published, cancer has remained a predominant health concern in this country and worldwide. In fact, the social costs and implications associated with cancer are actually growing and expanding, despite the remarkable scientific advances in its diagnosis and treatment. This has occurred along with a significant movement in the United States involving the increasing use of complementary and alternative medicine (CAM) therapies by millions of people, costing billions of dollars. Many hospitals and clinics are also now beginning to explore how these therapies can be integrated into mainstream care, and more than 60 percent of U.S. medical schools now include CAM topics in their curricula.

The revised and updated edition of *The Journey Through Cancer* addresses these trends and provides information on important scientific developments in the understanding, diagnosis, and treatment of cancer. Numerous updated resources for information and support are also included. The fundamentals of the Seven Levels of Healing—and the inspiring true stories of patients who directly experienced them—remain intact, and indeed are ever more relevant.

One in three people alive today will be diagnosed with cancer at some point in their lives. Clearly, the need for a powerful, holistic approach to responding to cancer has never been more urgent. The Seven Levels of Healing program described in this book is an effective, tested model for healing and transforming the whole person. It could be widely adopted in hospitals, clinics, offices, cancer centers, and medical schools throughout the United States and beyond. It can also inspire many more patients and families to discover and experience peace, clarity, and comfort, wherever they may be on their journeys. It is my wish that *The Journey Through Cancer* will contribute to this vision, and continue to serve as a beacon of light for all who feel the impact of cancer in their lives.

THE
JOURNEY
THROUGH
CANCER

INTRODUCTION

WHERE THERE IS NO VISION,
THE PEOPLE SHALL PERISH.

—PROVERBS 29:18

Early in my senior year of medical school, my father was diagnosed with stomach cancer. It was a cool fall evening— September 18, 1985—and I had just arrived home after a tiring day. Flopping down in a big chair to relax, I casually pressed the Play button on my answering machine and was surprised to hear my father's voice. He rarely called.

"Oh, Jeremy," he said with some hesitation, "I think I've got a little problem. I had an endoscopy today and the doctor said I have a tumor in my stomach. Unfortunately, it's malignant. Maybe you could give me a call."

With my heart pounding I picked up the telephone and dialed his number. I knew this was not going to be a little problem. Not at all.

My father's illness occurred at a time when—after many years of distance and great difficulty in our relationship—he and I were falling in love with each other. I was twenty-nine, and like so many men of my generation I had missed a close relationship with my father. He was a tough, distant, romantic dreamer who during my childhood years was so deeply involved in his own struggles that he was unable to function as a parent in any conventional sense. When I was twelve he left our family to pursue his own life and dreams. He eventually built a career in New York City as the owner of two respected repertory cinema theaters and married a French woman who was a film director. They lived a remarkably bohemian life and were well known in the film circles of New York and Europe.

Although I now understand so much more of what occurred during those years, his departure was extremely painful. Still, after many years of challenge and conflict, we had recently, magically, discovered a love for each other that felt as exciting as any love I had ever known. At last, I was finally finding my father. And in the process, a deep, old, and hurtful wound was starting to heal.

As it turned out, his newly discovered cancer was an aggressive one. When his stomach was removed the next week we learned that the tumor had already spread into his liver and lymph nodes. "I'm sorry," the surgeon said after the operation. "The tumor was very extensive, and I couldn't get it all. I took out as much as I could. There's nothing more I can do."

Thus from the beginning the situation looked quite bleak. Our entire family felt stunned and completely disoriented, as if we had all been suddenly thrown into a bad dream. I could hardly believe this was happening. And there was a knot in the pit of my stomach that would not go away.

As the gravity of the situation began to sink in, my father's agony and the pain in my own heart and soul penetrated in a way I can hardly describe.

From that time until just before his death three and a half months later, we were partners in trying to find ways to help him fight and live. There was no small irony in the fact that early on in medical school I had decided that I would become an oncologist and dedicate myself to helping individuals and families who were dealing with cancer. Now suddenly, and in a very personal way, I was about to learn more about oncology than I had ever imagined, and much more about the extraordinary journey taken by people with cancer.

As a senior at New York University School of Medicine, I had access to the best hospitals and cancer specialists. My father also could afford the best medical care available. As we made the rounds of New York's top cancer centers and oncologists, I became progressively more discouraged by what he was experiencing. He was almost always identified by his tissue diagnosis *(high-grade gastric adenocarcinoma)* and stage of disease *(pathologic stage IV, with extensive liver and lymph node involvement)*, rather than by who he was as a human being. He was not seen as a *person with cancer*. Rather, from the moment of his diagnosis he was instantaneously and forever more transformed into a *cancer patient*. I had somehow managed to get through three years of medical school without fully understanding how quickly and pervasively this happens, or the effects it can have on those who are sick and on their families. And because of my father's particular diagnosis, he was invariably regarded as someone who was basically already dead. The words *metastatic gastric cancer* hung like an unpleasant odor in the room each time they were spoken, producing the same unmistakable frown on the face of virtually every oncologist he saw. Chemotherapy was offered, but with little enthusiasm, and always with a similar, unmistakable message—spoken or unspoken—that it probably wouldn't do much good. Instead, it was often gently suggested that it might be best for him to "get his affairs in order."

At no time did anyone even hint that my father himself could influence the outcome of what was happening to him. Nor were any ideas offered as to how he could at least improve the quality of the life he had left to live, regardless of how short a time that might be. Perhaps most distressingly absent were any suggestions of what he might do to deal with the mental, emotional, and spiritual aspects of all that he was experiencing: the tremendous fear and sense of loss associated with losing control of his body, the horrible sense of never being able to feel normal again, the loss of his stomach and the radically diminished ability to eat, the loss of his energy and strength, the end of life as he had known it, and the impending end of his life altogether. Somehow, unbelievably, he was left totally on his own to deal with all of these issues.

All of his family members and friends rallied to his side. However, we were also dealing with our own pain, sadness, anger, grief, and disbelief. Despite our best efforts, we were unable to find peace of mind in the midst of this traumatic time.

Late one afternoon, after a particularly discouraging visit with his oncologist, my father and I were riding home through Manhattan in a taxi. Some tests had come back that day and the results were not good. Although his oncologist was well-intentioned, and I am sure he meant no harm, the clinical, matter-of-fact way in which he had delivered such devastating information was hard to believe. It betrayed precious little—if any—awareness of the impact this was having on my father. And as usual, no meaningful or coherent follow-up support was offered.

During the ride home my father was more quiet and withdrawn than I had ever seen him. As we rode on in silence, I remember how strangely distant and gray the city looked. It was drizzling outside, and the rhythmic sound of the taxi's windshield wipers was all I could hear above the pounding of my heart and the sense of foreboding in my gut. As we began to pass through Central Park, crossing Fifth Avenue at Seventy-second Street, my father suddenly looked at me and began to speak.

"Jeremy," he said, his voice quiet, "I can now see that my doctors have given up on me." He paused before continuing, almost in a whisper, "How can I have any hope if my doctors have no hope?"

There was a look of resignation and defeat in his eyes that filled me with unimaginable sadness. I remember choking back tears as the deeper meaning of his words sank in.

How can I have any hope if my doctors have no hope?

And in that moment, I saw the light go out of my father's eyes.

Looking back now, I understand that that was the moment when my father gave up. Although in the coming weeks he fought on in many ways, I now see how in that moment of despair he decided that his battle had been lost.

His physician's message was now echoing loudly in my own mind, with an unexpected intensity. I was learning—the hard way—how powerful a physician's words could be and the enormous impact they could have on a patient, particularly someone with cancer.

I was also learning, more clearly and more personally than ever before, how the mind, heart, and spirit can profoundly influence the course of a patient's illness, the course of his or her life, and all too often the course of his or her death.

Soon thereafter we began making the rounds of alternative medicine, embarking on a blind search for *anything* that might help my father have a chance to live. Prior to medical school I had spent six years exploring Eastern religions and philosophy. For four of these years I lived in an ashram, a spiritual community, where I studied yoga, meditation, and vegetarianism, and learned a great deal about a variety of holistically oriented healing approaches. In addition, between my second and third years of medical school I visited Nepal and India. On that trip, which would be the first of numerous subsequent journeys to the East, I began to study the ancient and profound medical traditions of India and Tibet—Ayurveda and Tibetan medicine. I saw the immense power of these traditions to prevent and treat disease and to alleviate the suffering of human beings who are sick. So the next step seemed obvious. If conventional medicine couldn't save my father, maybe Ayurveda could. Or perhaps Tibetan or Chinese herbs. Or perhaps acupuncture or homeopathic medicine. Or perhaps some special diet. There had to be *something* that would work. And if there was, I was determined to find it. After all, this was my *father*—the one I'd never had before, the one I'd longed for all these years. I couldn't just sit by and let him die.

After seeing a variety of alternative health practitioners, it became increasingly clear that they were well-intentioned but remarkably limited in their knowledge of cancer. As a group they also tended to be extremely critical of conventional medicine, as fixed in their own beliefs as they accused the medical profession of being. The herbalists, naturopaths, and Asian medical doctors that my father saw were also emphatic that the chemotherapy he was now taking was "poisoning" him or "destroying" his immune system. Most refused to treat him as long as he insisted on taking chemotherapy. Sadly, I realized that this was fundamentally no different from the cancer specialists who insisted that they didn't want my father taking any "useless herbs" that might "interfere" with the chemotherapy—even while freely admitting that chemotherapy couldn't cure him anyway.

It was unbelievably frustrating. I felt as if I were stranded in a medical Tower of Babel, surrounded by doctors and healers who were all speaking radically different languages, unwilling and unable to hear or understand one another. Despite our ongoing pleas, they could not or would not look beyond their own particular viewpoints to see if there was anything else that could be done to help my father. Nowhere, it seemed, was there anyone who could provide any meaningful, coherent guidance about where to go, what to do, or how to dig through the avalanche of conflicting information that was coming at us from so many different sources. No one, it seemed, could guide us all the way through the painful and confusing journey we were taking.

Meanwhile, my father was growing weaker. He no longer had any appetite. Every day he lost weight and became more fatigued. Soon it became hard for him to move from his bed. Despite pain pills, shots, herbs, and acupuncture treatments, he was having increased abdominal pain and was vomiting up almost everything he put in his mouth. Nothing was working. We were running out of options, and running out of time. Above all, it was heartbreaking and devastating to see such a vigorous, independent, energetic man deteriorating so quickly.

At this point I began to realize at a deeper level what was really happening. Slowly and reluctantly, I began to face what I had tried with all my heart and mind and soul to avoid: he was going to die, and in fact was already dying. My beloved father was dying, and there was nothing I could do to stop it.

This realization marked the beginning of a major transition in our journey together. For my father, there was a sense of even deeper resignation to the inevitability of his own death. Accepting it was almost a relief for him, because he didn't have to fight anymore. But for me, facing it was extremely difficult because I didn't want to let him go. Deep inside, my heart was crying out, "No! Not now! Not when we have finally found each other after all these years!"

But the reality was inevitable. I had to accept that any further attempts to "help" would only ease my own pain, not his. In fact, urging him to fight on would only add to his burden, not relieve it. He really did not *want* to struggle anymore. He was so exhausted, and life inside his ailing body had simply become too emotionally and physically difficult. Even the simplest things had become overwhelming, and he had finally given up. But I felt so frustrated, even angry. "How can you not want to keep on fighting to live?" my heart demanded. It often took every ounce of self-control not to scream these words out loud.

At this point, trying to hold on to him was like trying to hold water in my hand; like water, he was slipping through my fingers. This was agony.

Intellectually, I knew I couldn't hold on any longer, but emotionally I wasn't ready to let go. No, not yet.

Then one day, in a moment of grace, I saw, and understood, and *accepted* that there was only one thing for me to do. I had to surrender completely to what was happening. No matter how much I wanted to or how hard I tried, I could not change the inevitable outcome. I realized that my greatest challenge now was to love my father as deeply and as fully as possible, while at the same time letting him go. To be there with him fully but no longer pushing or pulling him in any direction. To let him do completely as he wished in the last days or weeks of his life.

What happened in those last few weeks was profound. It transformed me as a person—and as a physician—in ways that I could not have imagined. As my father's own surrender and acceptance of what was happening deepened, I watched him go through a remarkable transformation— a spiritual awakening that I now recognize as a true healing journey. Though he died soon thereafter, he died with his eyes wide open, embracing the unknown with courage, grace, and love. Most important, our experiences together during the final days and weeks of his life—and in particular one special conversation we had—left no question in my mind that he reached the end of his time on earth with a deep understanding of himself, of life, of death, and of the nature of reality itself.

The incredible intensity of what I had shared with my father propelled me forward in my own journey. I began a deliberate search for greater understanding of all that had happened. I was filled with so many questions, and I felt that I simply had to find the answers—for myself, and for the many patients and families I would see and try to help throughout my life as a doctor.

Just as my experience with my father's illness had been frustrating and painful, I knew other people must be enduring the same thing, or much worse. Few cancer patients have access to the resources that my father did: I was a senior medical student in New York and was knowledgeable about cancer and mainstream medicine. I was also well informed about alternative treatments and had access to many of the best. Furthermore, my father had the desire to explore any treatment option that could conceivably help him. Despite all these advantages, our journey had been excruciatingly difficult and confusing. What must other people go through, I wondered, when they do not have any of these resources to help them? I shuddered thinking of this, and felt a deep resolve in my heart to do something about it.

Through my father's experience, I had come to appreciate the profound and universal challenges faced by people with cancer, or any life-threatening disease. In the years since then, this has been repeatedly confirmed by the vast number of cancer patients and family members who have shared their lives, their stories, and their extraordinary journeys with me. So many important concerns had been left unaddressed by my father's physicians during his illness. For instance, there was no meaningful advice about diet and nutrition. Except for recommending more pain and nausea pills, there were no suggestions of things my father could do to help ease his physical discomfort. And there was virtually no discussion of the intense emotional and spiritual issues a human being faces during such a profoundly challenging illness. These are aspects of cancer that the medical profession is only now beginning to address.

I saw too how inadequately my father's problems had been handled by *both* the mainstream and alternative medical systems. It was extremely difficult to find care that was reliable, technically sophisticated, and medically sound—as well as caregivers who were open-minded and knowledgeable about other approaches to healing. Furthermore, it seemed even more difficult to find state-of-the-art medical care offered in an environment that addressed the needs and longings of the mind, heart, and spirit of patients and their families in ways that were meaningful, coherent, and responsible.

From the pain of that experience a conviction began to grow within me that one day I would become the kind of oncologist that I wished so much had been available for my father: someone who understood Western science, but who also understood Eastern medicine and spirituality, as well as other models of healing and consciousness; someone who could look into the mind, heart, and spirit of a human being as intently as he could gaze at an MRI scan or a pathology report; someone who provided love, support, wisdom, and hope. A physician who genuinely embraced and lived these philosophies, and who was a truly joyful, spiritually conscious, loving human being. This meant becoming not only a fully credentialed and experienced doctor but a true healer as well, a person dedicated to helping people awaken to their true selves—to the infinite and eternal aspect of their being that is timeless, dimensionless, and untouched by any disease or circumstance.

For more than twenty years, I have pursued that vision every day. The journey has taken me to many extraordinary places around the world, and through many inner landscapes as well.

Along the way I have been richly blessed. Among the blessings for which I am most grateful is the experience of an intense, extremely high-quality education. I received my undergraduate degree from Columbia University and my medical degree from the New York University School of Medicine. I then had three years of internship and residency training in internal medicine at the University of California at San Diego Medical Center. This was followed by three more years of subspecialty training in hematology and oncology at the University of California at San Francisco Medical Center. These are some of the finest centers of medical education and training in the world. I deeply appreciate and give thanks for the knowledge I gained, the professional training I received, and the many extraordinary people I met.

I have also been blessed over many years by meeting and studying with some of the great spiritual teachers and leading-edge thinkers of our time. Each of them contributed profoundly to my growth and understanding, and their guidance and example have influenced my journey in deep and compelling ways.

All these experiences have profoundly inspired my work and vision for truly comprehensive, integrative medical care. Dedicated to this cause, I founded the Geffen Cancer Center and Research Institute in 1994, and directed it until 2003. It was one of the first cancer centers in the United States created specifically to provide a working model of complete, holistic care for people with cancer and their loved ones. The Center seamlessly integrated a wide array of conventional and complementary healing modalities in ways that were safe, practical, meaningful, and inspiring. The lives of thousands of patients and family members were profoundly impacted, as well as the lives of our highly skilled and dedicated staff members.

In working closely with these individuals over a number of years, I began to see that every single question and concern encountered on the journey through cancer falls elegantly, and organically, into one of seven distinct but intimately interrelated domains, or levels, of inquiry and exploration. This is particularly true for those seeking a deep experience of healing and transformation in their lives.

I'll never forget the morning when I awoke in a state of inspiration and clearly saw the pattern of the levels—the Seven Levels of Healing. I wrote them down and began sharing them with my patients and staff. Their feedback was uniformly affirming; the levels described and mirrored their own experience. It was like being handed a crystal-clear map of the entire terrain of the journey through cancer. It also soon became evident that the map and its principles were indeed universally applicable, as well as being eminently practical and inspiring.

In the ensuing years, I developed the Seven Levels of Healing into a coherent, well-organized program that became the foundation of the care offered to our patients and their loved ones. I also had numerous opportunities to share the Seven Levels of Healing with a large number of groups and organizations around the United States. Through this process, and mostly due to the courage and honesty of so many heroic people navigating the journey through cancer, I discovered numerous, essential distinctions about medicine that further deepened and transformed my understanding of what it means to be human, and to heal.

The book you're now reading is the result of this entire journey. The pages that follow present the Seven Levels of Healing program, which specifically addresses *all* the dimensions of who we are as humans—body, mind, heart, and spirit. In short, it encompasses the *whole person*. It explores the critically important role that these dimensions of ourselves play in the healing process and the extraordinary opportunity we have to understand and embrace them. It also examines the significant role that complementary and alternative approaches to healing and wellness can, and should, play in the care of people with cancer. Finally, it explores the dimension of our true nature that is beyond what can be seen or named. As a physician and as a human being, I believe the vision of this program can truly benefit and inspire us in all areas of life. If you are a cancer patient, family member, or caregiver, you can use this program and draw upon its vision in your own journey, regardless of where you are physically, mentally, emotionally, or spiritually.

Ultimately, the insights I offer here are those I sought for myself—as well as for the countless patients and family members who have taught me so much, and whose journeys through cancer have given so much inspiration and meaning to my own.

1

WHAT IS THE

PURPOSE OF MEDICINE?

FOR THIS IS THE GREAT ERROR OF OUR DAY,
THAT PHYSICIANS SEPARATE THE SOUL FROM
THE BODY.

—PLATO

In my years of training as a physician and an oncologist, I encountered and absorbed a vast amount of information. I also learned and mastered many different tools, technologies, and clinical skills, and a great many questions were asked and answered. But in all those years of study and preparation, the most fundamental question of all for a physician was never once raised.

What is the purpose of medicine?

Why are we doing this? What exactly are doctors trying to accomplish with all their hard work?

Perhaps it was assumed that everyone knew the answers to these questions: the purpose of medicine is to *fix* people—to replace illness with health. When a patient presents with a problem or symptom of some kind, medicine ought to return the patient to the condition that existed before the problem or symptom occurred. With respect to cancer, the purpose of medicine should be to eradicate tumors, normalize blood tests, alleviate pain, create clear CT scans, and prolong life. These, I believe, are the unspoken, culturally sanctioned notions of what physicians are supposed to do—and as a corollary, these objectives should be accomplished with the least possible effort, expense, and sense of personal responsibility on the part of everyone involved.

Despite its great achievements, the success of modern medicine in accomplishing these goals remains limited. This is especially true in oncology and the journey through cancer, where the challenges encountered by patients and family members alike can be extreme. Partly because of these challenges, millions of Americans—and cancer patients in particular—are turning to alternative and complementary forms of medicine. This trend is not motivated simply by the inability of mainstream doctors to cure their disease. It also arises, I believe, from a fundamental shortsightedness in medicine's understanding of what its purpose should be.

At present, doctors focus primarily on the physical characteristics of their patients—bones and organs, tissue samples, test results, height, weight, and age. Yet in each of us there is a rich mental, emotional, and spiritual reality that influences and even directs the course of our lives. Often, for both patients and their families, cancer brings this inner reality vividly to life and to the surface. If the inner reality is devalued or ignored by modern medicine, the effects can be devastating.

When you are diagnosed with cancer, conventional medicine may respond with surgery, chemotherapy, radiation, or perhaps another leading-edge treatment—in short, whatever is necessary to try to "get rid of the cancer." Throughout treatment, your physical signs and symptoms are carefully monitored. But many other important areas of your life receive far less attention. How is the illness affecting your marriage, your work, or your ability to find meaning and enjoyment in every day? What are your thoughts, beliefs, fears, and expectations about what will happen to you?

For most doctors and in most hospitals, these questions are of secondary importance at best. Individual physicians may address these issues, but most feel inadequately trained to handle them competently. As a result, when patients feel anxious or depressed, doctors will often prescribe anti-anxiety or antidepressant medications. Certainly there are instances in which these medications serve a very important role in the care of people with cancer. But, out of frustration or habit, many physicians rely on them as substitutes for addressing deeper issues.

A doctor's ability to deal with the mental, emotional, and spiritual concerns of his or her patients is often further restricted by the economics of medicine. Even if physicians have the desire and the skill to spend an hour in meaningful discussion with patients, the health care system in which they are working may make this impossible. In the era of the ten-minute managed care follow-up visit, anything but the most cursory assessment is often not possible. The financial, administrative, and time pressures on doctors in the United States have increased exponentially over the last decade, and current trends in managed health care suggest that things may only get worse.

It's important to mention too that a physician who explores emotional issues with patients and families may be opening a Pandora's box of unresolved feelings, such as guilt, anger, hostility, and confusion. Patients' demands and expectations can at times be wildly unrealistic, and disputes with doctors can degenerate into costly, time-consuming, and exhausting litigation. In oncology, where issues of life and death are commonly at stake and where decisions regarding diagnosis and treatment options can carry huge costs and consequences, emotions often run high. In response, many physicians choose to deal only with technical issues that can be clearly defined, objectified, measured, and treated.

All this often leaves everyone feeling frustrated and dissatisfied. Many doctors simply shut down emotionally and do the best they can under the circumstances. Meanwhile, and in increasing numbers, patients seek out alternative, complementary, and often unproven forms of care.

What is the solution? I believe it's time to enlarge our vision of medicine for cancer patients—and for all patients. In this new vision, medicine has two distinct purposes. The *relative* purpose of medicine is to relieve symptoms and to cure disease, to the fullest extent possible. But there is also an *ultimate* purpose, which extends beyond the physical realm to include the mind, heart, and spirit of every patient, and indeed of humanity as a whole.

In this view, cancer patients are understood to be asking two things of their physicians. On the relative level, patients most definitely want their illnesses cured. But this is not the whole story. On a deeper level, the ultimate reason people want to be cured is in order to feel love and joy in their lives. Quite often patients are convinced that their capacity for this has been violently stripped away by their diagnosis. Many cancer patients believe that they simply cannot experience the deepest levels of love and joy again until the doctor has gotten rid of the cancer. They have made a decision, consciously or unconsciously, that this physical criterion must be met before they can partake of the profound human emotions we all seek. They feel fundamentally separated from the emotions of love, joy, and fulfillment that make life worth living, and they feel that bridging the separation depends on the clinical work of the doctor or other practitioners they may also be seeing, or the treatments they are receiving, conventional or otherwise.

In light of this, I believe the ultimate purpose of medicine must be to foster the emotional and spiritual fulfillment that is a shared aspiration of all human beings. Moreover, medicine must empower patients to find that fulfillment *within themselves*—regardless of their diagnosis, their current condition, or their clinical outcome.

Thus, I would describe the ultimate purpose of medicine as follows: *to assist all beings to experience unbounded love, joy, and inner peace, and to know this is the essence of who we truly are.* This purpose deserves attention fully equal to the relative purpose of treating symptoms and curing disease.

Our potential to experience love and joy is in fact unbounded, and I believe that fulfilling that potential is the underlying objective of all human activity. But the fullest realization of that objective can never be found in external circumstances—not in a salary, an award, a relationship, or even in a clear CT scan. All external things will eventually change, and sooner or later will disappear. We must recognize, then, that the deepest levels of love, joy, and fulfillment we seek can only be found *within ourselves,* and in fact can always be found there, if we know how and where to look.

Helping patients to discover this is the ultimate purpose of medicine. If this purpose were understood and embraced, so much pain, confusion, and misery could be alleviated, regardless of our success in fulfilling the *relative* purpose of treating disease. Certainly cancer care demands the most advanced technology available, and providing that technology for patients has been one of my highest priorities for many years. But

I also know that no advances in chemotherapy, radiation, surgery—or immunological, genetic, or other targeted therapies—can ever fulfill the larger needs and concerns of patients and their families. Even when medicine succeeds in its relative purpose, even when the tumor has been eradicated and the CT scans are clear, our task is not complete unless the ultimate purpose has also been addressed. We must serve every patient's physical needs to the very best of our ability, but we must serve every patient's mind, heart, and spirit as well.

In striving to fulfill both the relative and the ultimate purposes of medicine, I have come to appreciate a fundamental insight that is often overlooked in daily life. In every moment we abide simultaneously in two domains of existence. The domain of *doing* encompasses all our worldly activities, efforts, identities, and endeavors. It includes everything we *do* to try to heal ourselves when we are sick, including taking chemotherapy, radiation, herbs, vitamins, massage, or acupuncture. But there is another domain of existence—the domain of *being*—that is equally real and important. The domain of being encompasses *who we really are*—beyond our thoughts, our individual identities, our successes, our failures, our sickness, or our health. And the domain of being is where the ultimate purpose of medicine leads.

The chapters that follow present a comprehensive, holistic program, the Seven Levels of Healing, which explores and embraces both the domains of doing *and* being in our lives. The program is also designed to fulfill both the relative and the ultimate purposes of medicine. Most important, it will show you how to embrace *all* the dimensions of who you are as a human being—whether a patient, a family member, a caregiver, or a friend—and will promote healing and transformation at the deepest levels of your body, mind, heart, and spirit.

The program is preceded by a discussion of "The Basics of State-of-the-Art Medical Care," which I believe must be the foundation of modern cancer treatment. Although the Levels are then presented sequentially, feel free to explore them in any order you wish. Many people find themselves returning to different Levels at different times in their journey. It is helpful to know, however, that in general terms, Levels One through Three focus on the most direct, practical issues involved in responding to a diagnosis of cancer, including optimizing survival and improving quality of life. Levels Four through Seven explore the deeper dimensions of healing and transformation that are possible on the journey through cancer, and indeed all of life.

An overview of the Levels follows.

"Level One: Education and Information" provides basic information about cancer and current treatment options. This empowers patients to actively participate in and obtain the greatest possible benefit from their care.

"Level Two: Connection with Others" explores the importance of reaching out to others for comfort and support on the journey through cancer.

"Level Three: The Body as Garden" invites patients and family members to see the human body as a growing and evolving whole, a wondrously complex living garden, rather than a machine. This level explores the benefits of good nutrition, exercise, massage, acupuncture, and the full spectrum of other complementary and alternative approaches to healing.

"Level Four: Emotional Healing" enters the inner realm of the human heart, where fear, pain, and anger can be acknowledged and released, and the healing power of self-love and forgiveness can be embraced.

"Level Five: The Nature of Mind" looks carefully at how our entire experience of life—including life with cancer—is profoundly influenced by our thoughts, our beliefs, and the meanings we give to events.

"Level Six: Life Assessment" explores the aspirations, goals, and purposes of our lives. What are we living for? What do we want to accomplish, experience, and share with others while we are alive, regardless of how long that might be?

"Level Seven: The Nature of Spirit" embraces the spiritual aspects of the healing process, as well as the dimension of our being that exists beyond illness, and even beyond birth and death.

As a physician, I seek to bring this vision of medicine and healing to my patients and to the world as a whole. My intention is that through this book you will be able to participate in this vision here and now, regardless of where you live and where you may be on the journey through cancer. I am confident that the time is coming when all patients, and all of medicine, will settle for nothing less.

2

BEVERLY IS EVERY

ONE OF US

"Dr. Geffen, you have a long-distance call on line six."

Debbie Dickerson, CLNI, the new-patient coordinator at our cancer center, was paging me over the intercom. Since it was the middle of a very busy afternoon, I knew it must be important.

Hurrying back to my office, I picked up the phone and heard a frightened female voice.

"Hello, Dr. Geffen. Thank you for taking my call. I'm so sorry to bother you like this, but I just had to talk to you. My name is Beverly Martin. I'm forty-four years old, and I'm calling from New Jersey. *I've just been diagnosed with breast cancer, and I'm terrified.* I had a lump in my breast, and it turned out to be malignant. Last week I had a mastectomy, and the cancer has spread into my lymph nodes. My doctor told me it is a high-grade infiltrating ductal carcinoma, and thirteen of nineteen axillary lymph nodes are positive. He says I'm going to need chemotherapy and radiation, but I'm so frightened. I've heard such awful things about chemotherapy and radiation, and I don't know what to do. I've never been sick a day in my life. I don't understand why this is happening, or where

19

to turn. My friend Phyllis heard you speak at a conference in Los Angeles last fall, and she told me I just had to call you. She said you'd know what to do. Will you help me? Is there any way I can deal with this other than chemotherapy and radiation? I'm so frightened and confused."

Listening intently, I took a deep breath. This woman was a complete stranger, but I recognized her fear and pain all too well. I'd seen and heard it in hundreds of newly diagnosed cancer patients, all of whom had suddenly been presented with the greatest challenge of their lives.

Calls like this come in almost every day. Indeed, they seem to be increasing in number, for reasons that are clear.

Cancer is a growing presence in our society. If heart disease was the affliction of the World War II generation, cancer is the disease of the baby boomers—and more and more people like Beverly, ready or not, are suddenly being forced to confront it.

Cancer Statistics in the United States

It is now estimated that nearly half of all American men and more than a third of all American women who are alive today will be diagnosed with cancer at some point in their lives. Each year more than 1.4 million individuals learn they have cancer—more than 3,800 every single day. And every day more than 1,500 people die from the disease.

In 2002, cancer surpassed heart disease as the leading cause of death in the United States among those under age eighty-five. Reports project that cancer may soon become the leading cause of death in America among individuals of all ages. In 2005, approximately 560,000 Americans died from it.

A number of factors have contributed to the increasing mortality from cancer in our country, including a growing population, reduced deaths from heart disease, and the fact that more people are living longer than ever before. Another reason for the rising number of cancer deaths is the increased incidence of certain cancers over the last half of the twentieth century. Notable among these are lung and colorectal cancer (although in recent years these have begun to decline in incidence). The last several decades have also seen increases in non-Hodgkin's lymphoma, leukemia, bladder cancer, liver cancer, thyroid cancer, and melanomas of the skin.

The increase in prostate cancer—which in 1994 surpassed breast cancer as the most commonly diagnosed invasive malignancy in the United States—has been particularly dramatic. In 1985, there were 85,000 cases of prostate cancer diagnosed in this country. By 1995, the number of cases had climbed to over 244,000. A significant percentage of this increase has been attributed to improvements in prostate cancer screening, facilitated most notably by the introduction of the PSA blood test in 1986. Since 1995, the number of men diagnosed each year has declined, largely due to fact that the enormous original pool of men who had never been screened has now diminished. Nonetheless, in 2005, more than 232,000 men were diagnosed with prostate cancer, and more than 30,000 died from the disease. Today a man in the United States is estimated to have a one-in-six chance of being diagnosed with prostate cancer in his lifetime.

Awareness of the alarming incidence of breast cancer has also grown steadily in the United States in recent years. In 1999, more than 175,000 women were diagnosed with invasive forms of breast cancer, and nearly 44,000 women died from the disease. In that year, almost 40,000 more women were diagnosed with noninvasive forms of breast cancer. While highly curable, these cancers nonetheless often require treatment with surgery and radiation. In 2005, more than 212,000 women were diagnosed with invasive breast cancers, and an additional 58,000 were diagnosed with noninvasive breast cancers. In that year, more than 40,000 women died from the disease. Most American women are now well aware that they have a one-in-seven chance of developing breast cancer at some point in their lives.

In early 2006, the first-ever decrease in total U.S. cancer deaths was reported by the American Cancer Society. Careful tabulation of final 2003 data revealed a very slight decrease in the number of total cancer deaths compared with 2002. The decrease was miniscule, representing less than one-tenth of one percent. However, this was the first decrease in total cancer deaths seen in this country in more than seventy years. Experts attribute the decline to reductions in smoking as well as earlier detection and more effective treatment of cancer. It is too early to know whether this historic finding heralds the beginning of a new, long-term trend. Nonetheless, the overall number of new cancer diagnoses continues to increase each year, and the cumulative impact of cancer in our society remains enormous.

The Economic Impact of Cancer in the United States

In 1985, the National Center for Health Statistics estimated the total cost of cancer in this country at $72.5 billion. By 1990, this cost approached $100 billion, and since then it has continued to rise. In 1996, the cost exceeded $143 billion, and in 2005, the National Institutes of Health estimated that the overall costs for cancer had reached nearly $210 billion. Cancer now consumes approximately 10 percent of the entire health care budget in the United States.

The rising economic impact of cancer is attributable not only to the growing number of cases in this country. Many people are living much longer with the disease and require evaluation and monitoring with expensive technologies such as CT scans, MRI scans, PET scans, and sophisticated blood tests. Cancer treatments are also becoming more complex and often more expensive as well. For example, in recent years high-dose chemotherapy with peripheral stem cell transplantation has been used for an increasing number of hematologic malignancies—and it generally costs tens of thousands of dollars per patient. There has also been tremendous growth in the use of expensive drugs, including Neupogen (filgrastim), Neulasta (pegfilgrastim), Procrit (epoetin alpha), and Aranesp (darbepoetin alpha). These are synthetic forms of naturally occurring hormones, also known as *growth factors,* that stimulate the production of red and white blood cells. Originally these drugs were available only in universities and at major medical centers and were used sparingly. But they soon proved so beneficial that they are now routinely used in oncologists' offices all across America.

Over the past several years there has been an unprecedented increase in other drugs and technologies approved by the FDA for the care and treatment of cancer patients. Important examples include drugs such as Herceptin (trastuzumab), Tarceva (erlotinib), Avastin (bevacizumab), and Gleevec (imatinib mesylate), which are used for breast, lung, and colon cancer and chronic myelogenous leukemia, respectively. Hundreds of additional drugs are currently in the clinical research pipeline, and these will be steadily released in the future. New treatments for prostate cancer include *intensity-modulated radiation therapy* (IMRT), which is being utilized increasingly throughout the United States.

Almost without exception, all of these powerful modalities have been and will continue to be immensely helpful to many patients. But they will also continue to add to the overall expense of cancer care in our country.

All this illustrates an important point. If a new vision of medicine that honors and cares for the mind, heart, and spirit of human beings, as well as their bodies, could even slightly improve the incidence, morbidity, or mortality from cancer—or at the very least reduce the costs of cancer care, or the *suffering* experienced by cancer patients and their families—this would translate into tremendous benefits for millions of people in our country and across the world.

A significant and growing interest in complementary and alternative medicine (CAM) in the United States, particularly since the early 1990s, suggests that such a new vision is already coming into being. A landmark 1993 article in the *New England Journal of Medicine* pointed out that in 1990 approximately one-third (33.8 percent) of all Americans used some kind of CAM in their daily lives. Since then, the utilization of complementary and alternative forms of medicine has progressively increased. A follow-up to the 1993 article, published in the *Journal of the American Medical Association* in November 1998, revealed that by 1997 the utilization of complementary and alternative forms of medicine had risen to 42 percent of all Americans.

A 2004 report by the National Center for Health Statistics indicated that in 2002, some form of complementary or alternative medicine was used by 62 percent of American adults within the prior twelve months. The report also indicated that 75 percent of American adults had used complementary or alternative forms of medicine at some point in their lives. It was additionally noted that Americans spent between $36 billion and $47 billion on complementary and alternative therapies in 1997. Between $12 billion and $20 billion of this amount was paid out of pocket for the services of professional CAM providers. This exceeds the amount that the U.S. population paid out of pocket for all hospitalizations in 1997, and is about half that paid for out-of-pocket physician services.

While these trends continue to touch all areas of health care, they are particularly prevalent among cancer patients. The subject of unconventional cancer therapies has received extensive coverage in the media. From all the statistics and anecdotes, I believe two points are especially important.

First, a number of studies have shown that up to 80 percent of all cancer patients utilize at least one form of unconventional therapy at some point in their illness. The second point is very disturbing: *most patients do not fully disclose their use of complementary or alternative therapies to their medical oncologist.* They often pursue these treatments in secret. When trust between patients and physicians is eroded, this in itself can be a serious impediment to the healing process. In addition, lack of open and honest communication can be medically dangerous for patients who may not understand that adverse interactions can occur between various kinds of therapies.

Why is this happening? Why are so many people exploring complementary or alternative approaches to cancer treatment, often at great expense to themselves? Moreover, why are they so often not discussing it with their physicians? Some of the most compelling answers follow.

Despite the tremendous advances in cancer detection and treatment in recent years, conventional medicine is still unable to cure many patients with cancer. When confronted with what may be considered by conventional medicine to be an incurable disease, patients and family members will often turn to complementary or alternative methods in their search for hope.

Many patients are frightened by the rigors and challenges they may encounter as part of conventional cancer treatment, so they seek out forms of care that might be less arduous, less invasive, and less toxic—even if those alternatives might be less effective as well.

Quite a few patients explore complementary and alternative therapies to relieve symptoms associated with cancer and conventional cancer treatments.

Patients and family members frequently turn to complementary or alternative methods because they are seeking a system of care that is more sensitive to their needs as a whole person. They want care and attention for their mind, heart, and spirit as well as their body.

Patients are often reluctant to discuss their interest in complementary and alternative therapies because their oncologist has neither the time nor expertise to address their questions coherently. Even worse, patients are often fearful of having their interest in these therapies ridiculed or dismissed out of hand.

Despite these concerns, a new kind of cancer patient is beginning to appear. These are people whose expectations of medicine are very high—not only in terms of clinical treatment but also in their demand that physicians communicate clearly, honestly, and compassionately. When patients seek out complementary and alternative therapies, it is often because they long to be listened to, cared for, and *heard.* If there is one lesson that conventional medicine can learn from complementary and alternative therapies, it is the importance of listening attentively to patients and enlisting their participation at every level of the healing process.

The nature of the discussion between a cancer patient and his or her doctor has undergone considerable evolution in the last several decades. In the past the general consensus was that people were better off not knowing the whole truth about their condition. Even direct questions were often deflected with ambiguous responses from doctors and nurses. For a variety of reasons, the situation is now completely different.

One of the most important reasons for this change is a dramatic evolution in cultural beliefs, which now emphasize a patient's "right to know." The notion that a patient's informed consent must be unambiguously obtained before any medical procedures are performed is now the cultural standard as well as the legal one.

Another obvious reason for the changes in the nature of discussions between patients and doctors is the availability of so many more options. These include sophisticated and innovative surgical procedures, advanced radiation therapy techniques, and complex chemotherapy regimens. However, these carry new risks and potential side effects, which must be explained and discussed.

Finally, amid all these choices, and despite the clear advances in many areas of cancer treatment, the best option for a particular patient is often not clear. Along with the stress and fear of a cancer diagnosis, the resulting uncertainty can be extremely difficult for patients and family members alike.

Beverly, whom we met at the beginning of this chapter, found herself confronting this kind of situation following her surgery. There were a number of paths she could follow: no further treatment, complementary and alternative therapies, or conventional chemotherapy and radiation all the way up to the option of high-dose chemotherapy with stem cell transplantation, which was an accepted treatment at that time. She could also try to somehow integrate all these options. Although many people offered Beverly advice, no one could provide her with absolutely clear assurances one way or another. Ultimately she would have to consider her options, review the statistics and reports that were available, consider the advice and opinions of her doctors, family, and friends—and then . . . she'd have to make her own choice.

A week after our initial telephone conversation, Beverly came to see me for a consultation. She desperately wanted advice and counsel from a physician who not only was experienced and knowledgeable about conventional cancer treatments but also would be willing to help her explore other options. She felt frustrated because she hadn't been able to find anyone who would guide her through *all* the options. And she was certain of one thing: the stakes of making the "wrong" decision were high.

After we talked for a while, Beverly asked me a very direct question. "What would you do, Dr. Geffen, if this were you, or your sister, or your wife?"

Her question was a powerful one, but not unexpected. Whenever I counsel a person with cancer, this is a touchstone that I always use: *What would I do if this were me, or a member of my own family?* Fortunately, in Beverly's case, I felt clear about what I would do, so it was relatively easy for me to respond.

I could see that she was somewhat surprised by my answer. She knew by now of my strong belief that cancer treatment should include mental, emotional, and spiritual components, with a variety of appropriate complementary therapies for the body as well. She may have expected that I would suggest forgoing the conventional medical treatments. But, while acknowledging the limitations of chemotherapy and radiation therapy, I explained my strong belief that these modalities, when used skillfully and sensibly—and with love, compassion, wisdom, and humility—can be extraordinarily beneficial.

"I would pursue a number of options," I said. "I would do chemotherapy and radiation, and I would also closely monitor studies involving emerging new conventional treatments for breast cancer. There are also many complementary therapies I would explore, especially those relating to diet, nutrition, exercise, and stress relief. And I would do everything possible to explore the deeper dimensions of who I am as a human being, and the deeper dimensions of healing the body, mind, heart, and spirit.

"You see, Beverly," I continued, "it is true that you have a physical body, and your body needs love, care, and attention. There is no question that this is very important, and we will make sure that we accomplish this in a meticulous and elegant way. But you are a whole person, and you have a mind, a heart, and a spirit that need love, care, and attention as well. I believe that honoring and caring for these other dimensions of yourself is just as important as caring for your body.

"Whatever you do," I concluded, "in the midst of your treatment—including chemotherapy and radiation or whatever complementary therapies you might also use—don't forget to find out what is most important to you in life. And above all, don't forget to find out *who you really are.*"

Fortunately, Beverly had a bit of time before she had to make her decision, which is true for most, but not all, patients. She and her family had decided to take a brief vacation to think things over together. I thought this was a great idea, and I encouraged her to spend some of her time sitting quietly and listening to her heart. I suggested that she start writing her thoughts and feelings in a journal every day, including any questions that might come up, and I asked her to call me if she wanted to discuss anything further. At the end of our meeting she thanked me and promised to be in touch again soon.

Beverly embodies and expresses all the strengths and vulnerabilities of the contemporary cancer patient. In a later chapter, we'll meet her again and see how her fear and sense of isolation were transformed into a very different experience—mentally, emotionally, and spiritually. It is important that we learn from Beverly in this way, because as the statistics clearly show, cancer is an extremely widespread disease that will impact all of our lives in the years to come. Once we understand this, we'll see that Beverly is much more than a typical cancer patient. Beverly is every one of us.

3

THE BASICS:

STATE-OF-THE-ART MEDICAL CARE

EXCELLENCE, THEN, IS NOT AN ACT, BUT
A HABIT.
                                        —ARISTOTLE

This brief chapter exists to make a very important point. It is my absolute conviction that every cancer patient should receive state-of-the-art medical care, administered by a highly trained and thoroughly qualified team of caregivers, under the meticulous supervision of an experienced oncologist. This must be the foundation of every cancer treatment program.

Within that general conviction are several additional points that must be made. It is important to address the suspicion and hostility with which many cancer patients, particularly younger ones, approach conventional cancer treatment. A mythology of war stories has grown up around the triad of surgery, chemotherapy, and radiation therapy, which are often called "poisonous" or even "barbaric." There is no doubt that many people have indeed experienced a great deal of pain, frustration, and toxicity associated with these therapies. And this has led some patients to avoid or abandon conventional medicine altogether. However, I believe it is almost always a serious mistake for patients to rely solely on unproven alternative therapies as their primary cancer treatment.

First, there are many instances in the course of care for cancer patients when a decisive medical intervention—especially when performed early in the diagnosis—can literally mean the difference between life and death. Missing such an opportunity because of fears or mistaken ideas about conventional treatment is tragic.

Second, for all the drawbacks and limitations of conventional medicine, alternative or complementary modalities of care can offer nothing that even remotely matches the proven benefits of conventional medicine in treating cancer—particularly on a consistent, reliable basis. Even the great medical traditions of the East, including Ayurveda, Chinese medicine, and Tibetan medicine, clearly acknowledge their own limitations once a disease process has become well established, as it usually has by the time cancer symptoms are manifest.

This is not to suggest that alternative and complementary therapies do not have significant benefits to offer patients, which they most certainly do. But there is an important distinction between therapies intended to treat the *illness* directly and those intended to help treat the *person* who has the illness, as we will explore further in "Level Three: The Body as Garden" (page 95). At present there are few, if any, scientifically proven benefits of alternative or complementary therapies as a direct treatment for cancer, despite anecdotal evidence to the contrary. Thus, while it is possible that some patients may indeed benefit from alternative and complementary cancer therapies, to choose them exclusively over proven conventional treatment remains a risky proposition.

There is really no reason why conventional medical care and other approaches to healing should be considered mutually exclusive. In fact, it is becoming increasingly recognized that great benefits can be achieved when they are integrated in a thoughtful, rational way, in a trend known as *integrative medicine*. I firmly believe the proper role of these other approaches is as *adjuncts* to conventional care. It is nonetheless absolutely clear that the treatment options now offered by conventional medicine are safer, less toxic, and far more effective than ever before—and are getting better all the time.

For example:

• A number of cancers that were routinely considered deadly just twenty-five years ago, including Hodgkin's disease, testicular cancer, hairy cell leukemia, and childhood leukemia, are curable in the majority of cases, and up to half of all patients with non-Hodgkin's lymphoma can now be cured.

- Advances in screening and postoperative treatment of breast and colorectal cancer have resulted in a 30 to 40 percent reduction in deaths from these two common cancers.
- At one time a diagnosis of acute myeloid leukemia (AML) was virtually a death sentence. But now 65 percent of all AML patients treated with chemotherapy achieve a complete remission.
- Treatment of chronic myelogenous leukemia with newer agents, particularly Gleevec (imatinib mesylate), has also led to dramatic improvements in overall survival compared with just ten years ago.
- Recent advances in the treatment of non-small cell lung cancer with the combination of newer chemotherapy drugs, radiation, and advanced surgical techniques are now extending life in many patients beyond what was considered possible just a few years ago.
- Advances in the treatment of ovarian cancer and multiple myeloma over the past decade have led to significant improvements in survival of patients with these diseases.
- The preservation of anatomy and function has been greatly advanced in the treatment of many cancers, including those of the eye, breast, larynx, esophagus, rectum, anus, and prostate.
- The addition of chemotherapy to surgery has significantly enhanced survival in the treatment of osteogenic sarcoma (a form of bone cancer), and chemotherapy plus radiation or surgery can now cure a majority of patients with Ewing's sarcoma (another form of bone cancer).
- Significant advances have also been made in the area of pain control. New medications, implantable pumps, and more sophisticated surgical interventions give many patients more freedom from pain than ever before.

There is abundant reason to believe that progress against cancer will be even more dramatic in the near future. Entirely new classes of treatment are emerging, many of which are grounded in stunning breakthroughs in molecular and genetic technology. Over the past twenty years, important new understanding of cancer has been gained through research on:

- *Oncogenes,* which promote the growth of cancer cells
- *Tumor-suppressor genes,* which must function effectively if cancer growth is to be forestalled
- *DNA damage and repair,* which play central roles in the formation and longevity of cancer cells
- *Molecular cell biology,* which explains the underlying mechanisms of growth for both malignant and normal cells
- *Angiogenesis,* the ability of tumors to generate the blood vessels that are necessary to provide them with vital nutrients
- *Metastasis,* the process by which tumors spread throughout the body
- *Apoptosis,* the mechanisms that regulate the programmed life span of cells

Advances in these areas are now enabling physicians to attack the disease process at its most fundamental levels.

The Human Genome Project, which involved the mapping of the 3 billion units of encoded genetic information contained in every human cell, was completed in 2003. The information gained from this enormous endeavor is leading to an even deeper understanding of the genetic basis of cancer, and is contributing greatly to the general field of *genomics,* which studies the overall role of genes in human health and disease. This information is also leading to treatments that are closely matched to a patient's individual genetic makeup.

An international effort has also begun to define and map the more than 1 million different proteins that are estimated to be present in the human body. This emerging field is called *proteomics.* The Human Proteome Organization, comprising hundreds of scientists all over the world, is coordinating leading-edge research that promises the ability to identify cancer at a far earlier stage than is currently possible. This research may also lead to even more novel and dramatic improvements in cancer prevention, diagnosis, and treatment.

Significant advances have occurred in a variety of diagnostic technologies that greatly enhance our ability to detect cancer, including high-resolution spiral CT scans, positron-emission tomography (PET) scans, digital mammography, and more powerful MRI scans.

In addition to the significant number of new and more effective chemo-therapy drugs that have been released in recent years, great gains have also been made in controlling the side effects of chemotherapy. When chemotherapy is carefully administered and monitored, nausea and vom-iting now only rarely occur. Sophisticated techniques—including the use of growth factors and stem cell transplantation—allow oncologists to safely administer higher doses of chemotherapy. This significantly lowers the chances of relapse in many patients and provides cures for many others.

Today there are more than 10 million living Americans who at one time have been diagnosed with cancer. Roughly 5 million of those people have been alive for more than five years since their diagnosis, and the majority of those 5 million are considered cured. Virtually all of them owe their lives to the achievements of conventional medicine.

New developments in gene therapy, immunotherapy, and other emerg-ing fields may soon race far ahead of current treatments. Gene therapy is an area in which extremely interesting developments are taking place, es-pecially with the discovery of increasing numbers of oncogenes and tumor suppressor genes. Likely hundreds of these genes are in every human cell, and the location and function of dozens have already been identified. Mutations of one important tumor-suppressor gene, called *p53*, have been linked to up to 70 percent of colon cancers and are very prevalent in a wide variety of other human cancers. Another well-known oncogene, *HER-2/neu*, has been found to be overexpressed in approximately 30 per-cent of breast cancers. Understanding of this oncogene has already led to significant changes in the way many patients are being treated for breast cancer.

Immunotherapy, which uses the body's own defense mechanisms against cancer, holds the promise of creating vaccines against malignan-cies similar to those for measles, polio, and other formerly widespread diseases. The ability of malignant cells to bypass the body's immune defenses is a key reason why cancer is such a dangerous illness, but sig-nificant progress is being made in understanding how and why this oc-curs. Effective immunotherapies require an ability to identify specific markers, called *antigens*, which differentiate between malignant and normal cells. Once these antigens are better identified, they can become targets for emerging and more effective immune-directed therapies.

One of the most significant areas of development in recent years involves what are called *targeted therapies*—new medications directed at specific antigens and other genetic and molecular mechanisms. One broad, emerging class of targeted therapies is *monoclonal antibodies*. These are drugs directed at a variety of different tumor antigens, and their use is becoming increasingly widespread. A well-known example includes Herceptin (trastuzumab) for breast cancer, which is directed at the HER-2/*neu* antigen. Rituxan (rituximab), now commonly used for non-Hodgkin's lymphoma and chronic lymphocytic leukemia, is directed at an antigen called CD20. Tarceva (erlotinib), used for non-small cell lung cancer, and Erbitux (cetuximab), used for colorectal cancer, are directed at an antigen called epidermal growth factor receptor (EGFR).

Avastin (bevacizumab), also used for colorectal cancer, is directed at an antigen called vascular endothelial growth factor (VEGF), which is involved in the formation of tumor blood vessels. Emerging drugs of this type are called *anti-angiogenesis* or *anti-angiogenic* therapies. They hold great promise for the treatment of many different kinds of cancer, particularly when combined with more conventional chemotherapy drugs.

As our knowledge of these all-important genes, antigens, angiogenic mechanisms, and other biochemical processes continues to advance, a true understanding of the molecular basis of cancer will become increasingly clear. As this is achieved, we will be dealing with the causes of cancer at a deeper level than ever before. This will not be just pouring water on the fire of a growing cancer. It will be removing the fuel that the fire needs in order to burn. In this way, many more cancers will be cured outright, and still others may be transformed into manageable, chronic diseases that patients can live with for years or even decades.

In addition to these advances, vastly more sophisticated techniques are now being used in the search for other entirely new anticancer drugs. Extremely powerful computers, along with new insights into the inner workings of cells, are enabling researchers to design specific drugs from scratch, rather than having to search for them in nature or among laboratory chemicals. This process, called *rational drug design,* is an extraordinary advance in the history of medicine. It holds great promise for the treatment of cancer and virtually all other diseases.

What is leading-edge research today will be routine cancer treatment tomorrow. The emerging modalities are so powerful and fundamental they are certain to shift the very foundations of medicine. As this process takes place, patients' basic perceptions and responses to cancer will also transform. There is no question in my mind that we are now at the threshold of this transformation—and, indeed, have already begun to step through the door.

4

LEVEL ONE:

EDUCATION AND INFORMATION

Nothing in life is to be feared.
It is only to be understood.

—Marie Curie

W hen you are diagnosed with cancer, questions instantly begin to flood your mind. At times, these can be overwhelming. . . .

What is this illness? How did I get it? What will happen to me? Where should I go for treatment? How am I going to pay for it? Does my doctor really know what's going on? Does he or she really care about me? Will I be in pain? Will I be disfigured? Am I going to lose my hair? Will my family and friends still care about me? Am I going to die?

On the journey through cancer, it is vitally important for these and many other questions to be answered accurately, sensitively, and appropriately for your individual needs. Intense fears and beliefs about cancer, even if they are not entirely accurate, can profoundly influence every aspect of the experience. The process is further complicated by the vast amount of information about cancer and cancer therapies that is now available.

In the midst of all this, there is a certain amount of basic information that can be of immense benefit to patients and their family members.

Level One of this program is intended to provide that information in a succinct and coherent way.

If your mind is filled with doubts and worries about basic aspects of your medical care, it will be impossible for you to make the best choices about your treatment or derive maximum benefit from it. At the very least, it is important for you to feel confident about the medical care you are receiving. Without this, you will be plagued by fears and anxieties that can adversely affect your healing. You may also risk side effects, treatment delays, or other complications that can be avoided by a basic understanding of your care.

Once these fundamental questions are answered, you can begin to explore the deeper dimensions of healing.

The disease we call cancer actually includes well over a hundred different illnesses, each with a different presentation, natural history, and treatment approach. Patients affected by one of the many different forms of cancer are themselves very different from one another. The point at which a diagnosis is made also varies from patient to patient.

Two patients, for example, may receive identical diagnoses, but the fact that their illnesses have the same name is often much less significant than the particular molecular, genetic, and biological features of their tumor and the extent to which the tumor has progressed. Differences in their overall physical condition, their emotional makeup, their support network, and their beliefs and expectations about cancer treatment are also important. These two patients may have entirely different experiences during their illness, and their outcomes may differ as well.

Although cancer is usually described as a war and is often discussed—by doctors, institutions, the public, and the media—using military terminology, I encourage people to think of cancer as a journey; say, a rafting trip down a river. Sometimes the river can be relatively easy and slow; at other times there are sharp turns and frightening rapids. Like all journeys, different travelers begin at different points on the river, with different levels of knowledge and experience.

In order to get to your destination it is essential to know what sort of river you are traveling on, and where on the river you are starting. You will also need an experienced guide who has navigated this river many times before: someone who knows its twists and turns, and how to best support you along the way. This guide, of course, is your oncologist, and the relationship between you and your doctor is extremely important. But the journey down the river also requires the participation of your companions and the crew of your raft. Your companions are your family members, friends, and associates. The crew includes the medical support staff who is involved in your care, including nurses, phlebotomists, laboratory and radiation technicians, receptionists, billing and insurance staff, and social workers.

As with your doctor, you should be very aware of the profound effect your companions and crew members can have on your journey. If the people beside you are angry or rushed, if they're impatient or distracted, or if they're not really loving their work, it will influence the quality of your experience in a significant way.

Be especially alert to the beliefs and feelings of your caregivers. Do they share the philosophy that cancer treatment is a journey, or at the very least an opportunity for learning and spiritual growth? Or do they see it as an ordeal, or a punishment to be endured? Although it may be challenging for a new patient to understand, the journey through cancer should not be rushed. It is important to take an appropriate amount of time to make informed, empowered decisions. It is also helpful to stop at various places along the way to look over the terrain, to reflect on what's really happening, and to see what you can learn from the entire experience.

I hope it's becoming clear that the experience of cancer includes much more than the technical aspects of medical care. Your relationships with family, friends, and caregivers will play a vital role. Careful choice of your doctor and awareness of the environment in which you are treated are also vitally important. Your medical team should certainly be technically competent, but they should also clearly demonstrate that they truly care about you as a unique human being.

"I've just been diagnosed with cancer. What should I do?"

Upon receiving a cancer diagnosis, you may find yourself facing this frightening experience without any knowledge or understanding of how best to help yourself. The sheer volume of information that is now available about cancer and various treatment options can make the aftermath of diagnosis even more distressing for you and your family. The appropriate answers to your questions are unique to you and your specific circumstances, and they should come directly from your oncologist. However, a few basic principles can help everyone who faces this challenge.

1. Recognize that fear is natural, and know that it can be overcome.

For the great majority of patients, there is a sharp and very understandable focus on the physical aspects of the illness and treatment process. An important message of this book bears repeating here: *the mental, emotional, and spiritual aspects of cancer are often as immediate, urgent, and challenging—if not more so—than the physical concerns.* By understanding and recognizing fear as a completely normal reaction, you can begin to develop the conviction that it can and will be overcome. Recognize your need for love, support, and highly reliable information, and know that you can and will find it. No matter how scared or confused you may be feeling, you must consciously choose to believe that you will get the care and support that you need and deserve. Decide right now to seek out and utilize the many sources of comfort and emotional support that can so greatly benefit you at this time. You will be amazed by the number of loving, caring individuals, organizations, and groups that are ready and willing to help. Information about these is provided in the appendixes at the end of this book. But you must be open and willing to receive what they have to offer. Once again: decide right now to give yourself the gift of love and support that can be so precious at this critical time.

2. Slow down the decision-making process.

In the initial phase of dealing with cancer, you may feel a sense of urgency to decide what kind of surgery, chemotherapy, radiation therapy, or other treatments you should have. You may also want to know about taking herbs, vitamins, and supplements; how you should change your diet; and what other complementary and alternative therapies might be of value—and you may want all this information *immediately*. Very few instances exist in cancer treatment, however, in which such urgency is warranted. The process can almost always be slowed down for at least a few days in order to gather information and support. Don't allow yourself to be frightened or pressured into making any decisions about your treatment until you have a clear understanding of your choices. Take time to explore your options. Take time to breathe—and breathe deeply!

3. Ask yourself this question: "Do I have trust and confidence in my doctor?"

In order to safely and effectively navigate your way through the diagnosis and treatment of cancer, you must have a qualified guide. In my opinion, this guide should be a well-trained oncologist who is experienced in dealing with your particular kind of cancer. In addition, you should feel assured that your doctor cares about you as an individual, and that he or she truly has your best interests at heart. Your doctor must also be able to readily take care of you if you become sick. What kind of hospital or medical center is the doctor affiliated with? What other specialists are available, if needed? Where will you go if you have problems or complications from your illness or treatment? Is this an environment in which you feel safe, comfortable, and genuinely cared for?

In many instances, dealing with cancer is straightforward, and the course to follow is clear. Sometimes, however, the best course is not clear at all—a wide array of options and treatment approaches exist for many cancers. Each has its own advantages, disadvantages, risks, benefits, and potential toxicities, and appreciating these distinctions will take time and careful consideration. In such cases, it is important to communicate openly and directly with your doctor, and to have all your questions and concerns adequately addressed. If you feel this is not happening, you should by no means compromise. You must find and choose a doctor you can talk to, who genuinely respects your viewpoint, feelings, and wishes. This may require interviewing a number of oncologists. Don't hesitate to get a second opinion, or as many opinions as you need, until you feel at ease with your doctor and the options presented to you. Your relationship with your oncologist may become one of the most important relation-ships in your life, so make sure you are comfortable and confident before you proceed.

4. Recognize that your physical body needs love and attention, but so do your mind, heart, and spirit.

Cancer is most certainly a crisis that is occurring in the physical body, and it is imperative that patients receive the best possible medical care for their disease. Once again, this care must be led by a competent, caring, and qualified guide, and administered in an impeccable manner. Inte-grating other modalities such as nutrition, exercise, vitamins, herbs, sup-plements, acupuncture, and massage can also be extremely important and valuable. But while you have a body, who you are is not limited to your body. You are *a whole person.* Thus, for healing to be complete, all the di-mensions of who you are as a human being must be addressed with equal skill and attention—including your mind, heart, and spirit. Take time every single day to honor and care for these other dimensions of who you are.

5. Recognize that life is a journey, and so is dealing with cancer.

All of life has a rhythm, a natural unfolding, and this includes the expe-rience of cancer. It is important to seek out the information and care that you need. But it is equally important to remember that you need time to rest, to relax, to experience silence, and to be still. Give yourself this time each and every day. It is also important to give yourself permission to feel what you feel. Don't judge yourself—in any way—for whatever you may be experiencing at this moment in time. Know that dealing with cancer is a process in which you can and will become skilled and masterful. Recog-nize the fact that right now more resources exist to help and guide you than ever before in history, and these resources are fully available to you. You can find what you need, and you will.

FOUR MAJOR CATEGORIES OF CANCER PATIENTS

There are four major categories of cancer patients, and they all have their own unique hopes, fears, needs, and concerns. Understanding which of the four major groups you belong to can help you and your family members resist the panic reflex that is so often activated by the word *cancer*.

1. Newly diagnosed patients who have not yet had surgery or begun other treatments

New diagnostic techniques, screening methods, and heightened awareness of cancer risks are changing not only the needs and concerns of cancer patients but also their clinical profiles. In an increasing number of new patients, cancer is far less advanced and far less life-threatening than in the past. Invasive cancers of the prostate, breast, lung, and colon are, in descending order, the most commonly diagnosed forms of the disease. In early stages, each of these, and many other forms of cancer, are potentially curable by surgery alone.

Currently about 50 percent of all people who are diagnosed with cancer will be cured with surgery. More than half of all colon cancer patients, for example, will have their early-stage tumors removed and the disease will not reappear. Other kinds of cancer may also become surgically curable following initial treatment with chemotherapy or radiation (called *neo-adjuvant* therapy).

This extremely positive news is tempered by two other realities. First, more than 600,000 people per year in the United States are not cured with surgery. Second, all too often surgically treated patients live in fear that the disease will return. Although their cancer is gone, they may be no better informed about how diet, exercise, and other factors can affect their health.

2. Patients who have undergone surgery and are being advised to have further treatment

Following cancer surgery, many cancer patients are advised to receive additional treatment with chemotherapy, radiation, or both (called *adjuvant* therapy) to prevent or diminish the chances of recurrence. For example, a woman who has undergone a lumpectomy for breast cancer is usually advised to have radiation to the remaining breast tissue. She may also be told that she needs four to six months of chemotherapy, and very likely at least five years of *hormone therapy* as well. Following surgery for colon cancer, a patient may be advised that he needs chemotherapy lasting up to six months. Similar therapies are now commonly recommended for patients who have undergone surgery for cancers of the head and neck, lung, ovaries, uterus, and bladder, among others.

Many patients regard these treatments with almost as much fear and anger as they have for the disease itself. Again, these feelings often appear reflexively, from associations with horror stories they have heard over the years. Perhaps a breast cancer patient has read an article describing chemotherapy as poisoning the body with chemicals to cleanse it of disease. Or a man with colon cancer may read that chemotherapy is like dropping a bomb on a battlefield in the hope it will kill more bad guys than good guys.

I would like to make three important points concerning these fears.

First, fear is a poor starting point for decision making. It can cloud your judgment and lead to decisions made in haste, without all the information you need to be truly informed about your options and their consequences. Even though others may have had a particular experience or outcome, it doesn't mean that you will, too.

Second, it is important to replace fear with knowledge, and ultimately with wisdom. Many of the things you fear about your diagnosis or treatment may simply not be true. Your physician should offer information about your illness, your condition, and the anticipated benefits of therapy. He or she should also explain the possible side effects that are part of many cancer treatments, even though many of them are much less debilitating than they were just a few years ago. You should also have a clear understanding of all your options for different kinds of treatment. If real data about your condition suggest that a particular therapy can have clearly defined benefits, you should strongly consider going ahead with it. Finally, attention must also be given to the mental, emotional, and spiritual aspects of your well-being. Later in this chapter (on page 79) you will find a very effective five-step process to help you make decisions about your treatment.

Third, the unique nature of each patient—not just the specificity of your diagnosis but your essential individuality as a human being—must be addressed.

Every person responds to treatment differently. What is challenging for one person may be easy for another. Attitudes and beliefs can also play a big role in how different individuals approach their care. Many patients, for example, have built their identity around health, nutrition, and exercise. They want their cancer treatment to be congruent with the healthy lifestyle they've followed for years. While I wholeheartedly believe in following a healthy lifestyle, that lifestyle did not prevent these patients from getting cancer, and it may not prevent cancer from coming back. Once that point has been made, though, decisions can follow on the basis of patients' personal feelings, combined with an accurate picture of their condition.

3. Patients with unresectable or metastatic cancer

A third group of patients are those whose cancer is not curable by surgery because the tumor is technically unresectable, or has spread from the primary site. When cancer spreads to other locations in the body, it is known as *metastatic cancer*. In some cases the original, primary site is never identified. Except in very rare instances, surgery is no longer a meaningful option. Therefore, it is not surprising that most patients with unresectable or metastatic tumors are generally less resistant to beginning chemotherapy or radiation treatment, particularly if there is a recognized benefit they can reasonably expect from their therapy. But here, as at every other stage of the journey, no one should focus only on the strictly clinical elements of cancer care. There are many other things you can do to promote healing in body, mind, heart, and spirit, and we will be discussing these throughout the remainder of this book.

For most patients with cancer, but especially those with metastatic cancer, the illusions of immortality that we all tend to harbor are profoundly shaken. This can be emotionally painful and frightening, but it can also be one of the genuinely illuminating effects of the cancer experience. It is an opportunity to have a transforming experience of yourself and the world you live in. It is a chance to learn and grow in ways that you may never have imagined before. Even if your illness is eventually cured, your experience of cancer can make an enormous difference in how you live each day from now on. It can impact—at the very deepest levels—every aspect of the way you engage life, and how you face death as well.

4. Patients whose cancer has relapsed, or is no longer responding to treatment

When a relapse occurs and it becomes unlikely that a cure will be achieved, an entirely new set of questions arise. At present, approximately 40 percent of all cancer patients will eventually find themselves in this category.

In addition to the spiritual issues that emerge at this point, concerns such as pain management, nutrition, and maintaining everyday quality of life reassert their importance with a new urgency. When you or a loved one has cancer that has relapsed or is no longer responding to treatment, what do you do with yourself and how do you choose to spend the time you have left? The realization that life really will end at some point can bring new meaning to every moment and can open undreamed-of possibilities for love and growth. If that sounds sentimental, please be aware that I've made the journey through cancer with thousands of people, including members of my own family. I have seen cancer ignite pain, but I've also seen it kindle love, fulfillment, inspiration, and joy at the deepest levels. While few people are oblivious to the first possibility, it is important that they not ignore the second.

Though the explicit goal may no longer be to cure your cancer, there is still a great deal that can and should be done to enhance your enjoyment and quality of life. It is also important to carefully consider further options that might extend survival as well.

New anticancer drugs and therapies are appearing every day, and advances are being made in entirely new domains of treatment. Newspapers, books, magazines, television, and the Internet provide up-to-the-minute information on these developments. Many late-stage patients and their family members hope that a new experimental treatment will cure their disease. This belief often occurs whether the therapy is being offered at a major National Cancer Institute–designated cancer center or at an alternative medicine clinic in Europe, Mexico, or the Bahamas. It also occurs even if the therapy is an unproven herbal compound that can be purchased through the mail. Very few late-stage patients or their family members understand that only a relatively small percentage of patients will personally benefit in a significant way from experimental or unproven therapies. However, when an experimental therapy is offered at a legitimate cancer center, as part of a legitimate clinical trial, the information gained from the trial can be potentially invaluable for the lives of others, and many patients find this meaningful and comforting. Such a benefit is rarely possible at clinics that offer completely unproven, and often completely irrational, alternative therapies.

As someone who has spent the majority of his adult life dealing with cancer in a clinical setting, I've found that the true miracles of cancer rarely take the form of drugs, potions, or herbs. More often than not, the true miracles take place in the minds, hearts, and spirits of patients and their families.

CANCER QUESTIONS AND ANSWERS

What is cancer?

As stated earlier, *cancer* is a broad term that encompasses well over a hundred different diseases. Although varying degrees of difference and similarity exist among these diseases, they share certain fundamental characteristics. All cancers involve abnormal cells that differ in two important ways from other cells in the body.

First, cancer cells divide in an uncontrolled, disordered manner. When this happens, they form tumors that can grow, impinge upon, or even invade adjacent tissues and structures in the body.

Second, most cancer cells have the capacity to spread from their original point of origin to other sites, where they can continue to grow. This process is called *metastasis,* and for most cancers it is what causes the most serious problems for patients.

What causes cancer?

This is one of the most controversial and perplexing areas in our understanding of the disease. Contrary to some popular misconceptions, human beings are not the only species to be afflicted with cancer. Virtually all animal species, including mammals, fish, birds, reptiles, and amphibians, have the potential to develop cancer. Tumors have been documented in all of them.

Nor is cancer solely a product of the Industrial Age. Evidence of tumors has been found in Pleistocene cave bears and dinosaurs from the Cretaceous Period, as well as in Egyptian mummies from 3000 B.C. Cancer is even mentioned in one of the world's oldest medical treatises, the Edwin Smith Papyrus, which originated in Egypt between 3000 and 2500 B.C. Here, eight classes of tumors or ulcers of the breast are described that are believed to have been treated with primitive forms of surgery. Even Hippocrates, one of the giants of ancient medicine, wrote extensively about cancer in the fourth century B.C. and postulated about its possible causes.

One of the most remarkable and challenging aspects of cancer is that it arises from cells within our own body that were previously normal.

Current medical science describes the origin of cancer as a sequence of events at the cellular level that culminates in the appearance of cancer cells. The sequence begins with changes in the genetic material of normal cells brought about by so-called cancer *initiators.* These can include *external* factors, such as cigarette smoke, exposure to other carcinogenic chemicals, exposure to ionizing radiation, or, rarely, viruses and *internal* factors such as abnormal hormonal activity or inherited genetic abnormalities. One of the effects of these initiating factors is to activate certain cancer-causing genes, called *oncogenes.* Just as important, initiating factors can also cause other genes that suppress the development of cancer, called *tumor-suppressor genes,* to become inactive. When the normally fine-tuned balance of activity between oncogenes and tumor-suppressor genes has been disrupted, cancer cells can begin to grow. Once cancer development has been initiated, it can be furthered by the presence of a variety of cancer *promoters,* including alcohol, chemicals, and dietary factors.

Since the discovery of oncogenes in the 1970s, a challenging philosophical question has been raised: Why do human beings have genes in their DNA that can influence the development of cancer? The answer is still unknown. One theory proposed is that—under normal circumstances—these genes may play an important role in the regulation of development of the human embryo. It is when these genes become altered in some way, or are inappropriately activated or over-activated, that they lead to abnormal cell growth and multiplication, which can eventually result in cancer.

While it is tempting to attribute the cause of cancer to events or substances in the external world, or to internal physiologic or genetic changes, an important distinction has to be made between the true *cause* of cancer and the *mechanisms* by which cells become cancerous.

For example, while many people who smoke and drink do get cancer, many more do not. Genetic factors have been cited as a possible explanation for this, but inadequately so. Thus, it remains unclear why individuals can have such widely different manifestations of health or disease. Viruses have also been implicated in the origin of some cancers, though rarely and without a complete understanding of exactly how this can occur. Just as with smoking and drinking, it is still unclear why most people infected with certain potentially cancer-causing viruses never get the disease.

Scientists generally postulate that the difference between individuals will be found in specific deficits or changes in their immune function, or in other constitutional factors. However, the nature of the specific differences in immune function or constitution from one individual to another are still poorly understood.

In recent years, a great deal of attention has been focused on the fact that some people have cancer that appears to run in their families. These inherited predispositions have led to a great deal of research on the possible specific inherited genes that might be causing the problem, such as the

BRCA1 and *BRCA2* genes in breast cancer. While we now understand much more about these genes and the role they may play in the development of cancer in certain individuals, their role in the development of cancer as a whole remains far from clear. However, overall, the percentage of cancers that can be clearly identified as being genetically inherited is recognized as being relatively small.

Another area of great interest has to do with the role of the immune system in preventing cancer from appearing, or spreading, in different individuals, whether or not they are infected with certain viruses or exposed to potentially cancer-causing substances. Many scientists postulate that cancer cells—which are known to spontaneously appear in the body on a microscopic level—only rarely grow into full-blown tumors because they are cleared by various cells of the immune system. This idea is the so-called *immune surveillance theory,* which has found its way, in various forms, into the public eye. It is now clearly understood that the relationship between the immune system and cancer is highly complex. Unfortunately, the complexity of this relationship is often not fully appreciated by individuals with cancer, leading many to assume that they got cancer simply because their "immune system is weak." Even more unfortunately, this notion leads many individuals with cancer to mistakenly believe that all they have to do is "boost their immune system" with herbs, mushrooms, vitamins, or other supplements and their cancer will go away. If only it were so simple!

Despite clear evidence that in some instances dysfunction of the immune system is related to the development of cancer, this is by no means a universal phenomenon. Many people with completely normal, functioning immune systems develop cancer. And many more patients with damaged immune systems do not develop cancer. Boosting the immune system of cancer patients with simple methods such as herbs and vitamins—or with aggressive methods such as alpha-interferon or interleukin—has not yet proven to be a reliable or effective form of treatment.

One of the major reasons for this has to do with the nature of cancer cells themselves. Since they arise within our own bodies, from our own previously normal cells, it is often hard for the immune system to tell the difference between a normal cell and a cancer cell. Unless the immune cells can accurately identify and distinguish exactly which cells to kill—

which is, once again, often hard to do—"boosting" the immune system even to superhuman levels will not help.

Ironically, this same ambiguous quality of cancer cells is one of the things that so often limits the effectiveness of chemotherapy and radiation. The cancer cells frequently retain so many of the characteristics of their normal progenitor cells that it is very difficult to kill them all without also causing unacceptable damage to normal cells and tissues of the body.

A final important point to mention in this discussion is that cancer has long been thought of as a disease of the elderly. This is because the risk of developing cancer has always increased significantly after the age of fifty. A majority of cancers occur in people over the age of sixty-five, although it is also true that more younger people are being diagnosed with cancer in recent years than ever before. The reasons for this trend are not entirely clear, but dietary, lifestyle, and environmental factors are likely contributors. As to why cancer still occurs most commonly in the elderly, the answer also remains unclear. One theory postulates diminished immune function, with decreased immune surveillance as a significant cause. More recent scientific discoveries suggest other possible contributing factors, including one or more abnormalities in the cells' ability to regulate their own normal life cycle.

There is no question that modern science will continue the search for a deeper understanding of the cellular, molecular, and genetic changes that lead to the development of cancer in humans. And there is no doubt that as scientific tools and technologies progress, newer and more powerful insights will emerge. But for now, a definitive, single cause of cancer has not been established.

How does cancer harm the body?

As cancer cells reproduce, they can form larger and larger tumors, which may displace normal tissue. The displacement of normal tissue can cause organs to function improperly or to stop functioning altogether. For example, a collection of cancer cells within the liver may initially form small nodules that can increase in number and size. If untreated, these can eventually overwhelm the liver, leading to liver failure and possibly even death. Similar events can occur in virtually every organ and system of the body. When this occurs in the lung, it can cause obstruction of a person's airway, along with cough, pain, or shortness of breath. When it occurs in the colon, it can cause obstruction of the bowel, resulting in abdominal pain and bloating.

When these kinds of obstructions occur, not only is the organ's ability to function impaired, but severe infections can also develop. Bulky tumors can themselves also serve as hiding places for bacteria, be inaccessible to antibiotics, and lead to infections.

Sometimes cancer cells infiltrate important lymph node regions of the body and cause obstruction of the lymphatic channels. When this occurs, the normal flow of lymph fluid can be impaired, and fluid collections can build up around the lungs or heart *(pleural or pericardial effusions),* in the abdomen *(ascites),* or in the extremities *(edema).*

Tumors can also invade other structures surrounding their site of origin and cause additional problems, including bleeding, ulcers, and pain.

Many types of cancer cells secrete chemicals that can cause a variety of metabolic problems in the body, often called *paraneoplastic phenomena.* Since cancer cells derive from normal cells, these chemicals are usually normal proteins that are now being produced in either excessive quantities or in an inappropriate manner. A common consequence of this phenomenon is the dramatic loss of appetite *(anorexia)* and weight loss *(cachexia)* that some cancer patients experience. Other common manifestations include significant elevations in blood calcium levels *(hypercalcemia),* abnormalities in blood sodium levels *(hyponatremia),* nerve damage *(neuropathy),* and severe muscle weakness *(myopathy).*

Some cancers also secrete chemicals that interfere with the blood in such a way as to cause blood clots to form. This is commonly called *Trousseau's syndrome,* or a *hypercoagulable disorder.*

Despite the numerous problems and challenges that the original, primary tumor can cause, it is rarely the direct cause of death. By a sequence of extraordinarily complex molecular and cellular processes, cancer cells can invade into and spread through the circulatory or lymphatic system and form new tumors in multiple locations in the body. As mentioned earlier, this process is called *metastasis.* It is the most serious aspect of cancer, and the one that causes the most problems for patients and oncologists alike. Physicians also use the verb *metastasize* to denote the spread of cancer cells. When a patient's cancer has spread to more than one site, the tumors are called *metastases* and the patient is said to have *metastatic disease.*

Why is metastatic cancer so difficult to control?

In cancer treatment, a basic distinction is made between cancers that are curable by surgery and those that are not. In general, when a cancer metastasizes from its primary site, it takes root in one or more new sites. Unfortunately, the location of all of these sites may not be detectable by even the most sophisticated diagnostic procedures, including blood tests, X-rays, bone scans, CT scans, MRI scans, or PET scans. Since metastases often involve multiple sites in the body, it is usually impossible to surgically remove them all. Furthermore, other microscopic sites of disease that are not yet detectable can eventually appear as well. For these reasons, surgery by itself only rarely cures patients who have cancer that has spread to other sites.

When a cancer spreads, it retains much of its original identity, regardless of its new location. Thus, prostate cancer that has spread to the bones is not bone cancer, but *bone metastases of prostate cancer.* Similarly, breast cancer that has spread to the lungs is not lung cancer, but *lung metastases of breast cancer.* As mentioned, cancer cells that have spread to other locations in the body will often form new tumors in these locations. And since these can rarely be removed surgically, other forms of therapy are generally required, such as chemotherapy, hormone therapy, or radiation. Here, carefully determining the primary cell of origin of the metastatic tumor is critically important in deciding which kind of chemotherapy or hormone therapy, or what dose of radiation, will be required.

One of the most fundamental challenges in oncology is the difficulty in eradicating metastases from the body once they have developed. Once again, a primary reason for this is that cancer cells, though different from normal cells in a number of important ways, are in many other important ways not different enough. Thus, conventional treatments such as chemotherapy or radiation that are used to kill cancer cells often damage or kill many other normal cells in the body at the same time. This is what causes many of the most severe side effects that are associated with conventional treatments. Furthermore, as powerful as conventional treatments are, they are often not powerful or effective enough to eradicate every last cancer cell, so the cancer can eventually grow back.

What are the main groups of cancer?

The overwhelming majority of cancers can be broken down into three main groups: *carcinomas, sarcomas,* and *leukemias/lymphomas.*

The first group, carcinomas, are by far the most common forms of cancer. *Carcinoma,* meaning "cancerous growth," was introduced into the Latin language by the Roman physician Aurelius Celsus around A.D. 25–50. He derived the word from the Greek *karkinoma,* meaning "crab," which Hippocrates had first used to describe the condition around 400 B.C. The group of cancers called carcinomas arise principally in the gland-forming cells found in virtually all the organs of the body.

The second group of cancers arises from the body's bone and connective tissues. These are called sarcomas, which is the term the Roman physician Galen first used to describe fleshy tumors, around A.D. 200. Sarcomas are much less common than carcinomas, but there are still many different kinds of sarcomas.

One of the hallmarks of carcinomas and sarcomas, which oncologists refer to as the *solid tumors,* is that they usually form discrete masses that can often be surgically removed if discovered early enough.

The third major group of cancers are the leukemias and lymphomas. These arise from the blood- and lymph-forming cells of the body, including the bone marrow and lymph nodes. Surgery is almost never an option in these cancers because they rarely form discrete, solid masses that can be resected.

While these three groups do not account for all cancers, they constitute the vast majority.

How do oncologists describe a patient's particular type of cancer?

A number of features are always assessed when oncologists evaluate a particular patient's cancer. Three of the most important features are the specific *type* of tumor, its *grade*, and the cancer *stage*. These features play a very important role in determining what kind of treatment will be recommended. They can also help predict what kind of response patients might expect from their specific therapy, as well as their prognosis.

Tumor Type

The vast majority of cancers can be classified under the three major groups described above (carcinomas, sarcomas, and leukemias/lymphomas). Within each of these three groups, or classes, of cancer, one finds a large number of specific *types*.

The specific type of cancer corresponds directly to the specific kind of cell from which it has arisen. Type is most commonly determined by analyzing a biopsy specimen taken from the tumor. The analysis is usually performed by a specialized physician, called a *pathologist*. The pathologist will look at the tissue under a microscope and scrutinize its appearance to determine as best as possible the specific kind of cell or tissue from which the tumor arose.

For example, a large number of different kinds of cancers arise from gland-forming cells that occur in the various organs of the body—the lungs, esophagus, stomach, pancreas, liver, colon, breast, and prostate, among others. Gland-forming cells perform a variety of functions that specifically define the organ. The gland-forming cells in the colon, for instance, secrete various lubricating molecules and also absorb fluids and nutrients. When the gland-forming cells become cancerous in a particular organ, a carcinoma is said to have occurred in that organ. Specifically, when a gland cell becomes cancerous, it is called an *adenocarcinoma*. If cancer arises in the gland-forming cells of the esophagus, it is called an *adenocarcinoma of the esophagus*. If it arises from gland-forming cells of the prostate, it is called an *adenocarcinoma of the prostate*.

Other kinds of cells are found in the various organs and tissues of the body. The esophagus has cells in its inner lining that are called *squamous cells*. When these become malignant and form a tumor, it is referred to as a *squamous cell carcinoma*. Another example is found in the bladder, which has *transitional cells*. When these become malignant, they are referred to as a *transitional cell carcinoma*.

The majority of breast cancers arise from specialized cells that make up the milk ducts. When these cancers invade through the milk ducts, they are called *infiltrating ductal carcinoma*. Approximately 70 percent of all breast cancers are of this type. Another, much less common form of breast cancer arises from tissues called breast lobules, which produce milk. When cancers of this type invade through the lobule, they are called *infiltrating lobular carcinoma*.

Two other important types of breast cancer are distinguished by their tendency to grow in place without invading into deeper tissues; these are called *in situ carcinomas*. When these arise from duct cells, they are called *ductal carcinoma in situ* (DCIS, or sometimes *intraductal carcinoma*). When they arise from lobular cells, they are called *lobular carcinoma in situ* (LCIS, or sometimes *intralobular carcinoma*). A major factor in how these are treated involves their uncertain potential to develop into full-blown invasive cancer.

By carefully identifying exactly which cell a tumor has arisen from, along with a variety of other features, doctors and scientists have learned to categorize the different types of cancer more precisely. Newer and more sophisticated tools and technologies are being developed that allow distinctions between cells to be made at increasingly specific molecular and genetic levels. As this occurs, new types and forms of cancers are being described that were not recognized before, and this process will also undoubtedly continue in the future.

Tumor Grade

Once the pathologist has defined the specific type of cancer involved, the next step is to determine its *grade*. The grade of a tumor is an indication or reflection of how aggressive it is. The grade is primarily determined by a further analysis of the tumor's specific appearance under the microscope.

For example, cancer cells that are similar in appearance to their normal cell of origin are likely to behave in a less aggressive way and are generally classified as *low-grade*. Cancer cells that appear significantly different compared with their normal cell of origin are more likely to behave in a more aggressive manner and are generally classified as *high-grade*. These kinds of cancer cells often have bizarre distinguishing features that make them relatively easy for a pathologist to identify under the microscope. Cancer cells that are intermediate in appearance, and often in their clinical behavior as well, are referred to as *intermediate-grade*.

An individual with a high-grade adenocarcinoma of the prostate will likely have a significantly different clinical course than an individual with a low-grade adenocarcinoma of the prostate. Similarly, the issues involved in treating a woman with a high-grade infiltrating ductal carcinoma of the breast are potentially quite different than for a woman with a low-grade infiltrating ductal carcinoma of the breast.

Tumor Stage

This is often one of the most important factors in determining the kind of treatment that will be recommended for a specific cancer, as well as a patient's prognosis.

Tumor stage is a representation or description of how far a cancer has spread in the body. In the majority of cases, cancers are described as occurring in one of four different stages.

Stage I tumors, in general, are small and localized to the area in which they were discovered. Thus, they are tumors that have not spread.

Stage II tumors, in general, are larger than Stage I tumors, and may involve nearby lymph nodes.

Stage III tumors, in general, have grown more than stage II tumors, and usually involve nearby lymph nodes.

Stage IV tumors are those that have spread widely, including to other organs.

A variety of different staging systems have been used by oncologists to describe the extent of spread of different cancers. Most oncologists are familiar with most of the different staging systems and routinely use them interchangeably. For example, it is still common for many doctors to refer to the Duke's staging system of colon cancer. Another example involves small cell lung cancer, which is still commonly described in clinical practice as being either "limited" or "extensive" stage.

But the most widely utilized and internationally recognized staging system is called the TNM staging system. Here, *T* refers to the size of the primary *tumor; N* refers to whether the lymph *nodes* are involved with the tumor; and *M* refers to whether the cancer has *metastasized* to other organs or tissues.

Regardless of the staging system used, all of them describe the same basic clinical features of the specific cancer, including—most important—the extent to which it has spread. In all of the staging systems, including the TNM system, the higher the stage of the cancer, the more widely it has spread.

Finally, several other factors are often important in the characterization and treatment planning of cancer. One well-known factor, the *hormone receptor status*, is involved in the assessment and treatment of breast cancer. This refers to the presence or absence of estrogen receptors (ER) and progesterone receptors (PR) in the breast cancer cells. The reason this is so important in a particular woman's breast cancer is that tumor cells in which these receptors are absent often behave more aggressively than when they are present. This may influence treatment recommendations as well as prognosis.

Another feature of cancer cells that has been gaining attention in recent years is called *antigen expression.* Antigens are special proteins found on tumor cell surfaces that help distinguish them from normal cells. For example—once again in breast cancer—tumors that express more than the usual amount of the HER-2/*neu* antigen have important characteristics that can greatly influence treatment recommendations and prognosis. In recent years, antigen expression has also led to a greater understanding of the origin of many of the different types of lymphoma and can influence treatment recommendations as well.

Finally, another significant area of interest and research in oncology has focused on specific gene abnormalities, which are being found with increasing frequency in a wide variety of cancers. Understanding of these is now beginning to influence the clinical management of different cancers, such as bladder and colon cancer, among others. These are often found to have characteristic abnormalities involving the well-known tumor-suppressor gene p53. Similarly, specific abnormalities in the well-known cancer genes BRCA1 and BRCA2 are associated with increased risk of breast and ovarian cancer, and may play a role in how these cancers behave clinically in individual patients.

What are tumor markers?

Cancer cells sometimes secrete specialized proteins into the bloodstream that can serve as a marker, or indicator, of tumor growth. These are called *tumor markers,* and they can be specifically associated with a particular type of cancer. Sometimes the same tumor marker can be secreted by a variety of different cancers. In other instances, identical proteins can be secreted by normal tissues, but usually in much lower amounts.

Not all cancers secrete tumor markers into the bloodstream, but when they do, they can be very helpful in early detection of cancer, monitoring response to treatment, or identifying relapses. In general, when concentrations of a specific tumor marker are found to be significantly elevated, the likelihood is increased that cancer is present. Very often, the blood levels of the marker will fall in response to successful treatment, or not fall if the treatment is not working well. If the marker falls to a very low level after successful cancer treatment, its subsequent rise can indicate that the cancer cells are once again growing—even before any specific symptoms appear.

The most well-known tumor marker today is the PSA, which stands for *prostate-specific antigen.* The PSA is a highly specific protein that is secreted only by cells of the prostate gland. It is one of the most widely utilized screening tests for cancer, and will be discussed in greater detail in the section on prostate cancer on page 64. Another well-known tumor marker in use today is the CA 125, which is important in the diagnosis of ovarian cancer, as well as monitoring its response to treatment. Other clinically useful tumor markers include the CEA (*carcinoembryonic antigen,* for colon cancer), CA 15-3 (for breast cancer), CA 19-9 (for pancreas cancer), AFP (*alpha-fetoprotein,* for liver cancer and testicular cancer), and beta-HCG (for testicular cancer).

Research is currently under way on a wide array of newer and more useful tumor markers. These may prove helpful in a variety of ways, including selecting specific treatments and predicting responses to them with much greater precision than ever before.

What are the forms of cancer treatment?

Currently surgery, radiation, and chemotherapy are the three principal categories of cancer treatment. As research continues, a variety of drugs targeted at increasingly specific genetic and molecular mechanisms are gaining wide attention and utilization (see "The Basics: State-of-the-Art Medical Care," page 28). Further developments in various forms of immunotherapy, gene therapy, and tumor vaccines are also under way and hold great promise for the future.

Surgery

Surgery is by far the oldest form of treatment for cancer, and it remains the most widely used today. It is still one of the most effective treatments for a variety of different cancers—particularly when they have not yet spread to other parts of the body. Despite the skill of the surgeons, as well as ingenious advances in the operations themselves, surgery is still essentially akin to pulling weeds out of a garden. It does not deal with what caused the weeds in the first place or address how to prevent them in the future. Yet half of all cancer cures result from surgery, so its importance can hardly be overstated.

The standard practice in cancer surgery has been to remove the tumor itself and as much of the surrounding tissue as deemed necessary to try to prevent the tumor from spreading or growing back. In recent years, the trend has been toward less aggressive surgeries. Medicine is learning that in dealing with cancer, more is not necessarily better. The best-known example of this is the replacement of *radical mastectomy* for breast cancer (removal of the entire breast as well as the underlying muscle and tissue) with *modified radical mastectomy* (removal of most of the breast tissue and only a limited amount of underlying tissue). Over the last two decades this trend has been advanced further by *lumpectomy* (removal of just the breast tumor itself, with only a small amount of surrounding tissue) followed by radiation.

Another form of "downsizing" in breast cancer surgery that has gained attention in recent years involves the use of a new technique called *sentinel lymph node biopsy*. Here, surgeons are able to identify and remove just one or two of a patient's axillary lymph nodes, rather than multiple lymph nodes, as has been the standard practice, and still obtain the information necessary for prognosis and treatment recommendations.

In contrast to this trend, as surgical techniques continue to advance, many patients with lung and other cancers that were previously considered inoperable are now being successfully treated with more extensive surgeries.

Radiation

Radiation is also an important treatment modality in cancer care. Its beneficial effects are generally restricted to a specific area of the body where the radiation is focused. In this way, radiation is similar to surgery in that its potential to cure is generally limited to cancers that have not spread to other sites. Radiation occasionally can be just as effective as surgery, while often being much less disfiguring.

Certain types of cancer are very amenable to radiation, such as anal cancer, esophageal cancer, and tumors of the head and neck. Radiation is also effective for certain types of lung cancer, prostate cancer, cervical cancer, tumors of the bone, and lymphomas. For some malignancies such as inoperable brain tumors, it may be the only treatment available. But very often radiation is one element in an overall treatment plan that also includes chemotherapy and/or surgery. It may be used prior to surgery to shrink a tumor, or after surgery to prevent the regrowth of any remaining tumor cells.

Radiation is believed to cause genetic damage to cancer cells, which cannot easily repair themselves. In contrast, normal tissues that are exposed to radiation are generally better able to repair themselves and heal. That is why radiation can be administered without completely destroying the area surrounding the tumor.

Today radiation therapy is applied using extremely sophisticated techniques, often guided by advanced computer programs, which can focus the radiation beam to a small area that is composed predominantly of tumor cells. A well-known example of this is intensity-modulated radiation therapy (IMRT). In recent years significant advances have also been made in the implantation of radioactive materials directly into tumors, called *brachytherapy* or *seed implant radiation therapy*. These techniques are most commonly used in prostate and cervical cancer. They are also now being utilized in breast and lung cancer as well.

Another specialized form of radiation therapy is called *gamma-knife, CyberKnife,* or *stereotactic radiosurgery*. This is used predominantly to treat small brain tumors that are inaccessible to conventional surgery.

An additional, exciting new development in recent years is *radio-immunotherapy*, which allows radiation to be delivered directly to tumors. This is accomplished by linking radioactive substances to monoclonal antibodies that are administered intravenously. The monoclonal antibodies travel through the bloodstream and attach to highly specific antigens found on cancer cells. When this occurs, the radioactive substances are brought into direct proximity to the cancer cells, causing them to die. Examples of FDA-approved radioimmunotherapy drugs include Zevalin (ibritumomab tiuxetan) and Bexxar (tositumomab), both of which are used to treat non-Hodgkin's lymphoma. A number of additional agents of this type are under development for use with lymphomas and other types of cancer as well.

Chemotherapy

Chemotherapy is the third element in the standard approach to cancer treatment. It is the youngest of the three modalities, with origins as recent as the 1940s.

Although a certain amount of controversy surrounds chemotherapy in the popular literature on cancer, it is not controversial in the minds of experienced oncologists. In fact, chemotherapy is the foundation of treatment for a very large number of cancer patients. Despite its obvious limitations, when used with great care and skill its benefits are unmistakable and can be extraordinary.

Different anticancer medicines work in different ways, but all ultimately work by interfering in some way with the division and replication process of cancer cells. Some of the older drugs, such as Alkeran (melphalan), Cytoxan (cyclophosphamide), Adriamycin (doxorubicin), and

Platinol (cisplatin) cause the destruction of malignant cells through direct damage to the cell's genetic material, the DNA. Others, such as 5-FU (5-fluorouracil), disrupt cancer cells' ability to replicate by inserting unusable material into the DNA. Several drugs that are derived from plants, notably Oncovin (vincristine), Velban (vinblastine), Taxol (paclitaxel), and Taxotere (docetaxel), interfere in unique ways with specialized proteins within cells that are important for cell division.

Steroid medications such as Deltasone (prednisone) and Decadron (dexamethasone) are also sometimes used in the treatment of cancer. They are particularly toxic to lymphoid cells, in ways that are not entirely clear. A variety of different hormones is sometimes used in cancer treatment as well. They suppress the growth of tumors by blocking certain hormone receptors inside the cancer cells, especially in cancer of the breast or prostate.

Chemotherapy has contributed to many extraordinary advances in cancer treatment, especially over the last twenty-five years. However, it remains saddled with three fundamental limitations: side effects, eventual drug resistance by cancer cells, and the inability to reach every cancer cell in the body. Let's deal with each of these directly.

1. Side effects of chemotherapy. These are legion, and well known: fatigue, nausea, vomiting, diarrhea, hair loss, suppression of the bone marrow, nerve damage, kidney damage, loss of appetite, and mouth sores are some of the most common. The primary reason for these side effects is that chemotherapy drugs generally kill cancer cells more effectively when they are dividing rapidly than when they are not. Unfortunately, they also kill normal cells in the body that are also dividing rapidly, such as those found lining the gastrointestinal tract, in hair follicles, and in the bone marrow. It is damage to these normal tissues that usually accounts for the majority of the side effects encountered with chemotherapy.

It is important to recognize that not all patients will suffer from these side effects. Some will experience a number of them, to varying degrees—and others will experience none at all. The side effects also vary with the specific drug being used, the interval of time between treatments, the specific dosage, and the nutritional status and overall condition of the patient.

Fortunately, oncologists are now able to give chemotherapy in a manner that minimizes side effects while still deriving maximum benefit from the drugs. Many new chemotherapy drugs have significantly fewer side effects than older ones, and many other medications have been released in recent years that can minimize, if not eliminate outright, a number of the side effects previously associated with chemotherapy.

2. Drug resistance. Cancer cells can sometimes have very devious and efficient ways of resisting the effects of chemotherapy, known as *drug resistance*. Over the years, oncologists have employed a number of different strategies to try to overcome this problem, with only limited success. Another aspect of the problem involves the fact that cancer cells may sometimes become resistant to chemotherapy drugs even if they initially responded to them very well. This is one of the reasons it can be so hard to actually cure cancer—especially solid tumors—with chemotherapy. If only one cancer cell is not killed by the therapy, it can grow back and cause more problems.

3. Chemotherapy's inability to reach every cancer cell in the body. This occurs in two major ways. First, some tumors grow so large that blood vessels no longer carry blood to their deepest, innermost regions. Since chemotherapy is carried in the blood, it sometimes can't reach all of the cancer cells that are buried deep inside the tumor. When this happens, those cancer cells survive and can continue to grow, spread to other sites in the body, and develop more resistance to chemotherapy, as described above.

A second way this problem occurs involves what are called *tumor sanctuaries*. These are special areas of the body that are naturally protected from the effects of drugs and toxins in order to keep us well. The two most important areas that are considered to be tumor sanctuaries are the testes and the brain. When cancer cells are found in these organs, it is hard for the chemotherapy drugs to reach them, and cancer will often regrow there if not treated with some other means, such as surgery or radiation.

How are chemotherapy drugs administered?

Chemotherapy drugs are administered in a variety of ways, but usually via an intravenous infusion or oral tablet. The intravenous infusions can range in duration from a few minutes to many days continuously, depending on the drug and the kind of cancer being treated. Hormone therapies are usually administered by tablet, muscular injection, or by a skin patch.

Chemotherapy today is very different from even five years ago, to say nothing of twenty-five years ago. One goal of *The Journey Through Cancer* is to dispel the perception of chemotherapy as a toxic, reprehensible abuse of patients by uncaring physicians. In the 1970s and '80s, the number and efficacy of chemotherapy drugs were limited. But since then many new drugs have appeared that are significantly more effective, and in many instances much less toxic.

If there is a real problem with chemotherapy, it is often not in the drugs but in the level of consciousness, skill, and attentiveness with which they are administered. Successful use of these medications demands a real commitment to caring for the patients who receive them. Two patients may take the same dose of the same drug, but the manner in which it is given—including the environment, the care with which it is administered, the fears and expectations of the patient, and his or her overall physical status—are all very important factors in influencing the patient's experience. Meticulous follow-up is also extremely important. A doctor who fails to closely monitor a chemotherapy patient is like a driver who takes his or her eyes off the road. It only takes a split second for a serious accident to occur.

What are the most common forms of cancer?

By far, the most common form of cancer in the United States is skin cancer, including basal cell and squamous cell carcinomas. The overwhelming majority of these skin cancers are noninvasive, however, and are easily cured by surgery. Melanoma is another form of skin cancer, which has been increasing in incidence in recent years. While this form of skin cancer can be invasive and deadly, it is still relatively uncommon, with about 59,000 cases in 2005.

Other than skin cancer, cancers of the prostate, breast, lung, and colon account for the majority of invasive cancer diagnoses in the United States. Each of these diseases has a number of subtypes, and their characteristics vary among individual patients.

In 2005, these four major types of cancer accounted for approximately 55 percent of all invasive cancer cases in the United States (prostate, 232,000 cases; breast, 212,000 cases; lung, 172,000 cases; and colorectal, 145,000 cases)—a total of 761,000 cases out of approximately 1.4 million cases of invasive cancer overall. After colorectal cancer, the most common types of cancer are lymphoma (64,000 cases), bladder cancer (63,000 cases), melanoma (60,000 cases), uterine cancer (40,000 cases), kidney cancer (36,000 cases), leukemias (34,000 cases), pancreas cancer (32,000 cases), and ovarian cancer (22,000 cases).

In the pages that follow, some of the important issues in prostate cancer (below), breast cancer (page 67), lung cancer (page 70), colon cancer (page 72), ovarian cancer (page 72), and lymphoma (page 73) will be addressed in greater detail.

What are the important issues in prostate cancer?

Prostate cancer arises from gland-forming cells of the prostate gland, a walnut-sized organ adjacent to the urinary bladder in men. The specific cause, or causes, of prostate cancer remain unknown, though there are several well-recognized risk factors for developing the disease.

By far, as with the majority of cancers, the most well-established risk factor is age. Diagnosis of prostate cancer is rare before age fifty, but thereafter incidence as well as mortality rates increase dramatically—prostate cancer is actually a common disease in elderly men. Estimates from different studies suggest that undetected prostate cancer may be present in as many as 43 percent of men by age eighty. In many of these men, however, the disease will never become clinically significant. This important fact has contributed greatly to the current debate about the best way to manage prostate cancer, particularly in elderly men.

A strong family history of prostate cancer can increase a man's risk of developing the disease by a factor of two. Another well-accepted risk factor is race. The incidence of prostate cancer in African American men is higher than among Caucasian men. African American men also tend to have more aggressive tumors and a higher mortality from the disease. For reasons that are not yet clear, prostate cancer is less common in Asian men, and rarest of all in Chinese men. Dietary factors—including a high intake of animal fat and a deficiency of vitamin D—have also been implicated in the risk of developing prostate cancer. However, these risks are still less well defined compared with other risk factors, and remain somewhat controversial.

Widespread screening for prostate cancer began in earnest in the mid-1980s, utilizing both digital rectal examination of the prostate gland and the serum PSA test. (PSA stands for prostate-specific antigen, as described earlier.) By early 1997, data collected from numerous clinical studies suggested that since prostate cancer screening could lead to earlier detection, it might also lead to decreased mortality. This has not been conclusively proven, and a great deal of controversy remains regarding the overall benefits of widespread screening for prostate cancer.

False positive screening tests can lead to unnecessary biopsies and other costly and/or uncomfortable diagnostic studies. Annual screening of millions of men without a proven reduction in mortality will add further costs to a society and a health care system that are already heavily burdened. In light of these controversies, additional studies are under way to define the benefits of widespread screening for prostate cancer.

In the meantime, the American Cancer Society recommends that beginning at age fifty, men who have a life expectancy of at least ten years should undergo an annual digital rectal examination of the prostate gland and a serum PSA test.

Normal as well as cancerous prostate cells produce and secrete PSA into the bloodstream, but cancerous prostate cells do so much more readily than normal prostate cells. In the absence of prostate cancer, the blood level of PSA is usually less than 4 nanograms per milliliter (ng/ml). When the level of PSA in the blood increases above 4 ng/ml, the likelihood of cancer being present increases.

It is important to remember that not all men with PSA levels above 4 ng/ml will have prostate cancer. Other benign conditions can cause an elevation of the PSA level without cancer being present, including *benign prostatic hypertrophy* (BPH) or *prostatitis* (inflammation of the prostate gland, usually caused by infection). Also, a man with a PSA level of less than 4 ng/ml can occasionally have prostate cancer, particularly if the tumor is poorly differentiated.

Screening should begin at a younger age—for example, forty-five—for men who are in a high-risk group for developing prostate cancer. Examples of this group include men with a strong family history of prostate cancer and African American men.

Digital rectal examination of the prostate gland should be performed by health care professionals who are skilled in the procedure and experienced in recognizing subtle abnormalities of the gland that might suggest the presence of cancer.

As with almost all other forms of cancer, prostate cancer has a wide spectrum of presentations, and the issues involved in treatment vary widely as well. Some of the major forms of treatment that are currently used for localized (i.e., nonmetastatic) tumors are:

- *Radical prostatectomy,* or surgical removal of the prostate gland, along with regional lymph nodes
- *Nerve-sparing prostatectomy,* which can greatly reduce some of the most troubling long-term side effects of prostatectomy
- *External beam radiation therapy,* which involves radiation targeted at the tumor
- *Seed implant radiation therapy,* in which small radioactive "seeds" are implanted directly into the prostate gland of patients, usually under ultrasound guidance
- *Cryosurgery,* which involves inserting probes containing liquid nitrogen directly into the prostate gland, in order to freeze and kill the cancerous cells
- *Combination therapy,* in which patients are treated with hormone therapy along with radiation or surgery
- *Watchful waiting,* in which patients are followed prospectively by

their physician and monitored closely for any signs of progression of their disease before any specific treatment is initiated

When prostate cancer has spread to other parts of the body, the initial treatment usually involves some form of hormone therapy. In recent years, various kinds of chemotherapy drugs have also been used, particularly in patients whose cancer has become resistant to hormone treatments. When this occurs, the patient is said to have *hormone-refractory disease.*

Prostate cancer is an enormous public health issue in the United States, and its impact in our culture will undoubtedly be felt for years to come. With increased awareness of this disease, however, and with continued advances in diagnosis and treatment, the prognosis of men who are diagnosed with prostate cancer should continue to improve in the future.

What are the important issues in breast cancer?

Breast cancer is one of the most readily treatable cancers in humans. It is an area in which new treatment protocols are rapidly appearing and established ones are continuously being revised. There is also no doubt that breast cancer is one of the most controversial and politicized health issues in the United States.

A number of risk factors for breast cancer have been identified. Age is clearly important, as incidence increases significantly in women over fifty. A family history of breast cancer is also associated with a higher predisposition to developing the disease.

Increased exposure to estrogen over many years is believed to heighten a woman's chance of developing breast cancer. This can occur in women who experience early menses or late menopause, become pregnant for the first time after age thirty, never have children, or have never breast-fed. Numerous studies have demonstrated a higher risk of breast cancer among women in these groups. It is also believed that drinking alcohol may result in higher estrogen activity, and several large studies have indicated that risk of breast cancer increases with increased alcohol consumption.

Interestingly, exercise has been shown to be helpful in reducing the risk of breast cancer in women. This is presumed to be related to decreased estrogen levels in women who exercise for substantial periods of time, particularly more than four hours per week.

Many attempts have been made over the years to link breast cancer with specific eating habits and to recommend foods that would reduce risk or even prevent the appearance of the disease. Although it's tempting to search for these dietary benefits, conclusive evidence has been difficult to establish. At the present time, the role of dietary factors in cancer risk remains hotly debated, although evidence does suggest that eating a plant-based diet provides some protective benefits. Further research may lead to even more specific recommendations for women to follow.

In addition to the shifts in our understanding of specific risk factors for developing breast cancer, the conceptual paradigm of the biology of breast cancer has also changed. In the early years of the twentieth century, breast cancer was thought to spread in an organized, predictable manner: beginning with an enlarging mass in the breast, then extending to the axillary lymph nodes before spreading throughout the body. This view prevailed for a long time. Over the last several decades, however, as our understanding of breast cancer has advanced, we have recognized that there is often not an orderly progression of the disease. For example, a small tumor in the breast of one woman may have already spread at the time of her diagnosis, while a larger tumor in the breast of another woman may remain localized for a long period of time.

Several significant developments in the treatment of breast cancer have emerged as a result of this understanding. The first relates to the surgical management of breast cancer, as mentioned earlier in this chapter. Clinical trials have shown that lumpectomy with radiation confers the same survival benefits to many women as mastectomy would, and with much less disfigurement. This controversy extended over several decades but has been clearly resolved.

An extension of the evolving role of surgery in breast cancer concerns axillary lymph node dissection, which in a significant percentage of women can lead to debilitating swelling in the arm, known as *lymphedema*. Sentinel lymph node biopsy is advancing in utility, and is now routinely used in evaluating the lymph node status of women with breast cancer, particularly those with early-stage disease.

A second significant development in the management of breast cancer involves the use of adjuvant chemotherapy. This has been proven to reduce the risks of recurrence in virtually all women with invasive breast cancer. However, the degree of risk reduction depends upon a number of factors, including the patient's age, the size and grade of the primary tumor, the tumor's hormone receptor and HER-2/*neu* status, and the number of lymph nodes involved at the time of diagnosis.

A third important development involves the use of emerging new hormone therapies to treat breast cancer. After completing surgery, many women are advised to receive adjuvant treatment with a hormonal drug, either alone or in addition to chemotherapy and/or radiation. Hormone therapies are also used to treat women with breast cancer that has metastasized. For many years, tamoxifen—one of the most widely utilized cancer drugs in the world—was routinely used for these purposes. In recent years, a new class of hormonal drugs known as *aromatase inhibitors* has become available for breast cancer. These new drugs work by a mechanism of action that is different than that of tamoxifen, and are approved by the FDA for use only in postmenopausal women. Examples include Arimidex (anastrozole), Femara (letrozole), and Aromasin (exemestane). Studies have shown these drugs to be more effective for postmenopausal women than tamoxifen, and with fewer toxicities. As a result, they are gaining widespread acceptance.

Another important issue in breast cancer surrounds the question of screening. While the PSA blood test has become a safe and important screening technique for prostate cancer, there is no comparable screening tool for breast cancer. Currently, the methods of detection for breast cancer are still limited to *breast self-examination* and *mammography*.

It is clear that mammograms for women over fifty save lives. Studies show that women over forty also benefit, but to a smaller degree. Recent improvements in mammography techniques, most notably *digital mammography*, offer the promise of even greater benefits. The number of lives saved by mammography, however, comes at a high cost. As with prostate cancer, considerable burden on society and the health care system results from regularly testing millions of women who do not have and will never develop breast cancer. This is compounded by the significant anxiety, inconvenience, and expense often encountered by the women themselves.

These remain hotly debated issues, and women over forty should speak directly with their physician about appropriate mammography screening.

Again, breast cancer is one of the most treatable, if not always curable, forms of cancer. It is an area in which new drugs are rapidly appearing, including the anticancer drugs Taxol (paclitaxel), Abraxane (nanoparticle albumin-bound paclitaxel), Taxotere (docetaxel), Navelbine (vinorelbine), Gemzar (gemcitabine), and Xeloda (capecitabine); hormone therapies such as the aromatase inhibitors previously mentioned; and the monoclonal antibody Herceptin (trastuzumab).

As new and even more sophisticated diagnostic tests, screening modalities, and treatments for breast cancer continue to emerge, even further progress will be made in improving the lives and care of patients with this disease.

What are the important issues in lung cancer?

Lung cancer, which was almost unheard of a hundred years ago, is one of the greatest public health travesties ever to befall humankind. This disease could be virtually eliminated if the dissemination of cigarettes were to stop. And if lung cancer were eliminated, 30 percent of all cancer cases in the United States would also be eliminated.

Lung cancer is most often diagnosed when patients present with symptoms such as cough, weight loss, or shortness of breath. Sometimes the diagnosis is made from a chest X-ray done during a routine physical examination or prior to a surgical procedure. Screening for lung cancer with X-rays or sputum cytology has not conclusively been proven to save lives and thus remains controversial. A number of studies have suggested that screening with CT scans of the chest—which are able to detect lung cancers at a much earlier stage than routine chest X-rays—leads to improved survival in people who are at high risk. These results, however, are not yet considered to be conclusive. Furthermore, considerable costs and potential complications are associated with pursuing abnormal but noncancerous findings that appear on the CT scans of many individuals. These factors have thus far precluded the widespread acceptance of CT scans as a routine screening tool.

Until recently, lung cancer was one of the least curable forms of cancer. But the paradigm is shifting in the treatment of lung cancer, particularly in recent years with FDA approval of drugs such as Taxol (paclitaxel), Paraplatin (carboplatin), Gemzar (gemcitabine), and Navelbine (vinorelbine). Once unthinkable numbers of people are now living for as long as five years. This is a very significant advance in a disease that not long ago was commonly fatal within six to twelve months. As with most other cancers, a fundamental issue in lung cancer is whether the tumor can be surgically removed at an early stage. When that is the case, five-year survival rates are fairly high. An important clinical trial published in 2004 confirmed that survival rates are enhanced even further in patients who receive adjuvant chemotherapy for their resected lung cancer, and this is now accepted as the standard of care.

The disease is divided into two main categories: *small cell* and *non-small cell* lung cancer.

Small cell lung cancer, which accounts for about 25 percent of total cases, has been divided into two subgroups, called *oat cell* and *intermediate cell,* based on their microscopic appearance. The remaining 75 percent of lung cancer cases are of the non-small cell variety. These occur in three main subgroups, called adenocarcinoma, *large cell carcinoma,* and *squamous cell carcinoma,* based on their cell of origin.

At the time of diagnosis, small cell lung cancer is much more often disseminated than the other forms. Small cell lung cancers are also relatively sensitive to radiation and chemotherapy. They respond extremely well, and a significant percentage of limited-stage tumors, and even some advanced-stage ones, can have remarkable—even complete—responses to conventional treatment. Unfortunately, they also have a tendency to recur.

Non-small cell lung cancer has in the past been more resistant to chemotherapy and radiation. But when treated with the newly available drugs—by themselves, or in combination with radiation or surgery—the disease can respond more dramatically than ever before, prolonging life in many patients.

Lung cancer is no longer the uniformly dire illness that it was. With early diagnosis and proper treatment, the outlook is now much brighter.

What are the major issues in colon cancer?

A unique feature of colon cancer is that pre-malignant tissues can be clearly identified and removed in many patients. To take advantage of this fact, screening for colon cancer is very important in higher-risk individuals, including people over fifty and those with a strong family history of the disease. When colon cancer is detected early, it is highly curable by surgery. When the tumor has extended through the bowel wall or spread into local or regional lymph nodes, it is still often curable with surgery followed by adjuvant chemotherapy.

Most colon cancers develop from polyps, which are growths arising from mucous membranes in the wall of the colon. Polyps are common in adults and are usually benign. If they are detected early enough, they can often be removed with a fiber-optic scope (called a *sigmoidoscope* or *colonoscope*) on an outpatient basis. If the polyp grows too large, surgery may be required. Occasionally, benign polyps can become cancerous and begin to invade the colon wall. In these cases, surgery is usually required and a segment of the colon must be removed as well.

As with other kinds of cancer, treatment decisions for colon cancer are based on the staging of the disease in an individual patient. There are several staging systems in use (the Duke's system, the modified Astler-Coller system, and the TNM staging system), which describe various stages of the illness, from localized to metastatic. In addition to surgery, chemotherapy is an important aspect of colon cancer treatment, especially on an adjuvant basis. The drugs 5-FU (5-fluorouracil) and leucovorin have been the mainstays of colon cancer chemotherapy for decades. Recent advances include newer chemotherapy agents such as Eloxatin (oxaliplatin), Camptosar (irinotecan), and Xeloda (capecitabine), as well as the monoclonal antibodies Avastin (bevacizumab) and Erbitux (cetuximab). New applications of chemotherapy, radiation, and emerging targeted therapies are currently in clinical trials.

What are the major issues in ovarian cancer?

This disease has gained increased attention since the death of the popular actress Gilda Radner in 1989. Today there are roughly 22,000 cases of ovarian cancer annually in the United States. Ovarian cancer has been called "the silent killer" because it can develop and progress with no symptoms whatsoever, until it is finally discovered in an advanced stage. When this occurs, it is often difficult to cure. Screening the general population of women for ovarian cancer remains controversial. However, women who are at high risk for developing the disease may be screened with a pelvic ultrasound and the CA 125 blood test. It is important to be aware that the CA 125 blood test is not entirely reliable because there are a number of conditions that can cause false positive results. Accurate diagnosis usually requires surgery and a biopsy.

Standard treatment for ovarian cancer includes surgery and chemotherapy. In recent years, the drugs Taxol (paclitaxel) and Paraplatin (carboplatin) have significantly improved survival rates, allowing many patients to live for years longer than was true in the past. Even further improvement in survival rates has recently been demonstrated in selected patients who receive *intraperitoneal (IP) chemotherapy* in addition to standard treatment. IP chemotherapy is a technique that involves the infusion of chemotherapy directly into the abdominal cavity. It requires experienced practitioners to be administered safely; however, its benefits can be very significant. In fact, in early 2006, the National Cancer Institute issued a formal announcement urging doctors to offer the treatment to all women who meet the medical criteria for it.

What are the major issues in lymphoma?

The lymphomas are a diverse group of cancers that arise from various cells of the lymphoid system of the body. They can occur wherever normal lymphocytes are found, including lymph nodes, visceral organs, skin, bones, and even the brain. In general, lymphomas are divided into two main groups, Hodgkin's disease and non-Hodgkin's lymphomas.

Non-Hodgkin's lymphomas (approximately 56,000 cases in 2005) are far more common than Hodgkin's disease (approximately 7,000 cases in 2005). For reasons that are not clear, in recent years, non-Hodgkin's lymphomas have been increasing significantly in incidence in the United States. They are now the fifth most common cancer in this country and the fifth leading cause of cancer death.

Historically, a variety of classification systems have been used to define and describe non-Hodgkin's lymphomas. One of the most commonly used systems is known as the *Working Formulation*. It divides ten major subtypes of non-Hodgkin's lymphomas into low-, intermediate-, or high-grade groups, based primarily on specific aspects of their microscopic appearance and clinical behavior. In the 1990s, a new classification system began to emerge, called the *Revised European/American Lymphoma (REAL) classification system*. This system is based on a progressively deepening understanding of important genetic and molecular features of the many different types of lymphoma that are now known to exist. A further refinement of REAL, published by the World Health Organization in 1999, is now gaining widespread acceptance.

One of the hallmarks of non-Hodgkin's lymphomas is that they are usually highly responsive to chemotherapy and radiation. However, depending on the stage of the lymphoma, along with its specific grade, subtype, and molecular as well as genetic characteristics, non-Hodgkin's lymphomas can range in behavior from indolent (slow-growing) to highly aggressive. For this reason, it is important for oncologists to know precisely which kind of lymphoma they are dealing with, particularly when formulating a treatment plan. Cure rates for different non-Hodgkin's lymphomas are quite varied, but in general are lower than for Hodgkin's disease.

A significant advance in the treatment of non-Hodgkin's lymphomas in recent years involves the utilization of Rituxan (rituximab), both alone and in combination with conventional chemotherapy. This monoclonal antibody has been shown to yield significant improvement in response rates and survival for patients with a common type of lymphoma called diffuse large B-cell lymphoma. Significant clinical benefits have also been demonstrated in other types of lymphoma. Additional studies involving Rituxan combined with different chemotherapy regimens, radiation therapy, and even other monoclonal antibodies are under way.

Hodgkin's disease—which was first described in 1832 by the English physician Thomas Hodgkin—has characteristics that are distinct and in many ways quite different from non-Hodgkin's lymphomas. For example, it generally occurs in younger patients and progresses much more predictably than non-Hodgkin's lymphomas. It is also curable in the majority of cases. In fact, along with testicular cancer, Hodgkin's disease is regarded as one of the most reliably curable forms of cancer.

What is a clinical trial?

As we've discussed, there are many different types of cancer, and within each type there are often many variations. The standard treatment for each kind of cancer represents the culmination of both laboratory research and clinical experience with many patients over long periods of time. Standard treatments, however, are always subject to change based on new information. When a new drug or technique has achieved positive results in laboratory testing, it then becomes available for carefully monitored clinical trials with cancer patients.

Clinical trials are typically designated as Phase I, II, or III. Phase I trials are intended primarily to determine how new treatments affect human patients and specifically what range of doses is safe and acceptable. Because of the risks that may be associated with Phase I trials, they typically only involve patients whose illness is no longer responding to standard treatments. For patients who enroll in Phase I trials, there is usually a small but real potential for being helped by the new treatment. There is also the opportunity to advance medical knowledge, which may help others in the future.

Phase II and III trials usually involve larger numbers of participants than Phase I trials. The purpose of Phase II trials is to define more precisely the benefits of new treatments on specific types of cancer. Phase III trials compare new treatments—ones that were found to be effective in Phase II trials—with previously used standard treatments.

As a cancer patient, you may ask or be asked to participate in a clinical trial. However, you are never required to do so. You will be informed of all the risks and potential benefits of the trial. If you decide to participate, you will be asked to sign a document attesting to your informed consent. You can also choose to leave the trial at any time, and this decision will in no way be held against you.

Participating in a Phase III clinical trial does not guarantee that you'll get the new treatment being studied. By a process of random selection, a certain number of patients will receive the new treatment, while others will not. In some cases, neither you nor your doctor will know whether you are a member of the treatment group or the control group. These are called *double-blind studies*. However, you will at all times be carefully monitored for your response to treatment and for any potential side effects.

USING EDUCATION AND INFORMATION IN THE DECISION-MAKING PROCESS

In this chapter we have addressed many of the questions that typically rush through the minds of patients upon receiving a cancer diagnosis. Some patients are much less troubled by questions, however, or by a need for detailed, specific answers. They are content to allow their physician, or their family members, to guide a majority of their treatment decisions. For an oncologist, recognizing and responding appropriately to these two broad categories of patients—and everyone in between—requires good judgment and a clear understanding of the role of information in the treatment process.

Even though there is a broad spectrum of interest and need for information among patients and family members, everyone can benefit greatly by understanding the basic facts presented above. Many patients have an endless number of questions, each of which they often believe is a matter of life or death. This desperate hunger for information raises issues that go to the heart of the doctor-patient relationship, as well as the treatment process itself.

Experience has taught me that, in general, patients themselves should decide what information they need or want. They should certainly have all of the information necessary to make truly informed decisions about their care and to understand the effect of their illness and treatment on all areas of their lives.

Unfortunately, many patients often feel that they *do not* have all the information they need or want. Caught in fear or lack of understanding, they complain, "My doctor didn't answer all of my questions," or "My doctor doesn't spend enough time with me." All too often this is true, and their complaints are justified. If you feel this way, express your concerns directly to your physician.

In order to get the answers you want, it is best to be aware of the thoughts and questions that are running through your mind and to put them into words in a way that seems most comfortable. Avoid making any judgments about the questions you want to ask and make it a point to write your questions down so you don't forget them.

THE IMPORTANCE OF TRUSTING YOUR GUIDE ON THE JOURNEY THROUGH CANCER

With this in mind, we can return to the issue of trust between doctor and patient from a somewhat different perspective.

Level One of this program is not intended to provide a specific, complete answer to every possible question that a patient or a family member might have. Rather, it seeks to provide some of the basic information that you and your family need in order to make informed decisions about your care and then to move forward on your healing journey with trust, confidence, and faith in your guide.

As a patient, you must at some point find a way to suspend the unceasing activity of a doubting mind. This is not to suggest that you should abandon thinking or abdicate your sovereign right to know and understand what is happening to you. However, if the doubting mind is left unchecked, it can seriously undermine the treatment process.

George Fairfax was someone who seemed to be following such a self-sabotaging path. He was a fifty-one-year-old man with a relatively straightforward type of cancer, and he gave the impression of a deep unwillingness to trust. When I met him, he had already been to the Mayo Clinic in Minnesota, the M. D. Anderson Cancer Center in Houston, and Memorial Sloan-Kettering Cancer Center in New York for consultations about his case. At each of these institutions he was given the same general recommendations for treatment, but he was neither convinced nor satisfied. Now he had come to me for yet another consultation.

George was a cyclone of information need. He wanted to know

everything about all of the various chemotherapy drugs recommended as part of his treatment. Moreover, he wanted to know about every single possible side effect that could possibly occur, no matter how unlikely. He also wanted to know exactly what I was going to do, *in advance*, to prevent—or at least minimize to the greatest extent possible—all of these possible side effects. He further wanted to know everything about a variety of herbs, vitamins, mineral supplements, antioxidants, Essiac tea, and much more.

After a lengthy discussion about all of this, it became clear that his operative impulse was not really a desire to know about cancer or the details of cancer treatment. Instead, he was plagued by a deeply rooted fear of pain, and difficulty in trusting and letting go. As a result, a tremendous amount of valuable time and energy was being diverted into unfulfilling and clinically unproductive channels.

"Mr. Fairfax," I finally said to him, "it is very important that at some point you make a decision to trust someone to guide you in this process. Maybe that person will be me, and, if so, I would be honored to help you. But if it is not me, then you must find someone else whom you do fully trust. I don't need you to trust and have confidence in me for my sake. It's for *your* sake. If you don't make a decision to fully trust me—or someone else—as your physician, you'll never stop worrying and wondering. You'll burden yourself mentally and emotionally whenever a neighbor, a friend, or a relative tells you about something he or she saw on the Internet, or about a different chemotherapy protocol offered somewhere, or about some new miracle herb or vitamin."

Everyone involved with cancer must ultimately develop the ability to live with uncertainty. Cancer is an area of human experience in which we simply do not have all the answers we want. Caregivers as well as patients have a responsibility to accept the uncertainty that is inevitably part of this journey.

The journey will undoubtedly include unpredictable experiences, and we must recognize that its destination is, in many ways, unknown. By embracing this perspective, no matter what the outcome, you can find and experience love and joy at every step along the way.

HOW TO MAKE THE MOST ENLIGHTENED DECISIONS ABOUT YOUR TREATMENT

Many cancer patients make treatment decisions out of fear—fear of what will happen if they agree to the treatment, or fear of what will happen if they don't. I believe that it is critically important for patients to resolve, here and now, that they will not make treatment-related decisions based on fear. Those decisions—like all decisions in life—are best made when based on entirely different criteria.

The decision-making system outlined here defines the specific criteria that can be extremely helpful for patients and family members on the journey through cancer. It is designed to be used with the help of your physicians and other caregivers. For each of the categories, think about the questions listed, then write your thoughts in the space provided or on a separate sheet of paper. After a day or so, look over what you've written and see if your feelings are still the same. If so, you're probably getting close to the decision you truly believe in. If your feelings have changed, write down your new thoughts and give yourself more time to choose the best option. Finally, make sure that you discuss these issues with your physician.

1. Knowledge and information. *Do I really have the knowledge and information I need to make the best decision about my care? What does that knowledge and information suggest as the best thing to do in the situation I am facing?*

_____

_____

_____

_____

_____

2. Understanding. *Do I really, truly understand what this knowledge, this information, and all these statistics really mean?* Often there is a big distinction between *having* information and *understanding* what it means. Ask yourself: *Do I really understand the implications of choosing this particular treatment?* Or, *Do I feel I have a sufficient level of understanding to trust my doctor's recommendation, and feel good about going ahead?* If you are considering declining a particular treatment, ask yourself: *Do I really understand the consequences of declining this treatment? Do I know and understand what the alternatives are, and what is involved in pursuing them?*

_____

_____

_____

_____

_____

3. Wisdom. *What is the wise thing to do? What does my deep inner wisdom say to me about these choices? What is the wisest choice in terms of accomplishing my most important goals in life?* For this part of the process, you need to enter deeply into silence and listen for the voice of your inner wisdom. You may wish to be guided in meditation or into a deep state of relaxation in order to hear this inner voice. You must also have clarity about what your goals are. These issues will be addressed in more detail in "Level Six: Life Assessment" (page 180).

_____

_____

_____

_____

_____

4. Love and compassion. *What is the most loving and compassionate thing to do—for myself and for the people I love and who love me?* Be aware of the difference between what may seem most loving and compassionate in the short term, as opposed to what may be most loving and compassionate over a longer period of time. Be honest with yourself! This is your life, and your treatment.

5. Intuition. *What does my intuition say is best for me to do in this situation?* After all of the previous questions have been answered, it is time for you to tune in to your intuition for additional guidance. This is a part of your unconscious mind that can speak from a place beyond logic or rational thought. This final step should not be taken before the other steps have been completed. The reason for this is that inner voices of fear and doubt can often masquerade as intuition and steer you off track. Thus, it is important to clear away the voices of fear and doubt by first addressing the questions above.

5

LEVEL TWO:

CONNECTION WITH OTHERS

TRUE LISTENING IS LOVE IN ACTION.
                                              —M. SCOTT PECK

Connection with other people lies at the heart of healing. This is true for cancer or any other illness. Though it can take many forms, the need for human connection is as basic as the need for surgery or chemotherapy or any other medical treatment.

Strong scientific evidence shows that love and support from others translates into better health, not just emotional but physical as well. Multiple research studies have confirmed what we might intuitively expect: people with diversified social networks live longer and healthier lives than those who are socially isolated. These health-promoting social ties can take many forms, including marriage, family, friends, neighbors, and colleagues, as well as a variety of social and religious groups.

We now know with certainty that the nervous system, the endocrine system, the digestive system, the immune system—indeed, *all* the biological systems of the human body—are inseparably interwoven. While the precise role of stress, anxiety, depression, and other psychological factors in the origin of cancer is still unclear, there is no longer any question about the importance of these factors in influencing a patient's experience of treatment and recovery.

A wide variety of interactions involving connection with others are commonly referred to as *psychosocial interventions*. Assessing their impact in the overall care of cancer patients and their families is a major area of interest and research. These interventions can take a number of forms, including educational programs and various types of psychological counseling. Perhaps best known, however, are the numerous kinds of support groups for cancer patients and family members that have gained recognition and acceptance over the past decade.

It is now very clear that support groups *work*. It has been repeatedly shown, for example, that a variety of cancer support programs can reduce the need for pain medicine, sleeping pills, and medications for depression and anxiety. Patients commonly report improvements in their overall sense of well-being and their sense of control and understanding of their disease. Support groups also give patients the strength and confidence they need to adhere more fully to their treatment plans, which can often have a powerful and positive impact on the course of their illness.

Remarkably, not only do patients report these and other improvements in their quality of life, but *family members report them as well*, even if it was only the patient who participated in the groups.

Support groups can dramatically relieve the overwhelming sense of isolation that is so often experienced by cancer patients. Again and again, patients refer to the isolation they feel when they are diagnosed, even if they are married and have families. The disease causes them to feel cut off from the rest of humanity, separated from everyone in the world who doesn't have cancer. As painful as this is, it can lead patients to isolate themselves further, even from other patients, and this plays into the hands of the disease process. Isolation is both a cause and an effect of depression, and untreated depression can clearly and adversely affect quality of life, immune function, treatment compliance, and even life expectancy.

On the other hand, when a cancer patient uses the diagnosis for making new connections rather than losing old ones, the experience of the illness changes profoundly. Instead of imposing an enforced isolation, cancer can become a bridge to a larger world. For many patients, support groups are a big part of that positive transition. It is a matter not simply of getting support, but of giving it as well. Participants often gain strength by *providing support to others,* sometimes even more than by receiving it themselves.

For many individuals—including patients, clinicians, and researchers—an important issue in evaluating psychosocial support is whether it prolongs survival. I believe that focusing primarily on the survival value of psychosocial support is missing the point, particularly in light of its other significant and undisputed benefits. The question of whether or to what degree psychosocial support impacts survival has been controversial for some time. The debate accelerated, however, in the late 1980s to mid-1990s with the publication of several well-known and intriguing studies that suggested that psychosocial support may indeed prolong survival times among cancer patients.

The first of these studies was published in 1989 by Dr. David Spiegel of Stanford University. It reported on the effects of a support group intervention for women with metastatic breast cancer. In Dr. Speigel's study, eighty-six women with metastatic breast cancer were randomly assigned to two different groups. Both groups of women received standard medical care for their breast cancer, under the direction of their oncologist. In addition to receiving standard medical care, however, one of the two groups of patients also met once a week for ninety minutes over the course of a year.

When the study results were analyzed, those women who participated in the support group were found to have experienced significantly less anxiety, depression, and pain. They also felt better able to communicate with their families and their doctors, and enjoyed a greater sense of overall well-being.

However, Dr. Spiegel was greatly surprised to also discover that, on average, the women who had participated in the support group were also found to have lived *nearly twice as long* as those who did not participate (36.6 months compared with 18.9 months, respectively).

The findings of this study raised quite a stir among oncologists and other cancer researchers. Dr. Spiegel and his team had been careful to examine whether any variables other than participating in the support program might have accounted for the difference in survival between the two groups of women, and none could be found. Could it possibly be true that something as simple as one year of a weekly support group could improve survival so dramatically in people with cancer? For the participants of Dr. Spiegel's study, the answer was an unequivocal *yes*.

A second well-known study also suggested that psychosocial support for cancer patients may help to prolong life, as well as enhance it. In 1993, the UCLA psychiatrist Dr. Fawzy I. Fawzy and his colleagues published the results of a study involving sixty-eight patients who had undergone standard surgical treatment for malignant melanoma, a potentially deadly form of skin cancer. As in the Spiegel study, Fawzy's patients were divided into two groups. One group had surgery alone. The other group had the same surgery and also participated in a structured group program lasting ninety minutes a week for six weeks, beginning shortly after their surgery.

At the end of the six-week intervention, patients who had participated in the group reported feeling more vigorous than the patients who had not. At a six-month follow-up evaluation, the differences between the two groups of patients were even more pronounced. Those who had participated in the support program showed significantly less depression, fatigue, confusion, and mood disturbance, as well as better coping skills, compared with the group who had received surgery alone.

Even more remarkably, at the end of six years of follow-up, Fawzy and his colleagues discovered that patients who had undergone the six-week intervention program had lower recurrence rates and *significantly improved survival*. Specifically, thirty-one out of thirty-four patients in the intervention group were alive, compared with twenty-four of thirty-four in the surgery-only group. Careful analysis of all possible contributing variables yielded a compelling, unmistakable finding: *the only significant difference between the two groups of patients was the participation by one group in the six-week support program.*

A third provocative study on the importance of social support was undertaken by the Canadian epidemiologist Dr. Elizabeth Maunsell. Her research, published in 1995, involved 224 Canadian women who had undergone surgery for breast cancer that was localized or had spread to regional lymph nodes. Three months after their surgery, each of the women underwent an in-depth home interview performed by the same specially trained nurse. The interview included questions on a variety of psychosocial factors, including whether they had confided their feelings to or discussed personal problems with one or more persons in the three months following hospitalization. Confidants include spouses, family members, children, friends, neighbors, colleagues, physicians, nurses, psychiatrists, psychologists, priests, and others. Seven years later, survival data for the 224 women were carefully analyzed. Among the patients who had no confidants, the seven-year survival rate was 56 percent. Among the women who confided in at least one person, the seven-year survival rate was 66 percent. And the survival rate for women reporting two or more confidants increased even more, to 76 percent.

As the authors acknowledged, the results of this study achieved only borderline statistical significance and must be interpreted with caution. Nonetheless, no other variables among the women were identified to account for the differences in their survival.

It is important to mention that over the last decade a number of other well-designed studies have been published that did *not* show any survival advantage among cancer patients who participated in a variety of support groups or other psychosocial interventions. This is not surprising given the complexities of cancer itself and the numerous challenges, variables, logistics, and costs involved in research of this kind.

The results of all these studies are intriguing, however, and at the very least, they point to the need for and value of further research in this area. They also highlight the importance of shifting our attention from a focus that emphasizes *length of life* toward a broader focus on *quality of life*. Here the data are abundantly clear: numerous published studies document significant, unequivocal benefits in quality of life from a wide variety of support groups and other psychosocial interventions for people with cancer and their loved ones. Connection with others is, without a doubt, one of the most powerful choices under your control on your journey through cancer.

Indeed, there are many things you can do as a cancer patient to access the benefits of connection with others. As you get started, the following points are helpful to bear in mind.

1. Seek out multiple sources of support and connection. One of the most interesting findings of the Maunsell study was that improvement in survival did not seem to be related to the *type* of confidant the women reported talking to. Whether the confidant was a family member, a friend, a clergy member, a nurse, or a doctor, the important element was the trust the patient was able to place in another human being.

For the great majority of cancer patients, family is the foundation of the emotional support system, and there is no question that strong family ties can be tremendously beneficial in the journey through cancer. But cancer patients must realize their families can't "do it all." The intimacy and intensity of family relationships are often a great source of strength. However, the very nature of family ties can also inhibit patients from sharing difficult emotions including anger, fear, and despair. Sometimes it is much easier, and more helpful, to share troubling feelings such as these with more neutral listeners.

In a similar way, family members of cancer patients should not feel compelled to take on sole responsibility for their loved one's emotional well-being. Whether acknowledged or not, family members of cancer patients are often under great stress themselves. Support can often be as important, and vital, for them as for the patient.

2. Once your support network is in place, use it to the fullest. Confide in your confidants. Allow yourself to feel however you are feeling, even if it is weak, scared, or angry. Acknowledge the fact that you may need or want help, or simply desire a deeper sense of connection with others.

Even patients who seem stoically self-sufficient at the outset of treatment often come to realize their need for support. To the extent that they have denied this very human need, they can set themselves up for sudden and unexpected overflows of emotion that may be overwhelming. It is important while navigating the journey through cancer that you acknowledge the full range of your feelings, that you share them in appropriate settings, and that you use them to make yourself stronger and healthier. This is an opportunity to experience a kind of trust and growth that many people have never allowed themselves to experience before in their lives. It is also an opportunity to allow those who love and care about you to be able to show and give their love. As difficult as it may seem at first, allow yourself to take full advantage of the connection and support that others want to offer you at this critical time.

3. Even if you choose to hide your illness from others, don't hide it from yourself. Although great progress has been made in controlling the side effects of cancer treatment, many of them still remain. Hair loss still occurs with a number of chemotherapy drugs. Radiation may redden or burn the skin. Some patients may also experience nausea, fatigue, or weight loss during treatment. How to deal with these side effects is a personal matter. The choice of whom to tell about the illness is also a highly individual decision, even if there are no visible signs of the disease.

Whatever approach you take, it's important to be totally honest with yourself about what you are experiencing. Despite the obvious courage of cancer patients, some feel a real sense of shame about their disease. A kind of hiding instinct may appear, which can undermine emotional well-being and complicate the experience of treatment. It is important that you resist this instinct if it is causing you to feel isolated or limited in your options.

You may choose to wear a wig, a scarf, a baseball cap, or makeup—or you may want the world to see you exactly as you are. This is one time in life in which any choice can be the right one, as long as it comes from self-acceptance and a desire for self-expression.

4. Communicate with present and former cancer patients. Ultimately, no one—not family members, friends, or physicians—can know how the journey through cancer *feels* from a patient's perspective unless they have been through it themselves. Oncologists may have administered chemotherapy to thousands of people, yet after only one treatment a patient will know more about the experience than the doctor. That is why it is so important to make contact with people who have firsthand knowledge of what you are going through.

The best way to overcome a sense of isolation is to realize you really are not isolated. Many, many people have been exactly where you are now and survived. Many others state unequivocally that their lives were undeniably transformed *for the better* by their experience with cancer. Cancer patients have much to share with one another that can be found nowhere else. Despite the seriousness of this illness, there is no question that it can be an extraordinary opportunity to give and receive advice, wisdom, and love. The support of others who have "been there" can be vitally important in helping you seize and make the most of these opportunities.

FINDING THE CONNECTIONS AND SUPPORT THAT ARE RIGHT FOR YOU

Today hundreds of psychosocial resources are available to cancer patients. Some, like talking to a clergy member or other spiritual adviser, have existed for as long as human beings have experienced illness. Others, like support groups and other psychosocial and educational programs, have been around for years and are becoming more available and sophisticated every day. A list of helpful cancer support organizations is provided in Appendix 2, and I strongly urge patients and family members to take advantage of them.

Still others are quite new, such as online chat groups or message and bulletin boards. The Internet provides astonishing opportunities for many patients and their families. A few clicks of the mouse can bring you up-to-the-minute, firsthand information about your diagnosis. It can also put you directly in contact with patients, physicians, publications, and leading cancer centers around the country, if not the world. In terms of connection with others, you can instantly interact in real time with people who are exactly where you are right now in the journey through cancer—and it's a lot easier to go on a rafting trip with other travelers than to take off in a rowboat all by yourself. A list of valuable Internet resources is provided in Appendix 3.

One of the Internet's unique features is the anonymity of the participants, since there are many instances in which communication is easier if no one knows who you are. However, the Internet is no substitute for human contact.

Support groups may at times seem more challenging, but they offer something that can come only from sitting down and spending time with other human beings. How this works is a mystery, but it is true. The experience of human beings gathering together to offer each other love and support has existed for millennia. The benefits of that experience are clear and profound.

It is also no exaggeration to say that support group participation can sometimes make the critical difference between patients giving up or fighting for their lives. It can also save a spouse or a caregiver from becoming completely overwhelmed by the experience of a loved one's illness. This aspect of the healing process is so important that it is now becoming a standard component of multidisciplinary cancer care throughout the United States and elsewhere.

In view of all the evidence regarding the benefits of psychosocial support programs, why do a surprising number of patients still resist participating in them or in other forms of counseling? I believe there are several answers to this, and it is valuable to look closely at each of them. If you are a cancer patient, or if someone close to you has cancer, ask yourself whether you recognize any of these feelings:

- *Do you feel uncomfortable attending a support group because you're "just not someone who joins groups"?* Many people value autonomy and independence as an important aspect of character. They simply aren't at ease with "joining"—whether it's a political movement, a charitable organization, or a support group. Cancer, however, is something entirely new in a patient's life, and everyone can benefit from new ways of helping to deal with the illness. This is not a matter of forsaking basic identity. It is simply an opportunity to introduce some flexibility into a situation where flexibility can be of real benefit.

- *Do you feel that psychosocial support would violate your identity as someone who doesn't need help?* When cancer strikes, your sense of self-sufficiency can receive a sudden and shocking blow. This causes some patients to retreat from others just at the moment when others are needed. What is really called for is a recognition that *you do need support.* This is often as true for family members as for patients themselves. No matter how strong you are or how highly you value your independence, trying to go through cancer alone is a mistake. Often it is simply the fear of admitting this that causes patients or family members to avoid support groups or other forms of psychosocial support.

- *Do you envision a support group as a threatening, unsafe, or depressing environment?* When a cancer patient wants to stay away from other cancer patients, this might really be an attempt to get away from himself or herself. It is often a way of unconsciously saying cancer is still "the enemy"—and that being close to people with cancer might lead to a deeply unsettling recognition of "the enemy within me." This often consumes significantly more precious time and energy than patients appreciate. A much more effective approach is to accurately identify what or who the real enemy is. Or, even better, to abandon the notion that there is an enemy at all.

- *If you were to take part in a support group, do you fear exploring emotions that might come to the surface?* A typical response to cancer is to try to shore up our areas of weakness, because cancer is going to require all the strength and attention we can muster. However, it takes a lot of energy to keep anger, fear, pain, resentment, and frustration bottled up. Acknowledging these emotions and working through them can be intimidating. Nevertheless, doing so is extremely important and worthwhile—and, as we have seen, can yield numerous positive benefits for yourself as well as those you love and care about. This is especially true since unexplored feelings can intensify under the stress of illness and may express themselves in ways that are hurtful, not only to patients but also to those close to them.

- *Would a support group violate your rules about sharing your feelings with strangers?* If all the world is indeed a stage, cancer pushes patients right onto the center of it and challenges them to start reciting their best lines. Many patients, however, would rather remain in the wings. It is only in the past few decades that the idea of expressing thoughts and feelings has begun to gain acceptance in our culture. For the generations who grew up during the Depression or World War II, what is now called denial was known as toughness and the ability to keep your mouth shut. But those qualities, especially if cultivated over a lifetime, come at a price that a cancer patient can hardly afford, regardless of his or her generation. The notion that sharing your feelings somehow diminishes your strength is simply wrong. In fact, the opposite is true.

• *Would joining a support group make it more difficult for you to deny you have cancer?* Some patients try to deal with their illness as if nothing has happened. These are people who rush from the hospital or from a chemotherapy treatment directly back to their well-established routine, whether it be golf, gin rummy, or trading commodities futures. Of course, this is every patient's right—but it is also a missed opportunity. Tremendous insight and growth can be gained at this time, but the opportunity is lost when you run headlong away from your immediate experience back to the known and familiar. Cancer must be seen for what it is. It is much more than an annoyance or an inconvenience in your daily routine—no matter how much patients may at times wish to deny this. The risk of wearing blinders regarding cancer is that they can suddenly come off. Without becoming obsessed with cancer, therefore, it is important for patients to give the illness its proper place and significance in their lives.

TYPES OF SUPPORT GROUPS

Just as chemotherapy, radiation, and surgery have evolved to focus much more precisely on the needs of individual patients, programs for support and connection with others are evolving as well.

Cancer patients often respond quite differently to various kinds of psychosocial interventions. Some patients respond more readily to individual counseling while others prefer group discussion. It is important for everyone involved to accurately define their needs and to choose the kind of support that serves them best.

A variety of group settings are often employed for cancer patients, family members, and caregivers. The following are among the most widely used group formats.

- *Open-ended groups* are probably the most common setting for psychosocial support in cancer. These groups may include any combination of patients, family members, friends, and caregivers, or they may be limited to only one category. Typically, groups meet on a regular basis with social workers, clinicians, or even former patients acting as facilitators. Often a group will continue meeting for several years. Many patients prefer this continuity rather than a shorter-term arrangement. Although patients may initially feel apprehensive about joining a support group, the vast majority find the experience beneficial in terms of their ability to deal with fear and anxiety, to communicate their feelings and concerns, and to gain vitally helpful emotional support at critical times.

- *Patient education groups* focus on the clinical and practical issues of cancer. For some patients, mastering the facts of their illness and its treatment can provide therapeutic benefit even if emotional issues are never directly addressed. This may be especially true for patients with an intellectual orientation to life. One of the most difficult aspects of cancer can be the impression that your life is being taken over by something confusing and beyond comprehension. When psychosocial support is used to dispel that notion, a major obstacle is removed.

- *Cognitive-behavioral groups* teach coping techniques of mindful awareness and positive reinforcement. For example, patients may learn valuable ways to stop themselves from slipping into depressive thought patterns or to replace negative thoughts with a positive or uplifting affirmation. Even learning to monitor and be aware of thoughts that occur during the day can be very helpful.

- *Supportive-expressive groups* encourage shared feelings and empathy among members not only during formal group sessions but outside the meetings as well. This aspect of psychosocial support has also been effective in areas outside cancer care. Twelve-step programs, for example, have different goals and intentions than do cancer support groups, but they also encourage members to become part of one another's lives outside the formal meeting. The power of this approach cannot be denied.

As we gain greater understanding of how psychosocial interventions and connection with others can impact the lives of cancer patients and their family members in profound ways, attention to this dimension of healing will become increasingly emphasized as part of the care offered at any oncologist's office or certified cancer center. If a patient is having bone pain or mouth sores associated with chemotherapy, it is the physician's responsibility to provide a medication that brings relief. Similarly, when a patient is suffering from isolation, loneliness, or others forms of emotional distress, and especially when we know how this can adversely impact his or her experience, we have a responsibility to address this aspect of the patient's needs with equal skill and integrity. This is not "window dressing" on cancer treatment. It is an absolutely essential component.

6

LEVEL THREE:

THE BODY AS GARDEN

THE NATURAL HEALING FORCE WITHIN EACH OF
US IS THE GREATEST FORCE IN GETTING WELL.

—HIPPOCRATES

Years ago, when I first began to explore the great spiritual and healing traditions of the East, my travels took me to India, Nepal, China, and Tibet. One metaphor from the traditions of those countries captured my attention: the human body seen as a garden, and the physician as someone who tends it. I was particularly impressed by the contrast of these images with those from the West, in which the human body is often regarded as a machine and the physician as a mechanic. I fell in love with the image of the body as garden, and it still inspires me. It also serves as the inspiration for Level Three of this program.

For both patients and doctors, the idea of the body as garden opens up new ways of thinking about ourselves—and about medicine and healing as well. It opens up tremendous opportunities for us all to play genuinely positive roles in the healing process. It gives each of us a chance to ask, *What can I do to cultivate the garden of my being in such a way that the fruits and flowers of health, well-being, and self-knowledge can blossom and grow? What can I do to fertilize and till the soil of my being in order to accomplish this?*

Within each of us are deep and powerful mechanisms of healing that can make an enormous difference in getting well. One of your most important objectives as a cancer patient should be to cleanse and nourish your body in a way that allows those inner healing mechanisms to flourish as fully as possible.

When a garden is carefully tended, destructive life-forms such as weeds or parasites may still appear, but they are much less likely to take over. They can be dealt with while they are still in an easily manageable form. Making a garden healthy also requires giving it adequate nutrients and water, and turning the soil so the earth mixes with fresh air. Removing toxins and other harmful substances from the environment is essential, along with making sure the garden has plenty of sunlight. By tending to all these things, a gardener gives nature the fullest possible opportunity to come into congruence with his or her wishes.

If a garden is neglected, another side of nature is likely to assert itself. Weeds are just as natural as roses, but they're out of sync with our ultimate interests. They're also out of sync with all the other plants in the garden. They can quickly usurp the space and nourishment of the other plants, often killing them in the process. The weeds can also eventually choke out one another and cause their own death.

This is as close to a perfect analogy with cancer as we are likely to find. Good nutrition, exercise, and a life that is emotionally and spiritually fulfilled provide no guarantee that cancer will be prevented, let alone cured. However, actively pursuing all these can help—sometimes very significantly.

Level Three of the Seven Levels of Healing is an invitation to develop an entirely new, ongoing relationship with your body. This new relationship begins by seeing your body as a garden that needs nurturing and care, as well as sufficient space and sunshine in which to heal and grow. Your body is not a machine that was created simply to carry out the will of its owner. The idea that the body must do the bidding of the human ego rarely works in the journey through cancer—in fact, it can be counterproductive. Your body is a living, breathing organism, a focal point of energy, information, intelligence, and growth. And healing from cancer is, ultimately, an organic process that requires many ingredients. An element of mystery also accompanies this process. Consciously connecting with that mystery can be healing in and of itself.

But a new perspective is not all that is required for a successful journey through cancer. On a very practical level, a wide variety of viewpoints, philosophies, and treatments for cancer is now available. These compete for attention, and sometimes are even openly in conflict. For every patient, they also raise complex but vitally important questions:

- How can I gain maximum benefit from conventional cancer treatment while minimizing risk and discomfort?
- What are the proper roles for complementary and alternative therapies in my cancer treatment?
- Is there anything I should be eating during my treatment, and what should I not eat?
- What vitamins, minerals, supplements, or herbs should I take?
- Should I be taking antioxidants, and if so, what kinds?
- How much should I exercise, or should I just rest as much as possible?
- Is it okay for me to have a massage if I have cancer?
- What can I do to minimize the side effects of my cancer treatment?
- How can I talk to my doctor about my interest in complementary and alternative medicine?
- What about the Eastern healing traditions? Do they have anything to offer me?
- What else can I do to help myself on this journey?

This chapter sorts out the enormous confusion that patients and family members so often encounter in dealing with these questions. It provides a framework within which different approaches can find an appropriate place without overwhelming one another, and without interfering with the most important clinical aspects of a patient's care.

While I strongly believe that conventional therapies are the foundation of effective cancer treatment, I also believe there are important roles for many of the other approaches that are available.

Let's define some of the terms in greater detail.

- *Complementary medicine* refers to the wide variety of physical, mental, emotional, and spiritual techniques that can benefit patients at all points in the journey through cancer. These include diet and nutritional programs, herbs, supplements, aromatherapy, massage, exercise, yoga, relaxation, journaling, visualization and guided imagery, acupuncture, chiropractic, homeopathy, therapeutic touch, Reiki therapy, and many more. In general, these may be used along with conventional treatment, hence the term *complementary*.

• *Alternative medicine* encompasses methods that are sometimes used by cancer patients instead of conventional cancer treatment. A defining characteristic of these methods is that they are scientifically *unproven* to be of benefit as a treatment of cancer. Some are even potentially dangerous. If they are used at all, and particularly as primary therapy for cancer, I believe it should be with great caution, and only when there are no proven therapies available that can be of benefit.

 Alternative treatments include Burzynski antineoplastons, the Hoxsey Method, the Contreras Method, DMSO, Kelly metabolic therapy, live cell therapy, the Gerson Method, the Nicholas Gonzalez Nutritional Regimen, the Greek Cancer Cure (Alivizatos therapy), high-dose intravenous vitamins, shark cartilage, Essiac tea, hydrazine sulfate, CanCell (Entelev), hyperoxygenation therapies (e.g., ozone and hydrogen peroxide), immunoaugmentative therapies, Iscador (mistletoe extract), Laetrile (amygdalin), Livingston-Wheeler therapy, macrobiotic diets, "psychic surgery," and the Revici Method, among others.

• *CAM* is an acronym that stands for *complementary and alternative medicine*. It is a widely accepted term that embraces many different kinds of therapies from these two general groups.

• *Eastern healing traditions* refer to the ancient healing methods of India (Ayurveda), China (traditional Chinese medicine), and Tibet (Tibetan medicine), among others. Elements of these traditions can be used in either complementary *or* alternative ways, depending upon the circumstances and the intentions of patients and practitioners.

- *Integrative medicine* refers to a large and growing trend that is occurring in this country and elsewhere. It involves the safe and thoughtful integration of conventional and complementary forms of medicine for the treatment of many different illnesses, including cancer.

A working knowledge of these ideas and principles can be very helpful to cancer patients and their families. We'll now look at them more closely.

Complementary Medicine

Diet and Nutrition

In our image of the body as garden, diet and nutrition correspond to fertilization of the soil. The importance of this is fairly self-evident. "You are what you eat" is a phrase that is well known, and on a basic level our physical selves are indeed an expression of the material we take in. If we are ill, quite often (although by no means always) this may be in some way related to what we have eaten. Furthermore, by eating and drinking with greater knowledge and care, perhaps additional illness can be prevented.

The question of how this applies to cancer is one that scientists have been asking for a long time, and although some answers have finally emerged, many areas of confusion and uncertainty remain. As a first step toward eliminating this confusion, it is helpful to recognize that diet and nutrition play different roles at three distinct phases in a cancer patient's life: prior to diagnosis, during treatment, and after treatment has been completed.

Let's look at each of these areas separately.

1. The Role of Diet and Nutrition in the Prevention or Causation of Cancer

Cancer has plagued human beings for thousands of years, and the disease is found in populations with a wide variety of dietary habits and customs. It is now quite clear, however, based upon hundreds of studies in the medical literature, that diet and nutrition do indeed play a significant role in cancer. The American Cancer Society estimates that diet is a primary factor in a third of cancer deaths. Some of these deaths can be attributed to the well-established link between cancer and obesity. But the precise nature of diet's role has yet to be defined.

Several things contribute to this lack of clarity. Primary among them is the great diversity found among different cancers and the individuals in which they arise. Not only does everyone eat different foods at different times of the day, but the foods are prepared differently, combined differently, and metabolized differently by different individuals. Research on diet and nutrition is also costly, time-consuming, and logistically challenging. Nonetheless, it is possible to make some general statements about the role of nutrition in the prevention of cancer, or in contributing to its cause.

A plant-based diet is protective against some cancers. The majority of studies regarding diet and cancer published in the medical literature suggest a significant protective effect of diets rich in fruits and vegetables. The most conclusive evidence to date suggests a benefit for cancers of the mouth and pharynx, larynx, lung, esophagus, stomach, kidney, colon, rectum, ovary, and bladder. Fruits and vegetables contain substances known as *phytonutrients* (from the Greek word *phyto,* meaning "plant"), which are believed to protect against cancer by a number of different mechanisms.

One of those mechanisms involves highly active molecules known as *free radicals,* which are present in every cell of the body. These can damage cellular DNA and other molecules in ways that initiate tumor development. Fruits and vegetables are key sources of *antioxidants,* which play an important role in preventing the damage to cells caused by these free radicals.

Some of the best-known antioxidants are *ascorbic acid* (vitamin C), *alpha-tocopherol* (vitamin E), and *beta-carotene* (a form of vitamin A), which are found in a wide variety of fruits and vegetables. *Lycopene* is another well-known antioxidant; it gives tomatoes their red color. Other examples include *polyphenols,* which occur in green tea, and *glutathione,* which is found in fruits and vegetables and is also created in the body from amino acids.

As mentioned above, numerous research studies indicate that people who consume foods rich in antioxidants have a lower risk of developing certain types of cancer. It is important to note, however, that commercially prepared antioxidant supplements have not consistently been shown to provide similar statistical benefits. In fact, in the Beta-Carotene and Retinol Efficacy Trial, published in 1996, the combination of beta-carotene and vitamin A supplements was shown to significantly *increase* the risk of lung cancer among subjects who smoke. Similar findings were noted in the Alpha-Tocopherol, Beta-Carotene Cancer Prevention Trial, published in 1994. In the last decade, additional studies have also consistently failed to show a benefit from antioxidant supplements in preventing cancer. One of the largest of these, the Women's Health Study, was published in 2005. It involved nearly 40,000 women who received daily vitamin E supplements and were followed for an average of ten years. Again, no benefit in reduced cancer incidence was noted. Despite the lack of scientifically proven benefit, antioxidant supplements have nonetheless become one of the fastest-growing health-related industries in the United States.

A word should also be mentioned about *selenium*, another well-known antioxidant that is found in vegetables, as well as in fish, meats, and nuts. A 1996 study, the Nutritional Prevention of Cancer Trial, suggested that individuals who consumed a daily 200 mcg selenium supplement for an average of four and a half years had significantly lower incidence of and mortality from lung, colorectal, and prostate cancer. Subsequent reports with longer follow-up from this study, however, revealed that the reduction in incidence from lung and colorectal cancer seen in the initial report was no longer evident. The benefits noted with respect to reduction in prostate cancer risk were still seen, but only in those patients with low baseline (pretreatment) serum selenium levels. Of further note, individuals who had received selenium in the study were now found to have a higher risk of developing squamous cell cancers of the skin.

These results highlight the uncertainties and challenges that persist in understanding the benefits—and potential risks—associated with commercially prepared antioxidant supplements. Further research is under way.

Cruciferous vegetables such as broccoli, cabbage, Brussels sprouts, and cauliflower are rich in other phytonutrients, notably *indoles* and *sulfora-phane*. These are believed to protect against cancer by mechanisms that are different from those of other food-based antioxidants, including removing estrogen and other potentially harmful substances from cells.

Resveratrol, which is present in red grapes and red wine, is another phytonutrient that is believed to protect against cancer by inhibiting enzymes involved in inflammation.

Soy products, including tofu, miso, and soy milk, contain chemicals called *isoflavones*, which act as weak estrogens and are believed to help reduce the risk of hormone-related cancers. Studies have shown that women who eat soy products have a lower incidence of breast cancer. This may be part of the reason why Asian women are at lower risk for developing this disease.

Garlic contains chemicals called *allyl sulfides*, which are believed to lower cancer risk by influencing the metabolism of cancer-causing substances in the liver. Studies have suggested that people with diets high in garlic may have a lower risk of stomach cancer.

Based on the vast amount of research available on this topic, the American Cancer Society recommends eating five or more servings of fruits and vegetables each day as a way of reducing one's risk of cancer. It also recommends eating other foods from plant sources (for example, grains, rice, and beans) several times each day.

The role of dietary fat in cancer risk has been another area of great interest and controversy for quite some time. In the 1980s high dietary consumption of fat was believed to be a major contributor to the development of several cancers, notably breast, colorectal, and prostate cancer. Much of this thinking derived from epidemiologic studies that associated a Western high-fat diet with increased risk of these cancers. It was not clear whether these associations were directly causal or whether they were confounded by numerous other possible factors. Some of the potentially complicating factors include total caloric intake, overall body weight, exercise habits, possible contamination by pesticides and hormones, dietary fiber content, and cooking methods.

It was also unclear if the observed associations of fat consumption and cancer risk were related to specific types of fat (such as *saturated*, *unsaturated,* or *polyunsaturated*). Some research suggested that saturated fats (found in meat and dairy products) and *omega-6 polyunsaturated fatty acids* (found in corn and safflower oils) may be more closely linked with cancer risk than other types of fat. Other research suggested that *omega-3 polyunsaturated fatty acids* (found in flaxseed and cold-water fish) may be protective against cancer as well as heart disease. Olive oil, which contains a monounsaturated fat called *oleic acid,* has also been suggested to have a protective effect against some cancers.

Over the last decade, however, large prospective studies have failed to demonstrate a conclusive relation between total fat intake and risk of breast cancer, about which there was great concern and attention. Interestingly, an association with increased colon cancer risk has been noted with high consumption of red meat, but not with total dietary fat intake. The connection between dietary fat and prostate cancer is not clear, although some meaningful evidence does suggest an association, particularly with more aggressive forms of the disease. The link between dietary fat and other cancers also remains unclear.

Despite the unresolved controversies regarding the precise role of fat and cancer risk, numerous organizations, including the National Research Council, the National Academy of Sciences, and the American Cancer Society, among others, nonetheless recommend reducing fat intake, particularly from animal sources, as a way of improving overall health. They also recommend reducing alcohol consumption and increasing intake of fruits and vegetables, as mentioned above.

Alcohol consumption contributes to cancer risk. The link between smoking and cancer has now been so well established that it hardly needs to be repeated here. Although the link between alcohol and cancer has not received the attention that has been focused on smoking, it is also very well established. Drinking seems to amplify the effects of carcinogens, particularly tobacco smoke. It also causes irritation to tissues of the mouth, esophagus, larynx, stomach, and liver in ways that might contribute to the development of cancer in these organs. By other mechanisms, it also increases the risk of breast and colorectal cancer.

But perhaps the most significant effect of alcohol consumption is the fact that it tends to promote unhealthy eating and lifestyle habits in general. When people are drinking, they're usually not eating broccoli and carrots along with their cocktails. Individuals who drink heavily develop cancer at a rate *ten times higher* than the overall population.

Having made these general statements, it should be emphasized once again that the precise role of diet and nutrition in cancer still remains controversial. As often happens in science, in recent years another article of faith about the relationship between diet and cancer has been called into question.

Since the late 1960s, it was believed that a high-fiber diet helped to prevent colon and rectal cancer. In January 1999, however, results from a sixteen-year study involving more than 88,000 women (the Nurses Health Study) showed that those who consumed the most fiber—up to 25 grams per day—contracted colorectal cancer with *virtually the same frequency* as women whose daily fiber intake was only 10 grams or less. A similar lack of benefit from fiber in reducing the risk of colorectal cancer was noted in another study involving more than 47,000 men (the Health Professionals Follow-up Study). A subsequent European study, published in 2003, did show a reduction in colorectal cancer incidence associated with high fiber intake. However, a long-term follow-up analysis of the original Nurses Health Study and Health Professionals Study, published in 2005, again showed no reduction in colorectal cancer risk seen with dietary fiber in the more than 120,000 individuals involved. These findings were clear and were derived from repeated assessments of the study participants' fiber intake over eighteen years.

Aside from what these studies say about fiber and cancer prevention, they reveal the tenuous nature of even the most "certain" information about this disease. Although a reasonable amount of fiber remains an important component of a healthy diet, this lesson should be kept in mind by everyone who is concerned about cancer and its causes.

We want to believe we can avoid cancer by eating healthy foods, and indeed a good diet can make the difference for a sizable number of people. While I certainly advise people to eat plenty of fruits and vegetables—and even to consider taking daily vitamin, mineral, and antioxidant supplements—I do not believe this should be done simply in order to avoid cancer. Throughout this book we are making the point that *no decisions should be made from fear,* whether it is eating broccoli or taking chemotherapy.

In my opinion, the best reason to follow the principles of a healthy diet—and a healthy lifestyle in general—is because doing so will yield significant benefits in *every area of your life.* Along with greater energy, improved physical health, increased vitality, and an enhanced sense of well-being, you will have greater awareness, increased clarity of mind, and expanded opportunities to achieve your life's deeper goals.

2. The Role of Diet and Nutrition During Cancer Treatment

The role of diet and nutrition in the treatment of cancer has been hotly debated in recent years, particularly among patients who want to do everything possible to help themselves get well. Unfortunately, despite good intentions, this subject can become an area of great pain and confusion for patients and family members.

Adequate nutrition is an important concern for everyone. Quite often, it is even more important for people with cancer. But in many instances, nutritional concerns are not as important—particularly in the short term—as they might appear to the individuals involved, or as sometimes suggested by complementary and alternative practitioners. The urgency and fear felt by patients and their loved ones around issues of diet and nutrition are often magnified, burdensome, and unnecessary.

Balance and perspective are the key elements needed here. Nutrition is rarely a make-or-break issue for people in cancer treatment. In the majority of cases, nutrition has a *relative* importance that must be factored into a long list of other priorities and concerns. It should be given *appropriate* attention—not too little, but not too much either. Furthermore, appropriate attention differs among patients, the various stages of their illness, and the treatment they will be receiving.

Many patients have early-stage cancers that need only limited, defined periods of adjuvant treatment. For them, the short-term issue of what to eat during their care is usually far less important than what they eat during the rest of their lives after their treatment is completed. On the other hand, if a patient has metastatic cancer and will require chemotherapy or radiation over an extended period of time, issues of nutritional support become much more important.

There is no question that during all phases of cancer treatment the body needs adequate vitamins, minerals, and calories. For many patients this will not be a problem, but for others maintaining adequate nutrition is more easily said than done. This is particularly true for patients with cancers that can directly affect their ability to eat—most notably cancers of the head and neck and upper GI tract—or for those undergoing surgical procedures for these cancers.

Several forms of cancer are associated with loss of appetite and a diminished sense of taste. Cancer treatments themselves can also produce these effects. Nausea and mouth sores sometimes associated with chemotherapy do not inspire patients to eat big, healthy meals. Another common problem, called *esophagitis,* can occur in patients receiving radiation therapy for lung cancer, esophageal cancer, or lymphomas in the chest. This condition is a radiation-induced "sunburn" of the inner lining of the esophagus, and it can make swallowing food or even liquids extremely difficult or painful. Patients undergoing radiation treatments for cancers of the mouth, throat, or neck can have similar problems.

General Diet and Nutrition Guidelines During Cancer Treatment

With the above as a preamble, here are some simple guidelines that can be helpful to patients. They can be useful for spouses and family members as well.

- Adopt a more plant-based diet.
- Try to eat several servings of fruits and vegetables each day.
- Cut back on your consumption of red meat. You can replenish your intake of protein by eating beans, fish, lentils, or nuts.
- Start eating whole grains every day, including brown rice, lentils, and buckwheat.
- Buy a juicer, and start drinking fresh fruit and vegetable juices daily.
- Avoid fried, greasy, or fatty foods.
- Minimize your intake of refined sugar.
- Minimize your intake of alcohol.
- Keep yourself well hydrated. Drink at least six glasses of spring water each day.

- Consider supplementing your diet with a high-quality multivitamin once or twice a day. If you have difficulty swallowing pills, try vitamin powders that you can mix in fruit juices or water.
- Consider other nutritional supplements, including liquid trace minerals and protein drinks.
- Above all, avoid making your diet another source of stress. Don't feel guilty about eating foods you like, and don't feel obligated to eat foods you don't want.

Despite anecdotal accounts of the benefits of intensive nutritional programs, including high-dose intravenous vitamin regimens, cleansing diets, and macrobiotics, none of these approaches has been scientifically proven to be helpful. Sometimes they also pose real risks and potential adverse effects.

This is particularly true of antioxidants when taken concurrently with conventional cancer treatment. Studies have suggested that patients who take antioxidant supplements during chemotherapy or radiation may experience fewer side effects. This occurs presumably because of the antioxidants' ability to reduce the toxic effects of the treatment on normal cells and tissues. Unfortunately, the antioxidants may be simultaneously reducing the effects of the treatment on the cancer cells. Patients may think the antioxidants are helping them when in fact they may be causing harm. The answer is simply not yet known. For this reason, I generally advise patients to avoid taking antioxidants until their chemotherapy or radiation treatments are completed.

Remember, everyone is unique, and your needs may vary at different times during your treatment. If you have any questions about your diet, and especially about the appropriateness of taking vitamins, minerals, antioxidants, or other nutritional supplements, it is important to consult your oncologist.

Some Advice for Family Members. It is very difficult to see a loved one in the midst of a serious illness. Quite naturally everyone feels an instinctive desire to help. Suggestions about diet and nutrition are often the vehicle people choose for expressing their love and concern. Family or friends may recommend macrobiotic diets, teas, liquid herbal extracts, vitamins, pills, and other dietary options. But well-meaning people do not always understand the real needs of patients during treatment. And patients themselves may not be able to express their needs as clearly or as forcefully as they might wish.

Beyond helping the patient get the best possible medical care, perhaps the most important task for family members is to *accept and support their loved one's choices.* Consciously choosing to honor and respect a patient's decisions is one of the greatest gifts a person can give. This comes up frequently in the area of nutrition, where family members and friends often feel compelled to offer food or dietary suggestions, even when patients are clearly not interested.

Paul Delaney was a seventy-four-year-old man undergoing combined radiation and chemotherapy treatment for esophageal cancer. He was a robust, jolly person who had always loved to eat, and his wife loved to cook for him. He had hardly been sick in his entire life until a few months before I met him, when he began to notice food getting stuck in his throat. Medical evaluation revealed a tumor obstructing a good portion of his esophagus.

During the first month of his treatment, Paul did extremely well. He had no nausea or vomiting, kept active every day, and started swallowing food more easily soon after his treatment began. His appetite was good, and he even started gaining weight. Following his second cycle of chemotherapy, he began to feel run down and tired. His appetite began to diminish, and he started to feel a burning sensation in his esophagus from the radiation. He started eating less.

Careful medical evaluation of his condition showed no other worrisome findings or cause for alarm. His weight loss was minimal. I informed Paul and his wife that his symptoms were entirely in line with what one might expect in a man his age at this point in treatment, and I offered him appropriate medications to alleviate his symptoms and some dietary recommendations as well.

Paul, reassured, was confident about going ahead with his remaining treatments. But for Marie, his wife, a big problem had arisen.

"Doctor, what am I going to do?" she said with exasperation. "My husband won't eat! I try to feed him ten times a day, but he refuses everything. It's driving me crazy! You have to do something. If *you* tell him to eat, then he'll listen. But he won't listen to me."

I asked Paul if this was true.

"Well," he replied, "I just don't feel like eating too much right now. I'm tired, and I don't have much of an appetite. I don't want to eat any big meals, but she keeps on pushing me to eat more."

"You *have* to eat more, Paul," Marie interrupted. "You're eating like a bird, and you're going to waste away and starve to death if you don't eat more."

"See? She won't let up on me," Paul said. "I tell her to leave me alone, but she won't stop. All day long, it's 'Eat, eat, eat.' But I don't *want* to eat. What should I do?"

This is a scenario that oncologists encounter virtually every day. Responding most effectively to it requires insight into all dimensions of what is really going on.

I responded to Paul's question by once again examining him carefully and reviewing his chart, and I then gently reassured Marie that her husband's medical tests had revealed no other cause for alarm. He had lost only three pounds over the prior few weeks, and I reassured her that this small amount of weight loss was not dangerous. He was by no means at risk of "starving to death." Fifty years of her home cooking had boosted Paul's weight to over two hundred pounds.

Then I turned to Paul and said, "Mr. Delaney, may I ask you a question?"

"Sure," he said.

"Why do you think Mrs. Delaney keeps trying to get you to eat so much?"

Paul paused for a long time, and then he started to choke up. He was a proud man, and he almost never allowed himself to cry. Fighting back tears, he said, "I don't know."

"Really, Mr. Delaney. Why do you think your wife wants you to eat so much?"

After another long pause, he finally said, "Well, I guess she does it because she loves me."

"I think that's very true," I said. "And why else does she try to get you to eat so much?"

"Well," he said, after another long pause, "I guess she does it because she doesn't want me to be sick."

I looked at Marie and asked, "Is that true?"

She nodded in agreement.

I looked back at Paul and asked, "And why doesn't she want you to be sick?"

Paul paused for a very long time before answering softly, "I guess because she doesn't want me to die."

I then asked Paul to look at his wife. Her eyes were filled with tears, and she reached out and hugged him. "That's right, Paul," she said. "I love you so much, and I'm afraid to lose you. I want you to eat so you'll be healthy. I don't want to lose you."

This was a beautiful breakthrough in their journey together. It was also a moment of truth and a turning point of sorts.

"May I offer you a suggestion?" I asked.

"Yes, please," they both replied.

"Okay," I said. "First of all, I want to acknowledge you both for telling the truth the way you just have. It is so beautiful and moving for me to see this. Thank you.

"Now, Mr. Delaney," I continued, "do you realize that asking Marie to stop offering you food would be very difficult and painful for her?"

"Yes," he replied. "I can see that."

"And, Mrs. Delaney, can you see how your continuous insistence that Paul eat all the time, and that he eat bigger meals than he really wants, is only causing him pain and making him feel *worse* than he already does?"

"Yes," she said, with an obviously heavy heart. "I can see that now. I didn't see it before."

"I'm sure you didn't," I said, "because I know you only want to help your husband."

"Oh, yes," she said. "That's true."

"Great," I continued. "My recommendation is that you have an agreement with each other that looks something like this." I turned to Paul. "What I'd like to suggest is that you agree to allow Mrs. Delaney to offer you food, but no more than three times a day. Will that work for you?"

"Sure," he replied.

"And will you also agree that if you feel hungry, or if you want to eat something special, that you will ask her to make it for you?"

"Why, sure," he said. "That's easy."

"Terrific. I feel we're making progress here."

I then turned to Marie and said, "Now, Mrs. Delaney, if Paul says, 'No, thank you, honey. I don't want to eat right now,' are you willing to agree that you will ask him 'Are you sure?' only one time?"

"Well, I guess so," she replied cautiously. "But what if he doesn't eat at all? What am I supposed to do then?"

"If that happens, I want you to call me, and let me know about it. If I'm not here, speak to any other of the staff members, and they will let me know right away. I don't want you to be worrying yourself sick over this. We will keep a very close watch on Mr. Delaney right along with you, and make sure that he is not losing too much weight. Okay?"

"Okay," she said. "That'll be fine."

The Delaneys' experience is a very common, human, and understandable occurrence on the journey through cancer. Underlying Marie's pain and anguish with regard to her husband's nutritional status was not only her love for him and her fear of losing him, but also a mistaken belief that she was in some way responsible for whether he eats. I believe it is absolutely essential for family members and friends to recognize that they are *not responsible* for what their loved one eats or does not eat. Although this is sometimes hard to accept—and unless a clear agreement exists to the contrary—they are not ultimately responsible for *any* aspect of the patient's care.

Let me explain what I mean by this. Although you may be involved in administering medications, changing bandages, or assisting with other aspects of the patient's care, I believe your most helpful role is to be a confidant, family member, lover, or friend. If you can fully embrace this idea, you will help yourself—and your loved one—more than you can imagine. My strong recommendation for patients and family members is to make a conscious choice to let the patient's physicians and nurses be responsible for the patient's medical welfare. If you have any concerns or anxieties about what is happening to your loved one, medically or nutritionally, address those concerns directly to his or her medical team. Also, it is a very good idea to seek out other avenues of support for yourself, such as individual counseling, contact with friends, or support groups where you can find valuable information, insights, and advice.

Here is a summary of these important ideas:

- The helping intentions of family members need to be openly acknowledged. Family members deserve to be heard, understood, and appreciated.
- Family members must accept their proper role as sources of love and support for the patient, rather than assuming responsibility for the patient's nutritional status or medical care on their own.
- Family members should agree that they will offer food to the patient no more than three times a day. If the patient declines, they agree to ask "Are you sure?" *only once.*
- The patient agrees to ask for more or different food when he or she wishes.
- Finally, family members must recognize and agree that the patient is a sovereign being who deserves their *unconditional* love and support. This includes supporting their choices about eating whatever and whenever they choose. Family members must acknowledge that the patient can direct *all* aspects of the journey through cancer as he or she sees fit—*even in ways that are completely different from what family members might wish or choose for themselves.*

3. The role of diet and nutrition after treatment has been completed

A good cancer recovery diet includes the recommendations for diet and nutrition during cancer treatment listed on page 106. It is not surprising that these recommendations can be helpful for everyone, whether they have had cancer or not.

Certainly, there is much more that an individual could explore to maximize health after cancer treatment beyond the recommendations given earlier. Pursuing optimum health is a lifelong and potentially unlimited process. Neither asceticism nor overindulgence are in the best interests of any cancer patient, or any human being. So, after your treatment is completed, by all means eat fruits and vegetables, take vitamins, and drink plenty of water—but don't be afraid to enjoy other foods also. Enjoy life!

In discussing the areas of complementary medicine that follow, it is best to adopt the same approach we have applied to nutrition. The issue is not *Which herbs, relaxation techniques, homeopathic remedies, or acupuncture treatments should I take to get rid of my cancer?* The more appropriate questions are: *What can help me feel better? What can improve my digestion, benefit my sleep, and enhance my overall health? What makes sense for me at this time in my life?*

Once again, your intention should be learning to care for the garden of your own unique being—with the help, support, and guidance of your doctor, your family, and your friends—so that the fruits and flowers of health, well-being, and self-knowledge can blossom and grow.

Herbs and Supplements

For millions of Americans, herbs and dietary supplements have become full-fledged alternatives to prescription drugs. In this brief discussion, we will make a distinction between the way herbs and supplements are often understood, and used, by patients. While this distinction may not be precise in all instances, I believe it is most helpful from a practical standpoint.

Herbs and *herbal compounds* are usually taken with a specific medicinal intent. They are commonly used to deal with particular clinical problems, which may be chronic or acute and can range from tension headaches to advanced cancer.

For many people, one of the real attractions of herbal medications is that they are "natural" products. They come from trees and plants rather than from laboratories and chemicals. In the minds of many individuals, "natural" generally means good, not dangerous, and nontoxic. Most herbs are indeed safe and free of side effects. But no substance, including water, is without risk in every patient and under all circumstances.

Conventional chemotherapy is often criticized for its toxicity, particularly by adherents of natural forms of healing, but many people are not aware that some important chemotherapy drugs are derived from plants. Nor do many people realize that herbs can be very powerful and should not be used indiscriminately—particularly when undergoing cancer treatment. Herbs have been used for centuries by different cultures around the world for the treatment of cancer, although most herbal cancer remedies are unproven by Western scientific standards. In addition, herbs are sometimes used to ameliorate the side effects of cancer and cancer treatment. Examples include St. John's Wort for depression, ginger for nausea, and aloe for topical irritations related to radiation.

The fact that herbs are derived from plants does not mean they are without risks, especially when taken concurrently with chemotherapy or other prescribed medications. Many herbs are metabolized in the liver, where they can interfere with the metabolism of numerous commonly prescribed drugs. One example involves a drug called coumadin, a blood thinner used to treat blood clots. Oncologists are sometimes puzzled by the inconsistent effects of coumadin on a patient—until they learn that the patient has been taking one or perhaps several herbal preparations that are interfering with the metabolism of the prescribed medication. If you are taking, or are thinking about taking, herbs of any kind—for any purpose—during your cancer treatment, it is important to notify your physician.

I believe it is best to use herbal medications, as with nutrition and other complementary forms of healing, with the intention of bringing love and care to your physical being—nourishing the body as garden— rather than as a specific treatment for your cancer. Resist the temptation to think of herbs as magic potions or as external sources of a quick cure for your illness. Don't put the responsibility for your health on the contents of any bottle, regardless of whether they are "natural" or not. Instead, use them as a means of supporting the healing intention that is present in your mind and heart. This is as true for chemotherapy as it for herbs.

While herbal medications are commonly used for specific medicinal purposes, *nutritional supplements* are usually intended to restore or increase the overall energy reserves of the body. By this definition, supplements include vitamins, trace minerals, antioxidants, protein powders, and substances such as creatine and DHEA. The purpose of these is usually to strengthen general aspects of the physiology rather than to provide relief from specific symptoms. When taken in moderation, most nutritional supplements are harmless, and many individuals feel they are helpful as well. But on a practical level, it is important to be aware of the biological effects of specific substances, on both a short-term and long-term basis. DHEA, for example, has received attention as an anti-aging supplement, but both men and women should be aware that the body metabolizes DHEA into testosterone and estrogen. This could be problematic for individuals who are at high risk for developing prostate or breast cancer. Similarly, as discussed earlier, the interaction of anti-oxidants with chemotherapy drugs remains at best unclear, and diminished side effects may come at the price of reduced treatment effectiveness.

As with herbs and other forms of complementary therapy, remember to discuss the use of nutritional supplements with your physician, particularly when you are undergoing cancer treatment.

Aromatherapy

For centuries, many of the world's religious traditions have recognized the importance of scent as a stimulus to higher awareness and awareness of the inner self. Incense is a prominent feature of many Christian, Buddhist, Hindu, and other religious ceremonies. The healing power of different aromas has recently come under scientific investigation as well.

Physiologically, the human sense of smell is characterized by a direct connection between the organs of olfactory perception in the nose and the brain's hypothalamus, which regulates functions such as body temperature and growth as well as emotional responses. Aromatherapy uses particular scents to help promote awareness and inner healing responses. Using aromas during cancer treatment is an excellent way to nurture body, mind, heart, and spirit. There are many varieties of scented oils and incense from which to choose. Sandalwood, lavender, and patchouli are especially useful to foster relaxation and a sense of inner peace.

Massage

I have repeatedly been amazed by the benefits of massage for cancer patients. Well-documented physiological effects of massage include pain relief through the release of *endorphins*—the body's natural painkillers—into the bloodstream; heightened immune function; and improved blood flow to vital organs. But the emotional benefits of massage may be even more significant.

For many patients, the loving, conscious touch of a skilled massage therapist just before a chemotherapy treatment can transform the experience from something to be endured into a time they actually look forward to with serenity and gratitude. For loved ones and caregivers, massage can provide an equally important source of respite and rejuvenation.

When massage is administered by a professional therapist, it provides an important source of human contact outside the circle of family and friends. This is valuable not only for patients but also for their loved ones, who often feel that they alone must fulfill all of the patient's needs, often neglecting their own. Massage is an opportunity for tapping into a sense of total receptivity to loving attention from the environment. Anxiety and apprehension are replaced by openness and tranquility, and this fosters healing at every level, for everyone involved.

At one time patients shied away from massage out of fear that it might promote dissemination of cancer cells in the body. For the great majority of cancers this is a myth, but you should consult your doctor before beginning massage therapy. Common sense is also important. Do not massage known points of disease or inflamed areas of the body. Otherwise, there is usually no reason why you cannot enjoy this important, powerful, and enjoyable form of healing.

A number of different styles of massage can be explored by cancer patients and family members. These include the Western styles, which derive from Swedish massage and are usually performed with warmed oils; shiatsu massage, from Japan, in which the therapist applies pressure at various points of the body; Thai massage, which sometimes involves stretching; and Marma massage, from the Ayurvedic tradition of India, which involves a mixture of slow, gentle strokes and brisk, invigorating movements.

Exercise

Exercise can often play an important role in helping patients tolerate cancer treatment. For many patients, exercise provides a heightened sense of vitality that improves their energy level and overall quality of life. Even light exercise can provide real benefits, and just taking a short stroll in the park can build strength as well as offer a moment of spiritual renewal. Walking up a single flight of stairs can provide an enhanced sense of self-sufficiency for a patient who only recently could not even get out of bed.

Biochemically, exercise helps the physiology in much the same way that turning the soil benefits a garden. Both the earth and the healthy cells of the human body need oxygen, and even slightly elevated rates of breathing and heart rate during exercise can help fulfill this need.

One of the most immediate and universal benefits of even brief periods of exercise is relief of stress and tension. This can be extremely helpful for patients, even if their endurance is limited by the effects of their disease or treatment. Numerous studies have documented improvement in anxiety, depression, physical performance, and quality of life in cancer patients who exercise. Use common sense when considering any exercise program, and discuss any questions with your physician.

Yoga

Yoga is an almost magical technique for both the mind and the body. Although in the past yoga often has been associated with difficult or strenuous postures, it can be a powerful yet gentle approach to creating awareness of and ultimately union among the physical, mental, emotional, and spiritual aspects of ourselves. In fact, the word *yoga* is Sanskrit for "union."

Yoga exercises can be done by anyone at almost any time, even while lying in bed, sitting in a chair, or riding in a car. Elementary exercises are designed not to strain the body but to stretch and tone the muscles and joints, increase energy, quiet the mind and breath, and promote greater awareness and inner calm. Many patients feel deeply renewed and rejuvenated after a yoga session, and there is evidence that yoga can en-hance many physiologic processes of the body, including immune func-tion, digestion, circulation, and sleep.

Relaxation

Long periods of worry and harried activity, whether physical, mental, or emotional, are bound to impede the healing process. Few things can counteract this more effectively than deep relaxation. Thus, it is ab-solutely vital that time be set aside for this on the journey through cancer. The kind of relaxation I am referring to here does *not* include watching television, reading books or magazines, or talking with family or friends, because in all these activities your mind remains active. Deep relaxation is a process that involves consciously entering into a state in which the body, mind, and heart become quiet and tranquil, and are restored on a profound level.

Relaxation is one of the important components of healing that pa-tients and family members tend to overlook. While overlooking it is cer-tainly understandable in the context of cancer treatment and its many demands, I believe this is unfortunate. Healing on many levels is pro-foundly facilitated by deep relaxation. Aspects of healing are accessed in deep relaxation that are experienced nowhere else. It is one of the sim-plest yet most powerful, direct, and accessible things that a patient can do to consciously help themselves on their journey.

There are many ways to facilitate deep relaxation and to make it easier and more enjoyable, including guided relaxation tapes, inspirational pieces of music, yoga, or a variety of meditation techniques. The benefits from all these techniques are immediate, diverse, and long-lasting.

Journaling

At various times throughout history, keeping a journal was a widespread and important part of daily life. Instinctively, many people discovered that they felt better after writing about the events in their lives and their innermost thoughts, feelings, and impressions. This remains true today—and though there are a large number of journal writers at the present time, it is only recently that the health-related benefits of journaling have been scientifically documented.

A number of studies in the medical literature have explored the measurable benefits of writing about events in one's life, including improved immune function and overall health. One notable example is a 1999 study published in the *Journal of the American Medical Association.* Here, patients with asthma and rheumatoid arthritis were found to have significantly reduced symptoms after writing about stressful events in their lives for twenty minutes a day over a period of several days. These improvements were beyond those attributable to the standard medical care that all the participants received. Similar benefits from written emotional expression were found in subsequent studies involving asthma and fibromyalgia patients.

Although the medical issues of cancer are unique, and obviously different from those of asthma, arthritis, or fibromyalgia, there is no doubt that putting your thoughts and feelings into writing can have significant benefits on the journey through cancer. In fact, a 2002 study published in the *Journal of Clinical Oncology* reported that women with breast cancer who wrote about their deepest thoughts and feelings concerning their disease experienced fewer physical symptoms and required fewer medical appointments than those who did not. I encourage all of my patients—and their loved ones—to purchase a journal and spend some time each day writing in it. Even five or ten minutes a day is helpful.

Journaling on a consistent basis provides an outlet for completely honest, unfiltered expression of yourself. It provides a record of your thoughts, questions, and experiences that may surprise and inspire you in the future. It also provides a reference to draw upon during difficult moments and a place to record important milestones. Finally, it gives you a precious opportunity to contact that part of yourself that is the silent witness of all the events in your life.

Visualization and Guided Imagery

Visualization and guided imagery are two related techniques that have gained great acceptance among cancer patients in recent years. In both techniques, patients typically lie in a comfortable position with their eyes closed for a period of time. Patients are guided through the process by a facilitator, or they can do it on their own.

In visualization, patients intentionally create specific images in their mind's eye to facilitate healing. Examples include visualizing Pac-Man or a knight in shining armor destroying cancer cells throughout the body, or visualizing cancer cells dissolving into nothingness. The biochemical helpfulness of this technique remains controversial, but there is no doubt that patients benefit when negative thoughts are replaced by images of strength and empowerment. I prefer patients to visualize their bodies filled with love, light, and healing energy, but if someone chooses to imagine an army destroying cancer cells, I support them in doing so.

Guided imagery is similar to visualization, but it often includes a script or a narrative that is read by a facilitator or played on an audiotape. The narrative often involves guiding the patient's consciousness to scenes or places of serenity and peace, such as tranquil gardens, healing meadows, or a soft and gentle seashore. In these settings, the patient gains access to inner wisdom, guidance, intuition, and reserves of powerful healing energy within. A variety of outstanding guided imagery tapes are available that can help patients deal more effectively with specific concerns, such as fear, anxiety, depression, or even the side effects of chemotherapy. A list of some excellent guided imagery audio products is provided in Appendix 1.

Acupuncture

Acupuncture, an ancient healing technique that originated in China, has been increasingly accepted and utilized in the West over the last twenty years. In the practice of acupuncture, extremely thin, sterile needles are carefully placed by the acupuncturist at specific points on the patient's body to facilitate the natural flow of vital energy, called *chi*.

In China, acupuncture has been used for centuries as a successful treatment for a wide variety of ailments. In the West, it is becoming understood that acupuncture has many valuable applications for medicine in general, and for cancer patients in particular. Acupuncture can be helpful in relieving symptoms such as pain, fatigue, insomnia, and muscle and joint aches. In 1998, acupuncture was recognized by the National Institutes of Health as a proven, effective treatment for chemotherapy-related nausea and vomiting. Studies suggest it may be beneficial in ameliorating other treatment-related side effects as well, including anxiety and radiation-induced dryness of the mouth. Acupuncture is also an excellent way to mobilize subtle levels of energy throughout the entire body, promoting overall healing and wellness.

Chiropractic

In the United States, chiropractic is one of the most widely utilized forms of complementary medicine. It has proven value in treating back, neck, and shoulder pain, particularly when caused by misaligned vertebrae. By reestablishing proper alignment of the entire vertebral column, proper function of the vast network of nerves that extend from the spinal cord to all the organs of the body is facilitated. Chiropractic promotes not only pain relief but overall health and vitality.

For all its acknowledged benefits, chiropractic must be used with special care by cancer patients who may have bone metastases. As with other complementary modalities, it is important to discuss the use of chiropractic with your physician before proceeding.

Homeopathy

Homeopathy is a system of medicine that was founded in the eighteenth century by the German physician Samuel Hahnemann. It is widely accepted in Europe, and in recent years has been gaining recognition in the United States.

Homeopathy is based on the principle that illnesses are specific to individuals and that "like cures like." Homeopathic remedies are composed of minute amounts of substances that in larger amounts would cause the very same symptoms that a patient is currently experiencing. The theoretical basis of vaccines is similar. In homeopathy, however, the substances are sequentially diluted with pure water or alcohol, almost to the point of disappearance. This is based on another homeopathic principle: remedies *gain* potency the more they are diluted.

Remedies are prescribed by a homeopathic physician after an extensive interview process and are highly specific to the individual. Although the precise mechanism of action of homeopathic remedies is not scientifically understood, many patients report significant responses and benefits. Homeopathic remedies may be particularly useful for cancer patients in dealing with a variety of symptoms, including depression, anxiety, insomnia, loss of appetite, and treatment-related nausea and vomiting, among others.

Therapeutic Touch

Therapeutic touch combines insights of ancient healing practices such as "laying on of hands" and contemporary theories of energy transfer drawn from physics and neurochemistry. The modern system of therapeutic touch was organized by Dolores Krieger, a professor of nursing at New York University. Therapy sessions include procedures to focus the therapist's attention on the patient, assessment of underlying energy imbalances in the patient's body, and finally rebalancing the patient's energy field. To accomplish this, the therapist passes his or her hands, held two to six inches over the patient's body, down the length of the body, past the toes, and away from the body. Sessions usually last twenty to thirty minutes and conclude with the practitioner transferring energy to the patient to further promote healing at all levels.

Reiki Therapy

Reiki is an ancient healing technique brought to prominence in Japan during the nineteenth century. Reiki therapy uses touch to stimulate the body's inner healing energy, but it is not simply a physiological procedure. Rather, it is a spiritual modality whose effectiveness is based on love and inner wisdom rather than clinical diagnosis and treatment. Reiki practitioners are trained by masters to perform the technique and teach it to others over a short period of time. Although therapy sessions may last for an hour or more, Reiki is not a difficult or esoteric therapy. Recipients of Reiki report positive benefits in alleviating anxiety, stress, and perception of pain and in promoting feelings of physical as well as psychospiritual well-being. It can be easily learned and used by patients themselves, and this is part of its appeal.

ALTERNATIVE MEDICINE

The use of alternative forms of cancer treatment is a source of great concern and confusion for patients and oncologists alike. Many different forms of alternative cancer therapies exist, often with openly conflicting theoretical bases. None of them has undisputed, scientifically proven benefit. Almost all require significant out-of-pocket expenses. Many have hidden costs and potential risks. And yet their appeal remains broad and understandable, particularly in the face of a potentially life-threatening illness.

In his outstanding and highly informative book *Choices in Healing*, Michael Lerner makes many valuable and important observations regarding so-called alternative or unproven cancer therapies.

- He states that he saw "no decisive and scientifically documented cure for any type of cancer among the unconventional therapies."
- He suggests that patients must distinguish between "the plausibility of the therapy, the credibility and character of the practitioner, and the quality of the service itself." Highly ethical and charismatic healers may sincerely believe in treatments that have no scientific basis. Often the treatments are available only in certain hard-to-reach locations, and these may be outside the United States. Patients may be eager to receive the treatments despite the difficulties involved, simply because of their own desperation or the convincing presentation of the provider. This can be a dangerous situation for patients who may already be weakened by cancer.
- He describes a psychological phenomenon in which "an inverse relationship exists between the openness of the alternative pharmacological therapies and the level of public interest in the therapy." In other words, the more exotic and esoteric the treatment, the greater the mystique in the minds of some patients. The idea of a conspiracy on the part of the government or pharmaceutical companies to

suppress cures for cancer has a long and colorful history. As with political conspiracy theories, this line of thinking appeals to people
who feel their urgent needs are not being met by the establishment.
But choosing treatments based on anger or frustration with mainstream medicine can be a perilous course.

These are important considerations, but I don't intend them to be a
global, unqualified rejection of alternative therapies. High-dose vitamins,
Essiac tea, antineoplastons, and other treatments have been described by
numerous patients as being beneficial. In the absence of proof to the contrary, it is reasonable to assume that for some patients, this may indeed
have been true. Some patients even believe they have been cured by alternative therapies. As implausible as this may seem from a conventional
viewpoint, this too may have occurred on occasion. It is important to remember that our approach to cancer can change at any time with a new
discovery or a completely unanticipated form of treatment. Such things
have happened repeatedly in the history of medicine. At the present
time, alternative therapies have *not* been proven effective in accordance
with the definitions of science. While some therapies may have value or
benefit, the magnitude and reliability of that benefit is still unknown.
Currently, these benefits seem relatively small at best, and unreliable. Some
of the therapies may actually be harmful. All too often, using them can
cause a patient to forgo a proven and potentially life-saving treatment.

To illustrate some of the issues that arise with unproven cancer therapies, it is helpful to look at a well-known case in point: shark cartilage,
which was one of the most popular and highly publicized alternative
cancer therapies not long ago.

It is an interesting fact of the natural world that sharks rarely get cancer. Despite being one of the oldest surviving forms of animal life (or
perhaps because of this), something about sharks' biology seems to make
them resistant to developing malignant tumors. What, then, are the implications of this anomaly for the treatment of human cancer? Or *are*
there any implications?

From the observation that sharks rarely get cancer, a multimillion-
dollar industry of books, Web sites, and shark-based medicines developed

in the 1990s—despite the absence of any reliable, scientifically proven benefit to cancer patients. One of the claims for shark cartilage is that it works by inhibiting the growth of tumor-supporting blood vessels. In medical terminology this is known as *anti-angiogenesis* (from the Greek *angio,* meaning "blood vessel," and *genesis,* meaning "to form"). As discussed in "The Basics: State-of-the-Art Medical Care" (page 28), anti-angiogenesis is an active area of mainstream cancer research. Laboratory tests have revealed that cartilage from sharks and other animals can inhibit the development of blood vessels under experimental conditions. However, positive results in laboratory tests, even assuming they can withstand the scrutiny of scientific review, by no means guarantee a viable anticancer treatment in humans.

The history of oncology is filled with stories of potential cancer cures that reportedly worked well in laboratory animals or petri dishes but failed in human subjects. In the case of shark cartilage, there are many reasons why a similar scenario would occur.

For example, shark cartilage treatments are usually administered orally. As with food and other substances, ingesting shark cartilage powder should lead to the enzymatic breakdown of the very proteins that are purportedly the active ingredient of the treatment. Thus many scientists believe it is extremely unlikely that any anti-angiogenesis factors present in the cartilage would be absorbed into the bloodstream in amounts sufficient to effect any activity against tumors. A second claim regarding the activity of shark cartilage is that it functions as an immune stimulant. However, no scientific evidence for this exists. Even if it were true, stimulation of the immune system by natural substances has rarely, if ever, been an effective means of cancer treatment.

Only limited clinical studies of shark cartilage have been performed, with mixed results. One study, performed under careful, scientific conditions and reported in the *Journal of Clinical Oncology* in November 1998, involved sixty patients with a variety of previously treated, advanced cancers who were given oral doses of shark cartilage as their only therapy. After twelve weeks of treatment, no patient achieved a complete or even partial remission. Ten patients showed no progression in their cancer over the duration of their treatment. To mainstream researchers, this observation was not significant, since many cancers do not progress consistently or rapidly. But to people predisposed to believe in shark cartilage, it was a highly significant development. Unwilling to accept the negative results of the study, shark cartilage advocates also criticized the types of patients selected for the study, the quality of the shark cartilage that was used, and the way it was administered.

Perhaps only repeated, overwhelming scientific evidence will dissuade fervent believers in alternative therapies. In the past, rigorous studies of many of these treatments have only reluctantly been undertaken by mainstream medicine or been allowed by the adherents of alternative therapies. Fortunately, this situation is now changing. In 1992, under mandate from the United States Congress, the National Institutes of Health established the Office of Alternative Medicine (OAM) as a resource for research on alternative forms of medicine. In 1998, the OAM was expanded into the National Center for Complementary and Alternative Medicine (NCCAM) in order to "facilitate the evaluation of alternative medical treatment modalities" and determine their effectiveness. The NCCAM now funds research on many aspects of complementary and alternative medicine (CAM) and the training of CAM researchers as well. The NCCAM's budget for 2005 was $121.1 million, increased from $50 million in 1998.

Scientific studies of different alternative forms of cancer therapy are now under way, with increasing frequency. Until the results of these and future studies are available, and clear guidelines for the safe and appropriate utilization of specific alternative therapies has been established, I recommend that patients use them with great caution, and only if no scientifically proven therapies are available to help them.

EASTERN HEALING TRADITIONS

Ayurveda

The traditional life science of India is one of the world's oldest and most comprehensive healing systems, and has been practiced for more than three thousand years. Ayurveda (the term means "science of life" in Sanskrit) perceives the universe as a whole—and human beings in particular—as a dynamic interplay of three principles that pervade all levels of creation. These principles, called *doshas,* exist in all living things, and are called *vata, pitta,* and *kapha.* They correspond to specific metabolic functions in the body, as well as to more fundamental forces of nature.

Good health depends upon maintaining a balance of the *doshas* that is appropriate for each individual. Ayurveda understands disease as a deviation from this natural state of balance and provides an interesting alternative to the Western mechanical model of illness. When a patient is sick, the Ayurvedic physician seeks to identify the underlying cause and nature of the *dosha* imbalance, and offers a variety of natural therapies that are specifically tailored for the individual. These therapies are intended not only to relieve symptoms but, more important, to restore the *doshas* to their natural state of balance, thus restoring health.

As an eminently practical and inclusive approach to sickness and health, Ayurveda makes use of herbal supplements, yoga and meditation, and cleansing techniques designed to clear toxins from the body as well as eliminate destructive impulses from the mind and spirit. One of the most profound aspects of Ayurveda is its understanding that physical health is not an end in itself. According to legend, the ancient physicians who formulated Ayurveda did so with the understanding that the pain and suffering of disease could impede life's deeper purpose, which is spiritual realization. Once the physical body is healed, we can begin to achieve our full spiritual potential.

Traditional Chinese Medicine

Traditional Chinese medicine dates back nearly three thousand years and is still used by one-fifth of the world's population. While the Western idea of longevity refers fundamentally to length of life, in the Chinese medical tradition longevity includes what the West calls "quality of life," so merely living for many years is meaningless without health, vitality, and joy.

It is a principle of Chinese medicine that illness arises from disruptions in the flow of chi, or life energy, within the body. Under conditions of good health, chi flows naturally through an extensive network of invisible channels, or *meridians,* that flow through the body and connect all of the internal organs and glands. Disruptions of the flow of chi can occur from blockages in the meridians caused by a variety of mechanical or physiological processes in the body. Chi can also flow in amounts that are excessive or deficient, thus contributing to illness.

Traditional Chinese medicine recognizes two complementary but opposing qualities of the universe, *yin* and *yang.* These principles correspond to polarities observable throughout nature, including male and female, hot and cold, and day and night.

Yin and yang are central to both diagnosis and treatment in Chinese medicine. Certain illnesses are associated with yin, while others are considered yang disorders. The five elements (fire, earth, metal, water, and wood) also play an important role in health and disease. Imbalances in yin and yang, as well as in the five elements, cause disruptions to the flow of chi, and disease results.

To restore proper balance in the body, Chinese medicine uses herbal preparations, massage, *moxibustion* (the burning of special herbs over particular points of the body), cupping, *qigong* (energy exercises), meditation, and acupuncture. Like Ayurveda, traditional Chinese medicine is a highly evolved and coherent approach that emphasizes treating the whole person rather than focusing on the particular illness. This is true for the Chinese medicine approach to cancer as well as other diseases. A large body of research exists on the use of Chinese herbs in cancer, either as primary therapy or in combination with more conventional treatments. Most of this research has been performed in China, and it is now attracting increasing attention in the West.

Tibetan Medicine

The origins of the 1,300-year-old science of Tibetan medicine are rooted in the teachings of Buddha, which emphasize the intimate relationship between body and mind. In the central text of Tibetan medicine, called the *rGyud bzi,* or the *Four Tantras,* physical disease is understood to originate from one primary cause: ignorance of our true nature. From this fundamental ignorance arises what are called the "three poisons" of desire, hatred, and confusion. Over time, these three poisons cause disturbances in three fundamental energy systems of the body, called *lung, tripa,* and *bad-ken* (the three *nyepa*). These disturbances ultimately manifest as physical illness.

As in Ayurveda and traditional Chinese medicine, Tibetan doctors endeavor to understand the cause and nature of the imbalances that are causing the patient's problems, and then to restore them to proper balance. Tibetan diagnosis relies upon extensive questioning of the patient, physical examination, examination of the tongue, urinalysis, and an extremely elaborate method of analyzing the pulse. In combination, these yield exquisitely detailed information about the underlying physiologic as well as mental and emotional conditions of the patient. The physician then prescribes a variety of natural remedies intended to restore harmony and balance to the three *nyepa.*

Tibetan medicines are largely based on combinations of herbs but can also contain animal products or even precious gems or metals. Dietary changes, physical exercises, moxibustion, cleansing practices, and a Tibetan form of acupuncture may also be prescribed. Finally, a variety of spiritual practices are recommended, if appropriate, to facilitate even deeper levels of healing. By combining sharply focused clinical knowledge with profound spiritual understanding and intention, Tibetan medicine provides an extraordinary model for individual health care as well as for Western medicine as a whole.

SOME PRACTICAL SUGGESTIONS

There are so many things you can do to nurture the garden of your body. The suggestions below are just a preliminary list, and you can surely come up with more. A useful guiding principle is to think of your body as a garden that needs sunlight, water, oxygen, nourishment, and loving care and attention. Once you've embraced this idea, exercise is no longer just a matter of physical exertion; it is an opportunity for bringing oxygen to the deep soil of your being. Similarly, eating nutritious, healthy food is no longer done simply to prevent or eliminate cancer; it is a way to fertilize and nourish the garden of the self. In all your activities, try to remain aware of this powerful and profound metaphor. When you keep the idea of your body as a garden in the forefront of your consciousness, you will naturally begin to live in ways that ensure your garden's continuing healthy growth.

- Look at your diet. Are you eating healthy foods every day? Refer to the nutrition guidelines listed on page 106.
- Eat foods that you enjoy. Try to become aware of the difference between satisfying a momentary craving for a particular food and eating something that is genuinely nourishing and satisfying to you—and your body.
- Consider giving yourself the gift of a massage at least once a week, more if you are able. Encourage your caregivers to do so as well.
- Begin an exercise program, but use common sense. If you are tired, consider a simple walk for a few minutes each day, or for a longer time if comfortable.
- Join a yoga class. Experience the joys of gentle stretching and deep relaxation.
- Drink six to eight glasses of spring water a day. Remember, it is important to water the garden of your being daily if you want it to be healthy.
- Make sure that your bowels are moving regularly. Eliminating toxins from your body is very important. If you are having any difficulties in this area, discuss it immediately with your physician.
- Breathe deeply for ten breaths, at least three times a day. Inhale for a count of two, hold for a count of eight, and exhale for a count of four. On the exhalation, push all of the air out of your lungs. This will deeply oxygenate your blood, improve the flow of lymph throughout the body, and help you to relax, think more clearly, and become more focused.
- Consider seeing an acupuncturist for a general evaluation.
- Explore the benefits of therapeutic touch, Reiki therapy, or other forms of energy healing.
- Remember that the garden of your being needs sunshine! Spend some time each day in nature. Even if you live in a city, take at least a few minutes a day to appreciate the sun, the sky, and whatever trees and plants are around you.

- Get a journal and spend at least five to ten minutes a day writing down your thoughts, feelings, and impressions. Keep a record of important events, questions, ideas, or inspirations that come to you as well.
- Take time every day to rest and relax. Explore the benefits of deep relaxation on a consistent basis.
- Try some guided imagery audio programs and discover new resources of healing, creativity, intuition, and inner wisdom.

7

LEVEL FOUR:

EMOTIONAL HEALING

WE SHALL NOT CEASE FROM EXPLORATION.
AND THE END OF ALL OUR EXPLORING WILL BE
TO ARRIVE WHERE WE STARTED, AND KNOW
THE PLACE FOR THE FIRST TIME.

—T. S. ELIOT

An important transition takes place between Levels Three and Four of the Seven Levels of Healing. So far our principal focus has been on the biological and clinical issues of the journey through cancer. We've explored the major issues involved in understanding cancer types, staging, and treatment, as well as the importance of having trust in your doctor—including his or her personal and spiritual qualities as well as technical expertise. We've looked at our common, human instinct and need for connection with others, and the important benefits that can be derived from a variety of psychosocial support programs. And we've considered an entirely new way of perceiving our body—as a garden, rather than a machine—and begun to explore the vast array of alternative and complementary therapies that can help facilitate nurturing and healing.

Now the healing intention turns inward. Many patients never make this shift in focus. If they don't, I believe that they have missed an important opportunity.

Any challenge in life—and especially a great challenge such as cancer—can ignite the mind and heart to search for deeper understanding.

Once you have made the decision to put your medical care in the hands of a trusted physician or a team of caregivers, you are then free to devote attention to any underlying human issues that may be unresolved but that will certainly affect your healing process. Now the journey through cancer becomes less about cells, chemicals, and diets and more about thoughts, feelings, and emotions.

Remarkably, an interesting paradox now appears. By turning some of your attention away from the clinical issues of care, you may actually increase the effectiveness of your treatment.

When cancer has been detected in the lung, breast, colon, or any other vital organ, medicine often fails to recognize that the heart is always involved as well. Here I am referring not to the physical pump located in the middle of the chest, but rather to the emotional and spiritual center of every human being. This metaphorical heart is invariably affected and often transformed by a cancer diagnosis. If that transformation is a positive one, true healing can take place at every level of being.

Robots and machines do not get cancer. Living and breathing human beings do. They develop malignant cells in their bodies and respond to the disease with thoughts and feelings that are a mix of chemistry, psychology, genetics, and the mysterious nature of consciousness itself. The interplay of all these factors in the journey through cancer is an authentic expression of the human condition—at times painful and frustrating, at other times heroic and inspirational, but always a mystery to behold. One thing, though, is absolutely certain: all cancer patients, as well as everyone close to them, will be exposed to a seemingly infinite variety of emotions along the way.

Trying to ignore or deny those feelings is fundamentally self-destructive. It only strengthens the repressed emotions and makes it more likely that they will eventually break through with doubled force. Make no mistake: cancer is an emotional roller-coaster ride. There are times when you'll want to scream, and there are times when you'll want to cry. Incredible as it may seem, there are even times when you'll want to laugh.

After serving as physician, friend, coach, mentor, and guide for thousands of patients and their family members over many years, I can say that *not one single person* has ever truly healed from cancer without undergoing a transformation and healing of their emotional self. This is a key point, and I want to make it clearly. The challenges encountered in the diagnosis and treatment of cancer are often intense and profound. The rigors of the journey are such that inner vulnerabilities can be laid bare and even exacerbated. Addressing these very real, understandable, and human vulnerabilities—and everything that often accompanies them— is therefore of vital importance.

THE EMOTIONAL PARADIGM

For most people, the flood of practical questions encountered during the initial phase of cancer treatment does eventually subside. When that happens, complex and often uncomfortable feelings can begin to assert themselves, and choices have to be made about how to deal with them. Sometimes the feelings are completely ignored, sometimes they're completely indulged, but they are almost always misunderstood unless they're given conscious attention. The roller coaster of feelings can have some steep ups and downs, for which few people are prepared. Fear is only the most obvious and accessible emotion associated with cancer. I've seen a full spectrum of rage, resentment, frustration, sadness, guilt, remorse, doubt, and discouragement in virtually everyone who has tried to deal with cancer, including myself during my father's illness. At the very least, these emotions deserve to be acknowledged. The real challenge, however, is working through them, and finding release and freedom from them in a safe and positive way.

Many patients actively bottle up their emotional responses to their illness. So often I've walked into exam rooms and found cancer patients trying with all their might to present themselves as cool, calm, and collected. Unresolved emotions are often expressed as irritation, impatience, and annoyance at even being in the presence of the doctor. All sorts of silent messages are beamed my way:

> *This shouldn't be happening. I resent it. I won't stand for it. I'm a CEO, and I'm used to being in charge.*

> *I'm not going to let anyone see I'm upset by this. Not you, and especially not my husband.*

Money is no object to me. I've always been able to buy my way out of anything, and I'll buy my way out of this, too.

I've eaten healthy foods, exercised, and meditated for years, and have never taken an aspirin! I can't believe this is happening to me.

But perhaps the most common message comes from the vast majority of patients who are struggling to deal with the significant logistical challenges of cancer, including day care for children, time off from work, and financial pressures. For these people, the impulse to suppress their emotions often has a different rationale:

I just don't have time for this. I've got more important things to do.

I don't have the time or energy to worry about my feelings.

Who cares about feelings, anyway? I'm just trying to survive.

As we begin the consultation, conversations with patients who are responding in this way are often stiff and abrupt. The focus is on getting rid of the problem and attending to other business. However, after completing the history and physical examination, I make a point of gently asking, "How are you feeling in all this, Mr. Jones?" "What's this really been like for you, Mrs. Smith?" Again and again, these simple questions trigger dramatic outpourings of emotion. In a heartbeat, Mr. Jones and Mrs. Smith become lost and lonely children, weeping uncontrollably. Deep pain and frustration, often suppressed for years, instantly rise to the surface.

For me, the saddest thing is how quickly patients who respond like this seek to reestablish the internal status quo. Men straighten their ties, women reapply their lipstick and makeup—and they depart *as if nothing had happened!* The feelings are so troubling that they must never be shown to the world, or even acknowledged. Yet by denying their emotions, patients often deprive themselves of the very experience of healing that they are really seeking when they come to me for help.

It is also unfortunate that mainstream medicine minimizes the importance of emotional work in the healing process. A major reason for this is that, with the exception of psychiatrists, doctors are not trained, honored, or paid to adequately address the emotional concerns of cancer patients and family members. Furthermore, distinguishing emotional factors that are functional and situational from those that are derived from an underlying neurochemical imbalance can be a subtle, complex, and time-consuming process. Depression—which occurs in *up to 50 percent of cancer patients*—may be mistaken for anxiety, or vice versa. Genuine and appropriate grieving is often tagged as depression and is frequently overmedicated or undermedicated. A number of factors contribute to this, including the training, experience, and practice habits of the physician, as well as the patient's wishes and willingness to explore and disclose his or her true feelings.

THE ELEPHANT IN THE ROOM

In some respects, cancer is like an elephant that suddenly appears in your living room. Certainly the first order of business is to get the elephant out, but that may take some time. Meanwhile, what should you do? Some people block everything out of their lives except the elephant. They don't think or talk about anything else. Other people try to pretend the elephant isn't there. "Elephant? What elephant?"

The best answer to such an urgent but unwieldy problem lies somewhere between the two extremes. Once you give yourself permission to deal appropriately with the emotional issues associated with your illness, you can become freed from the burdens that accompany both denial and preoccupation.

In helping people make the journey through cancer, one of my greatest priorities is to skillfully and gently help patients address and resolve the feelings that must be dealt with. If this doesn't happen, whether their tumor shrinks or even goes into complete remission, the deepest possible healing will not have occurred. In an important way, the damage done by cancer will still be present. In fact, it will remain until hidden emotional pain is brought out in the light of awareness and healed in the light of love.

* * *

When I first met Laura Hill and her husband, Steve, they had been dealing with Laura's metastatic breast cancer for four years. Laura was a bright, fifty-one-year-old woman who had originally presented with Stage II disease and undergone a modified radical mastectomy and axillary lymph node dissection, followed by adjuvant chemotherapy and tamoxifen. A year later, however, her cancer returned and was found in her lungs and liver and on her chest wall. She went through high-dose chemotherapy with stem cell support at a major cancer center, with excellent results. Soon thereafter, however, her cancer once again came back. There followed several rounds of "salvage chemotherapy," repeated radiation therapy treatments to her chest wall, and a variety of hormonal therapies for breast cancer. The disease always reappeared.

Laura and Steve started to lose faith in mainstream approaches. They began to spend their life savings traveling to treatment centers and holistic healing facilities in the United States, Mexico, and the Bahamas, searching desperately for a cure. Laura underwent diet therapies, cleansing programs, coffee enemas, high-dose intravenous vitamin infusions, shark cartilage, Essiac tea, and mistletoe extract. Nothing worked, although one practitioner after another promised relief from the assault of her cancer. Whenever it became clear that a new therapy was not working, Laura and Steve would be off to the next healing center, shaman, sweat lodge, herbalist, homeopath, chiropractor, naturopath, or acupuncturist. Laura was Rolfed, rebirthed, and energy-balanced, and her chakras were repeatedly aligned. Exotic crystals were placed on every part of her body, and she visualized her cancer cells being eaten by white knights in shining armor a million times. Nothing worked.

Laura and Steve came to see me through a friend's recommendation. I was described as a board-certified oncologist who also understood and appreciated the value of other healing methods and traditions, someone who would give Laura chemotherapy if I believed it could help her, and who would honor and support her desire to do everything possible to help herself live.

After their long, lonely ordeal, Steve and Laura were deeply discouraged but not yet ready to give up hope. They loved each other. They loved their two kids. They loved life and they wanted more time together. They weren't ready for her to die.

But they were frustrated, and they were angry at so many things—especially at the cancer that had destroyed the life they had known together. They were also angry about how they'd been treated at conventional cancer centers, and how they'd been ridiculed for wanting to explore other options. Yet they also felt they'd been misled at alternative healing centers, even if by sincere and well-intentioned people.

Laura and Steve came to my office with a box of medical records, the sad chronicle of two people fighting against a formidable challenge. As I sifted through the records, I admired their courage and determination. Even in coming to see me, they were willing to risk yet more disappointment because of their desire for Laura to live.

We began to talk, and I asked to hear their story in their own words. Laura spoke first, then Steve took over. They had reiterated the story many times and had become a well-synchronized team in narrating their experiences. I had the feeling that Laura was growing tired of talking about it. Steve, on the other hand, was intent on recounting every incident, every disappointment. In retelling the story, he became animated, angry, and even sarcastic and contemptuous about the people they had met. Before long he even became hostile to me, someone he had never met before, a doctor to whom he had brought his wife for help.

Soon Steve was almost yelling. "They told her this, and they told her that, and nothing worked! It's all bullshit! They tell her to take this chemo, or drink this tea, or do these enemas, or swallow these vitamins and minerals, and her cancer will go away! But it's lies! It's all lies! Nothing has worked!"

This was a man who had exhausted himself trying to save his wife's life. His love and devotion were so clear, but his frustration and despair were beginning to consume him.

Finally, there was silence. I asked Laura if I could examine her. As she removed her shirt, I saw lengths of gauze wound around her chest that were stained with blood and pus. Slowly, carefully, we began unwrapping the gauze together, revealing the disfigured body of a woman who had endured a truly heroic ordeal. Laura's right breast was gone, replaced by scar tissue. The underlying skin was thickened and discolored from the effects of radiation. Her right arm was puffed and swollen with lymphedema, and it was difficult for her to open and close her fist. Her left breast was also thickened, red, and swollen. Examining it more closely, I saw it was full of cancer. A small amount of blood was oozing from the nipple, and a mass of thick, red, nodular lesions—a number of which were also oozing blood and pus—covered her entire chest and extended around to the right side of her back.

Twice each day, Steve cleaned the wounds on Laura's chest, gave her antibiotics, and wrapped her with gauze. This had been going on for many months.

As I examined Laura, I recognized this as one of the most difficult cancer scenarios: the disease keeps reappearing, and nothing seems capable of making it go away. Still, patients and their loved ones hunger for life.

Fortunately, several new chemotherapy drugs were now available that had a real chance of helping Laura on the clinical level—not to cure, but definitely to provide some relief from what her body was going through. However, there were many issues here beyond Laura's physical condition. It seemed to me that simply opening a discussion about more chemotherapy would have completely missed the point. The elephant seemed to be consuming all the air in the room. It would serve no one's interests to deny that fact by focusing only on her medical treatment or the purely clinical concerns.

After I finished examining Laura, she got dressed. I then turned to Steve and said, "May I ask you a question?"

"Sure," he replied.

"Have you and Laura talked very much about how you're feeling in all this?"

"What do you mean?"

"Well, I can see that both of you have become very knowledgeable about the relative strengths and weaknesses of various treatment options for breast cancer. I'm also deeply impressed by your courage and determination to keep fighting this disease. But along the way, have you and Laura taken the time to really talk in depth about what you're experiencing in this process? Have you communicated about what it's really like—with your doctors, or with yourselves?"

"No," Steve said, after a long silence. "Not really."

"Why not?"

There was another long silence. Then he said, "There never seems to be time. There's always so much to do. And no one has ever asked us about those kinds of things. All they've ever talked about was what her next therapy should be."

I turned to his wife. "Laura, is that your experience, too?"

It took a long time for Laura to speak, and then she expressed an almost universal perception among cancer patients and their family members: no one had ever really asked them how they *felt*, because the focus was always on what they *should do*. Consequently, they had devalued and lost touch with their feelings. This was clearly an issue that needed to be addressed as soon as possible. Any further discussion about what they ought to do clinically would be misdirected until we addressed the turbulent, underlying emotions that had been ignored for too long.

"Laura and Steve," I said, "I recognize that Laura's body most definitely needs love and attention and medical care right now, in a very serious way. And we can do a lot to help in that regard. But both of you also have minds and hearts and spirits, and these also need love and attention and care. If we focus only on the cancer, or on what new chemotherapy regimen to follow, or what herbs, vitamins, minerals, and supplements to take, we'll be bypassing really vast and important areas of the process, and I don't want to do it."

This shocked them a little bit. "What do you mean, 'I don't want to do it'?"

"Well, I'm not here simply to treat cancer, which is a very mechanical process. We can and will do an absolutely first-class, impeccable job with that—but it is *only one aspect of what needs to happen.* I'm also interested in seeing how I can help you both as human beings. But I can only do so much. You've got to get involved. You've got to participate, perhaps in a way you never have before. Are you willing to do that? Are you willing to start looking at the other dimensions of what is going on here as well? It may not be easy. Do you want to do it?"

They were quiet for a while, and looked at each other silently. Then Laura asked, "Well, what's really involved?"

"A lot is involved, but we'll go slowly. We'll talk about everything, including what to do for your cancer. But we'll also talk about how you're feeling deep in your hearts, and about what is really most important to you in life—what you really want to live for."

As I spoke these words, both Laura and Steve started to cry. I have seen this response in so many patients and family members when the door to hidden feelings began to open. After some time had passed I gently asked, "Why were you crying? Will you tell me?"

They answered almost in unison. It was the same answer I've heard over and over again: *"Because no one ever asked us how we're feeling."*

This was the beginning of a long and magical part of Laura and Steve's journey. In our talks over the coming days and weeks, by writing in their journals, and by participating in our support groups, much was discovered and much was healed. Steve had a chance to recognize and express his own anger and frustration at having his life, as well as Laura's, utterly consumed by her disease. "For four years," he cried, "I have focused completely on Laura and her needs. I have always had to put my own needs aside. Everyone in the family, all the doctors, all the healers—*everyone*—focuses only on Laura. For four years, it has always been 'What does Laura need today?' 'What does Laura want today?' I love her so much, but I can't stand it anymore. What about me? Nobody says, 'Steve, what do *you* need today?' We haven't made love for over four years, and I miss it. I feel frustrated and angry. I also feel lonely, and so sad. And then when I hear myself say things like this, I feel so guilty. How can I feel pity for myself? Look at what she has had to go through. I should be ashamed of myself to complain. I am ashamed of my selfishness, and ashamed that I haven't been able to save her. Isn't that what a husband is supposed to do? I've tried everything I can, but it is never good enough. Despite everything I've tried to do, her cancer keeps coming back, and I can't save her. I feel like a failure. I've given everything I have, but in the end I can't save my beloved wife and friend."

Slowly, Laura also began to reveal her deepest emotions, which were just as powerful.

"I feel so tired, and so afraid. I'm not sure I can keep on going like this anymore, but I'm petrified to admit it. I'm afraid Steve will hate me if I say a part of me wants to give up. Look at all he's done for me. How can I abandon him? I would feel so guilty. In fact, I *already* feel guilty. This cancer has disrupted everything in our lives. Steve has had to give up so much to keep me going. It has nearly wiped us out financially. If I die, what will Steve have left? What will be left to give to our kids? I'm also mad, *really mad,* because this cancer has robbed me of so much, too. We worked so hard to have a life together, to raise our kids and then have fun, and it has all been lost. There were so many things I wanted to do and experience. Look at me—I'm not a woman any longer. I'm not even sure I'm a person any longer. I used to look great. I had great breasts and a great body. Men were always attracted to me. Now, no one would ever think of coming near me. Even Steve won't come near me anymore except to change my bandages. Who can call this living? I'm also mad at Steve because he won't ever leave me alone. All day long he is asking me what I want, what he can get me, what he can do for me. I just want him to stop sometimes, and leave me alone. Sometimes I just want to be left alone and cry. But I can't say it because he will feel hurt and abandoned, and I don't want to hurt him. I love him so much. I'm so lucky to have him, but I'm also so mad at him. He mopes and feels sorry for himself, and he thinks I don't know. How dare he feel sorry for himself? I'm the one with cancer, not him. At times I am so furious at him for this, and then I feel guilty again. Oh, God, I don't know how I can handle it all!"

As I watched Laura and Steve acknowledge and explore these feelings, my admiration for them, and my love for them, deepened even more. As they gave themselves permission to experience their feelings without judgment, and as they learned ways of expressing their feelings without attacking or blaming each other, their relationship began to blossom and expand as never before. They realized that all their feelings and emotions were understandable, and deeply human. They also began to realize that even though they had these feelings, the feelings were *not who they really are.* Even though the emotional waves could at times rage fiercely, there was a deeper part of themselves, and their love for each other, that was safe, protected, and untouched by it all. As they continued on this process of self-discovery and self-disclosure, they moved deeper and deeper into one of the most profound experiences of love and forgiveness that a human can have. They learned to *completely forgive themselves* and *accept and embrace themselves for who they are.* And then they slowly began to *forgive each other* and *forgive everyone they felt had ever wronged them in their lives.* Slowly, one by one, the overwhelming burdens of guilt, shame, anger, rage, and resentment began to lift, and they could focus on the gifts they still had for each other and the love they still had to share.

Laura and Steve had another nine months together, and then she died. Those months were not always easy, but they were rich and precious, and filled with great discoveries, growth, healing, and love.

It is time for the institutions of medicine to pay attention to the elephants in the room that are so often completely ignored in the urgent drama of clinical cancer care. Helping patients and families face the emotional issues of cancer—whatever they are, whatever form they may take, and wherever they may lead—must be one of our highest priorities. In the life-or-death context of cancer treatment, doctors, patients, and deeply concerned family members may have difficulty with my emphasis on addressing emotional issues. But seeing cancer only in terms of biochemistry and physiology is a gross oversimplification and a disservice to everyone. When I urge patients to direct their focus away from the specific details of their diagnosis and their treatment modalities, I'm not asking them to avoid or deny the serious issues of the cancer experience. Rather, I'm suggesting that the *really* serious issues encompass a much wider universe than they may have realized—and that *all* those issues must be carefully and fully addressed in order for healing to take place at the deepest levels.

Because these emotions can be intense, and because they're often difficult to separate from the physical dimensions of the illness, emotional healing requires insight, tact, and great sensitivity from all involved. The process is often easier to recognize than it is to define. There is also no "magic formula" for putting it into practice. But here is a true story that shows how it works.

One Saturday I went to see David Buchanan on my usual morning hospital rounds. He was a kind, courageous forty-two-year-old man with AIDS who had spent the better part of the previous nine months battling Kaposi's sarcoma (KS). In the first decade of the AIDS epidemic, KS was quite common, and David had a particularly severe case. He had a number of KS lesions scattered around his body, but his legs in particular had become so extensively involved that they looked like two wet, swollen logs that had been burned and scorched in a fire with the bark left on. The skin from the tips of his toes to below both knees was blackened and purple, punctuated only by a number of pink, open sores. He was in pain. *A lot* of pain. High doses of long-acting morphine given every eight hours barely kept him comfortable enough to lie still, and he couldn't even think about standing or walking around. Although he hated to use a bedpan, day after day the bedside commode went untouched. It was just two feet away, but it might as well have been on another planet.

His predicament that day was particularly discouraging because of all he had been through over the previous nine months. Remarkably, when I had first met him nine months earlier his legs had also looked like this. I'll never forget the day his partner wheeled him into my office for the first time with his legs propped up in a wheelchair. My heart sank as the bandages were cut away and I saw what they had been hiding. Extensive dermal-lymphatic invasion of KS was, at that time, one of the nastiest, most unyielding manifestations of AIDS. Unfortunately, I had seen it all too often, but David's legs were among the worst.

Over the next five months I saw David almost every week as we battled the KS in his legs. Quietly, fiercely, and without ever once complaining, he went through weeks of chemotherapy, radiation, and whirlpool treatments, followed by more chemotherapy. Little by little his legs got better, and then one day he shocked us all by walking proudly into the office on his own, announcing that he was here for his next treatment. He was limping badly and leaning on a cane, but for the first time in months he was walking on his own. The whole office staff cheered, and many of us cried. We were so proud of him and so happy to see him walk again. We felt as though a miracle had happened in front of our eyes. We were even more surprised when he continued on with treatment and got even better. Eventually the skin on his legs started turning pink again, and his legs finally began to look like normal human limbs.

Two months later he started having serious problems. Ten days after his last chemotherapy treatment his white blood cell counts plummeted. This had happened before, but they had always come right back up with Neupogen shots. This time he wasn't responding to Neupogen. Each day

I held my breath as his counts remained low, and I prayed that the antibiotics he was taking would hold him over until his bone marrow recovered again. Late one afternoon, David called and told me that his temperature had suddenly spiked to 104 degrees, and he was feeling very sick. As I made arrangements for him to be admitted to the hospital, I knew he might be in for some real trouble. When he arrived at the hospital he couldn't breathe, and less than three hours later my worst fears were realized. He was in the ICU with bilateral pneumonia, respiratory failure, renal insufficiency, and profound sepsis. This was awful. The day before, he had felt fine, but now he was in very real danger of dying. I was heartbroken. He had fought so hard and come so far.

Over the next few weeks he amazed us all once again. He fought back, little by little—"inch by inch, row by row," as the song goes. No matter what, he just wouldn't give up. Slowly, gradually, he continued to improve, and when he left the hospital more than six weeks later it felt as if we had witnessed another miracle.

The unfortunate thing was that during his time in the hospital we had not been able to give him any more treatment for his KS. As a result, his lesions had taken off again with a vengeance—like a bat out of hell, actually. His legs had once again become swollen and covered with the same sickening darkness he had started out with nine months earlier. After all that work he was back to square one all over again. Just a few days after going home from the hospital, the pain in his legs became so unbearable that he had to be readmitted to get his pain under control and think about starting more treatment. He was also very sad, because in the midst of everything else his mother had died just the week before.

That is what was going on when I went into his room that Saturday morning to see him and try to cheer him up. The situation was complicated still further by the fact that I was not going to be able to give him great news about more treatment for his KS. I had spent a lot of time in the previous days trying to think of another chemotherapy regimen that we could use. His KS had already been treated with virtually every known active, available drug, and he had already received all the radiation his legs could tolerate. To top that off, he had nearly died from bone marrow failure and sepsis after his last cycle of chemotherapy.

"Good morning, David," I said quietly as I entered his room.

"Oh, hi, Dr. Geffen," he replied. "Thank you for coming."

"How are you feeling today?" I asked.

"Well, okay, I guess. But my legs still hurt a lot. The morphine doesn't seem to do the trick like it used to."

I could see a great sadness and longing for rest in his dark brown, battle-weary eyes. They seemed to protrude from his thin, bald head, his face now drawn and fatigued from chronic illness and pale from anemia and lack of sun.

In the nine months since we had met, it felt as if we had walked a million miles together. At each visit we always paused for just a second to silently acknowledge each other. It was always a precious moment, since neither of us knew how many more miles we had left to go.

"You know, Dr. Geffen," David said. "I'm a Christian, and I love Jesus very much. We've talked about this before. But lately I've been feeling that I must have failed in some way. That inside I must be impure."

"What do you mean, David?" I asked.

"Well," he said quietly, almost whispering, "look at what is happening to me. I've tried so hard to make up for my past, but it's not working. I think that Jesus must not have forgiven me for my sins."

His words stung my heart. David was one of the most beautiful, gentle, caring souls I had ever met, yet he felt that he had failed—not just with other people, but even with his Savior.

In my life I have come to understand and see again and again how, like nothing else, shame and self-hatred can destroy the human spirit and shatter lives and dreams. If ever there was a poison that could kill people as certainly as any cancer or any sword, it is this.

David's words carried the unmistakable tone of these most lethal, destructive emotions. I felt sad and angry because I could see so clearly once again how shame and self-recrimination were hurting someone I cared for very much, someone who was as gentle and loving as a soft breeze.

We talked about his feelings for a while. He had never opened up so deeply before or shared something this difficult. I was moved by his honesty, his vulnerability, and his unspoken plea for help. I knew that we had to work on this or his healing would never be complete, regardless of what eventually happened to him. I asked him if he wanted to explore these feelings more deeply. I was relieved when he said yes.

This was one of those moments that are both the true test and the true reward of an oncologist's life. At times like these, I feel humbled and privileged to enter into another person's reality. I am invited into that reality by their deep need and drawn toward it by my own wish to love and heal. It is not just a matter of guiding the patient, and certainly not of manipulating him or her in any way. Serving another human being—especially someone with a fatal disease—involves allowing the false boundaries of ego, identity, and separation to melt and fall away. It involves giving the precious gift of your complete attention and focus, and merging so deeply in the heart that you become one. So much of modern medicine is a matter of turning dials, prescribing drugs, and reading charts and X-rays. Moments like these, however, are also part of modern medicine—or at least they should be. They are what healers have experienced for thousands of years all over the world. This is where the scientific and the sacred meet, and where the apparent contradiction between them is revealed to be an illusion.

"David," I continued, "we've talked about your love of Jesus before, and your experience of Him. Do you really believe that He has not forgiven you for the things you feel you have done wrong in your life?"

David was silent for a long time. Finally, he replied.

"Actually, I *know* that He has forgiven me. But I don't *feel* it. I've never been able to feel it."

"Would you be willing to feel it right now?" I asked.

David paused again, then said, "Yes."

"Okay," I said. "Close your eyes. I think we may be able to get this settled right here and now."

Holding David's hand, I asked him to keep his eyes closed and see if he could picture Jesus standing in front of him.

He finally replied, "Yes."

"Okay. Can you now feel Him in front of you as well?"

After a long silence David softly answered, "Yes."

"Good. Now, can you feel Him looking at you and can you feel His love for you?"

"Yes."

"Great. Now, David, I'd like you to look directly at Jesus and ask Him if He forgives you for everything you have ever done in your life that you feel was wrong. Okay? Are you able to do that right now?"

"No," he said. "I'm too scared."

"It's okay," I replied. "Just go slowly, and take your time. When you feel ready, go ahead and ask him if He forgives you. Do you think you might be able to do this now?"

"Yes," he whispered.

"Good. Now silently ask Him, and watch Him closely."

I paused to allow this process to happen at its own pace. I wanted David to have plenty of time to have his own experience, without feeling rushed in any way. Eventually, though, I could tell he was having a hard time, so I asked, "Can you hear His reply?"

"No," David said. "I can't hear Him. I'm trying, but I can't hear Him. I want to, but I can't."

"Okay. Don't worry. Just ask Him again silently, and listen with your heart. Just relax, and let Him speak to you in your heart."

Now David grew very quiet, and I could tell he was really asking now and really listening. I closed my eyes again and went deep into my own heart. I felt the presence of Jesus, Buddha, my own spiritual teachers, and all those beings throughout history who have given their lives to help relieve the suffering of humanity. I felt the presence of timeless awareness, and felt myself floating in and merging with the infinite ocean of love that is the essence of our true nature as humans—that which transcends and gives rise not only to the mind and the body but also to all form, all creation, all phenomena. The bliss of this silence went on and on, until sometime later I finally heard David breathing more deeply than before. I opened my eyes and saw him begin to smile. He looked at me, and his big brown eyes were filled with tears that rolled softly down his face.

My eyes instantly filled with tears, too. I hadn't seen him smile like this for so many weeks, and now he was actually glowing from within. His eyes sparkled with beams of light that filled the vast, timeless, silent awareness that surrounded and embraced us both.

As we looked at each other, blinking through our tears so we could keep seeing each other, David's eyes grew stronger and softer. And as I watched, he became filled with a deep, inner peace. The peace of one who has looked deeply into his heart and soul and discovered a profound truth about himself. The peace of one who has come to know himself as timeless, dimensionless, and eternal—and as not only the source of love but the very essence of love itself.

"*I heard Him,*" David whispered, barely able to talk, but hardly needing to. "I heard Him," he whispered again. "I heard Him."

David had only a short time left to live. Even within that short time, he may not have always remained in the transcendent state of awareness he experienced that day. But I know he kept the feeling of that awareness and the memory of it, and I know it was a great source of strength for him to call upon. It has also been a source of strength for me, and I'm honored to have been there with David to share it.

SOME PRACTICAL SUGGESTIONS

The purpose of this chapter has been to show the importance of emotional healing and the powerful effect it has on the lives of cancer patients and their loved ones. Here are some practical suggestions that can foster this emotional healing at any point on the journey through cancer.

- Get a journal and write about your experiences for at least a few minutes a day. This is as important for spouses and family members as it is for patients.
- Remember, this is your private journal. No one else will see it without your permission. Be honest with yourself. By putting your feelings—all of them—into writing, you will begin to make room for new feelings. You may also find out some surprising things about what your deepest emotions really are. Ask yourself the following questions on a regular basis, and write down your answers without editing or judging them:

  1. *How do I feel today? What emotions have I experienced in the past twenty-four hours?*
  2. *How do I feel about this cancer? What is it doing to my life?*
  3. *What am I willing to give up to heal this cancer?*

4. *What are the gifts that this cancer can bring to me and my family?*

5. *What can I do to help myself feel better today?*

- Join a support group. It is critical for you to have opportunities to share your feelings with others in a safe and healthy way. Remember that your spouse and family cannot meet all of your emotional needs. It is unfair and unwise to ask them to do so. You can help yourself, and them, by finding other places for support.

- Consider finding a private therapist to talk with on a regular basis. The emotional ups and downs encountered on the journey through cancer may at times call for a professional counselor to help guide you through the most intense periods. If you find you are struggling with depression, anger, despair, fear, guilt, or resentment, it is time to get some help and support. This is equally true for spouses and family members. You can't really help the one you love if you are tied up in emotional knots. Getting help for yourself is one of the greatest gifts you can give to your loved one.

LEVEL FIVE:

THE NATURE OF MIND

THE GREATEST DISCOVERY OF MY GENERATION IS
THAT A HUMAN BEING CAN ALTER HIS LIFE BY
ALTERING HIS ATTITUDES OF MIND.
—WILLIAM JAMES

Shakespeare wrote, "Nothing is either good or bad, but thinking makes it so." This is the essence of the ideas we'll be discussing in this chapter, and I emphasize that these thoughts must be applied with great care and sensitivity in the journey through cancer. I don't intend to suggest that cancer is caused by "wrong" thoughts, or that it can be cured by thinking "right" ones. And I absolutely don't intend to suggest that getting cancer is "good." However, the *experience* of cancer is always and absolutely a *subjective* one. Recognizing this, we can discuss some important ways in which the journey can be transformed by understanding how our mental processes profoundly affect our experiences in the real world.

THOUGHTS

Although many thousands of thoughts race through your mind during your waking hours, there is surprisingly little variation among them from one day to the next. It is true that what you think about on a fishing trip to Alaska will be different from your thoughts during a meeting at your office, but the vast background of memories, worries, and aspirations changes very slowly over the course of years. From day to day or week to week there may be virtually no change at all. In this sense, our minds are like rivers, streaming with thoughts that flow along preexisting ruts and rivulets.

Despite the sheer numbers of our thoughts, it is a fact of cognitive psychology that we can experience only one of them at a time. A classic demonstration of this involves asking someone *not* to think of the color green. If you really try this, you'll find that your intention not to think of the color green overrides your ability to focus elsewhere, and mental images of grass, trees, and dollar bills may crowd your thinking process. Actually, every one of our thoughts pulls on our attention in the same way, but we are generally unaware of this. Our thoughts also move along so quickly that we experience them as a continuous stream, rather than as discrete objects. This process is much like the single frames of film that portray fluid motion when projected in a moving sequence onto a movie screen. Here, each frame is an individual thought, the movie screen is the screen of our awareness, and the movie itself is our perception and experience of "reality."

A diagnosis of cancer has an instant and extremely powerful effect on these characteristics of the thinking process. The consistency that characterized your thoughts from day to day suddenly changes. As the well-worn course of your mental stream abruptly veers off in a new direction, the effect can be profoundly destabilizing. The habitual thought patterns with which you were so comfortable—perhaps even too comfortable— are overridden as the mind tries to orient itself in new and uncharted territory. Moreover, the content of your thoughts often changes from a sequence of vaguely related or completely random entities to a single preoccupation.

In the past, your mind may have made a series of quick mental leaps from wondering where to eat lunch to thinking about your children and then to considering a problem at your job. Now there are just variations on a single theme: "Why did I get cancer? Where can I get the best treatment? I'm terrified . . . what is going to happen to me?"

Another metaphor for the activity of the mind can be found in the

Eastern traditions of meditation. Here the mind is sometimes described as a monkey, jumping incessantly from tree to tree, never stopping except when we are in deep sleep. In normal life, the "monkey mind" jumps from thought to thought, covering a wide range of subjects. But with a diagnosis of cancer the monkey mind can suddenly seem trapped in a forest of ominous and forbidding trees. Wherever it jumps, only dark thoughts are found.

Just as it does in the body, cancer can metastasize in the mind.

Subjectively, the tendency of cancer to monopolize mental content is experienced as *intrusive thought*. In the midst of any activity, a thought related to the illness may suddenly appear, with disruptive effects. Most often these intrusive thoughts are dominated by doubts, judgments, fears, and anxieties, and because they can be so common and so compelling on the journey through cancer, it is important to recognize their effects and bring them under control. Here is an example of how this process works, and how it can be changed.

Sarah Caldwell was late for her appointment. When I came into the examination room, her eyes were downcast, and I immediately sensed that she was not doing very well.

"Hi, Sarah," I said. "How are you today?"

"Okay, I guess," she said, barely hiding her sadness.

Sarah was a fifty-two-year-old woman who had been diagnosed with Stage II breast cancer three months earlier. She had undergone a right modified radical mastectomy and an axillary lymph node dissection, and metastatic cells were found in four of her lymph nodes. She was now undergoing treatment with adjuvant chemotherapy with the aim of decreasing her chances of relapse.

This is the standard approach, one that tens of thousands of women in the United States go through every year. Depending on the drugs used, the schedules and doses given, and the individual person, the toxicity from various chemotherapy regimens can vary from virtually none to life-threatening. Sarah was receiving a moderately intense regimen of three drugs, and was tolerating them remarkably well; she had not suffered any fatigue, loss of appetite, nausea, vomiting, mouth sores, or fevers of any kind after two cycles. But one major problem had come up—and even though we had talked about it, and she knew it was coming, she hadn't expected it to hit her so hard.

The problem was alopecia, or hair loss. This occurs quite dramatically with a number of chemotherapy drugs, including one that Sarah was taking. Over the past few weeks, at first in small strands and then later in clumps, and finally in what seemed to her like an avalanche over a few days, all of her hair had fallen out.

I knew how devastating this could be—and also how devastating the *thought* of it and the *fear* of it could be. I knew women who had avoided chemotherapy, and had very likely shortened their lives, because they were terrified of losing their hair. Some were not able to admit this was the reason they renounced the treatments, and they looked for medical or philosophical reasons that seemed easier to legitimize. But the real reason was the pain, loss of control, and loss of self-esteem they associated with losing their hair. If that weren't painful enough, they often felt too afraid or ashamed to admit this and discuss it openly with the doctor to whom they had entrusted their lives.

Sarah was usually a cheerful person who loved to laugh and make light of whatever was happening, but today I could tell she was at a real low point. Together we had faced her diagnosis, surgery, and pathology reports head-on. We had also faced her fears about chemotherapy, and she had found the strength to go forward and successfully complete her first two cycles of treatment with virtually no problems. But the experience of losing her hair was something else altogether. She looked forlorn, stranded, trapped.

"I know this is hard for you," I said. "Why don't you tell me what's going on inside?"

Looking up at me, her eyes suddenly filled with tears and she started sobbing uncontrollably. "Dr. Geffen," she cried, "I can't stand it. Every time I look at myself in the mirror, I feel so ugly. I don't want to look like this. Without any hair, I look just like a man."

The depth of her pain was raw and clear; it was heartbreaking to see. But at the same time I was also very proud of her. She was beginning to confront what her illness and the effects of her treatment really meant to her. It took real courage to face this so directly.

"Basically I feel okay about the chemotherapy treatments," she continued. "But I'm horrified every time I look in the mirror and see I'm bald. I just feel so *ugly,* and *I feel like I'm going to die.*" As these thoughts and images reentered her mind, her whole physiology transformed. Within seconds she was crying and sobbing again.

"Sarah," I finally said, "may I ask you a question?"

"Okay."

"How many times a day do you look in a mirror?"

"I don't know," she said, turning away.

"Really, Sarah—how many times a day do you look in a mirror?"

She paused for a long time, fighting the question. Finally she answered softly, her eyes looking downward, "Well, maybe four times a day."

She then looked at me, and without speaking another word we both knew that the real answer was probably more like 40 times a day, or perhaps even 140. But the actual number was unimportant compared to the emotional pain she was experiencing and the effect it could have on her treatment.

"Sarah, do you have any idea what these thoughts might be doing to your energy level and to your ability to heal in this situation? What do you think happens to your heart, your spirit, and even your physical body when you look at yourself in the mirror and have these kinds of thoughts over and over again?"

"I don't know," she said.

"Well, maybe we can find out. Are you willing to try?"

"Okay," she answered.

"All right, then," I said. "Now sit up straight, and take a deep breath. I want you to close your eyes and imagine you are at home, standing in front of your mirror, looking at yourself like you normally do."

Sarah closed her eyes, and I watched her face closely. Soon, I could see that in her thoughts, she was approaching the mirror and the familiar tape was beginning to run: *"I'm so ugly, I'm so ugly, I'm going to die."* Suddenly, she started crying again, literally bent over in pain, suffering exactly as if the whole experience she was imagining was *actually happening.*

"Sarah, look inside your heart and take another deep breath," I said. "Now, focus your awareness for a moment away from your thoughts and into your heart, deep inside of yourself. Take yet another deep breath, and focus again on your heart. As you exhale let the thoughts go and settle even deeper into your heart. Now, let your awareness expand, and observe what you're experiencing."

As her thoughts shifted focus, her crying stopped and she calmed down considerably. But her face still wore a look of great sadness. Finally she opened her eyes. "It's awful, Dr. Geffen," she said. "I feel so hopeless and unlovable. Look at me, I'm so ugly, so *disfigured*. And I feel like I'm going to die."

"Sarah, can you see what these thoughts might be doing to you, and what effect they might have if they continue on like this for weeks and months?"

"Yes," she said, then paused for a long moment. "They might *really* make me die."

This was a moment of genuine revelation for her. She had just witnessed a profound truth about what she was doing to herself with her own thoughts. She had seen how powerful and destructive her thought patterns could be. Even if they did not actually make her die physically, she realized how they were standing firmly in the way of finding inner peace and a deep experience of healing.

I allowed some time to pass for the full impact of what she had discovered to sink into her awareness. Then I gently said, "Sarah, may I ask you another question now?"

"Okay," she said.

"Did you ever think of how extraordinary it is that you love yourself enough, and want to live enough, that you would go through all of this in order to stay alive? That you would face even your worst fears in order to save your life?"

The look on her face in the next few moments was precious beyond words. In an instant her mind and heart and body had suddenly begun to discover an entirely new meaning in everything she had been going through. It was as if some dark gray cloud in the sky of her mind was parting, floating away, and rays of sunlight were beginning to stream through, tentatively at first but then stronger and stronger.

"Did you ever think," I continued, "that going through all of this is a statement not only of how strong and courageous you are but of how *beautiful* you are?"

Sarah was now sitting up much straighter. Spontaneously, her breathing had become deeper and more confident. I asked her if she was willing to take this understanding one step further. When she answered yes, I asked her to stay still for a moment. Then I went out of the room and asked one of our staff members for a mirror.

Back in the examination room, I asked Sarah to hold the mirror in front of her and to look directly into it.

This was difficult for her to do, and she kept looking away. She wanted to look at anything other than the mirror. I gently encouraged her to take this important step, but she just couldn't do it.

"I know it's scary," I said, "but I want to help you anchor in this new meaning that you have for how you look. I'd also like to help you feel differently about mirrors. Are you willing to do this?"

Slowly, very slowly, she answered, "Well . . . okay." But she was still not able to look at herself in the mirror.

So I asked her again to close her eyes. "Sarah, I want you to remember now where you were just a few moments ago. Remember feeling your strength and courage. Remember feeling how much you love yourself, so much, in fact, that you are willing to fight hard to stay alive. Can you feel this now, and appreciate how extraordinary it is? Allow yourself the pleasure of feeling how much you really do love yourself, and how courageous and beautiful you are."

I watched as a new wave of love and appreciation for herself started to flow through her body. Something so life-giving was beautiful to see. After a while she was smiling again and opened her eyes.

"Okay, Sarah, I want you to look at yourself in the mirror now. Are you ready?"

This was still a bit scary for her, but after a few additional moments of hesitation, she broke through and jumped right in. Staring at her own sweet, round face and completely bald head in the mirror, she sat there, smiling away.

"Now," I said, "I'd like you to repeat the following words after me. *'Sarah, I love you.'*"

Still staring at herself in the mirror, Sarah again hesitated for a moment. Then, speaking softly to herself, she slowly repeated my words. After she finished, I continued on.

"'And I love you so much that I'm willing to fight hard to keep you alive . . .'

"'I'm not going to let anything stop you . . .'

"'I'm willing to go through surgery, and chemotherapy, and a lot of pain and inconvenience for you . . .'

"'And I'm even willing to lose all of my hair, if that's what it takes, because I love you so much, and I'm totally committed to you.'"

As she repeated these words, looking directly at herself in the mirror, her face became soft and radiant. Then we sat quietly together as she took a few minutes to absorb and appreciate the full impact of what she had just accomplished, and how far she had come. In this silence her eyes again filled with tears, but this time they were not bitter tears. They were the sweet, nurturing tears that cleanse, heal, and uplift the human heart and spirit.

"Do you feel ugly now?" I asked.

"No," she replied, looking at herself once again in the mirror. "I feel beautiful." Now it seemed that she could barely stop looking at herself in the mirror, smiling, her eyes sparkling in love.

"I feel so beautiful," Sarah said again, then paused before adding, "And I *know* that I'm going to live."

BELIEFS

We've just seen a clear example of how thoughts can have a life of their own, particularly under the stressful conditions encountered in the diagnosis and treatment of cancer. Thoughts are almost always involuntary. In the form of fears, doubts, or apprehensions, they can appear and disappear without any conscious intention on our part. Beliefs also usually arise without our conscious intention or consent, but they involve a higher level of commitment than our thoughts. They are, quite simply, thoughts we have elevated to the level of truth.

For example, we may randomly and momentarily think about the dangers of flying before we board a commercial airline, but we confidently *believe* that we will arrive at our destination safely. Similarly, random thoughts about cancer may go in many different and even contradictory directions over the course of a day. But *beliefs* about cancer are much more deeply ingrained and slower to change. The remarkable thing about these beliefs is that they will influence every aspect of your experience of cancer in a dramatic way. They will also influence virtually all of the decisions about the course of treatment you choose. And thus, they may—in a very real way—affect your ultimate outcome as well.

The hallmark features of our beliefs include how unconscious they are, how pervasive they are, and how precious we hold and regard them to be. The truth is, we have unconscious beliefs about *everything,* and these act like invisible filters through which we sift everything that occurs in the "outer world." These beliefs are not intrinsically bad; in fact, we could not function without them. But they can become deadly in the face of cancer—unless we are willing to see what they are and consciously choose whether they are grounded in fact or fear. One of the saddest commentaries on the human condition is that human beings will kill others or even themselves because of their most deeply held beliefs. I have seen this many times in people who are struggling between the direct, practical realities of their cancer and the conviction of some of their most deeply held and cherished beliefs.

Despite the attachment that exists between people and their beliefs, most of us are largely unaware of how they developed or how we might benefit if they were changed. Beliefs most often originate in childhood from the statements or the actions of individuals we regarded as authority figures. Parents are by far the most important. If your parents told you over and over again that "you can't trust anyone," and scolded you whenever you betrayed this, this very likely became an unconscious belief that will have an effect on your relationships with people throughout your life.

You might think, "Oh, I understand this, and it doesn't affect me anymore," and that may be true to a great extent, especially in normal daily activities. But if you or your spouse is suddenly diagnosed with cancer, and you suddenly feel that your life may be threatened, this deeply seated unconscious belief may suddenly be activated and influence how you interact with everyone—including your spouse or the doctors who are trying to help you. This may be one reason why some people need three, four, or even five "second opinions" before they are willing to accept a physician's recommendations and care.

Human beings have unconscious beliefs about everything, and these influence both our decisions and our experiences of the actions that result from them. I have found that it is extremely important and helpful for people dealing with cancer to take some time out toward the beginning of treatment and explore what some of their beliefs are about matters that will have a great impact on what comes next.

In dealing with patients' beliefs about cancer and cancer treatment, I've found that it's much more useful to ask questions than to make directive statements. Putting questions and answers in written form can be especially illuminating. The concentration demanded by writing allows a different and more objective perspective on beliefs to appear.

I have developed a series of questions for patients and family members to explore and answer. You are encouraged to do this in private, and you don't have to share the results with anyone if you don't want to. But it is helpful to see some of the beliefs you hold, usually unconsciously, so you can decide if you want to change some of them. Very often people discover that they have conflicting beliefs. Discovering this can be very useful and often helps reveal why some decisions seem so much harder to make than others. Here are those questions:

1. What are your beliefs about cancer?

(For example: *Cancer is a deadly process. Cancer is curable. Cancer will wreck my life. Cancer will be a challenge, but it won't destroy me.*)

_____

_____

_____

_____

_____

2. What are your beliefs about doctors?

(For example: *Doctors are knowledgeable but uncaring. Doctors are knowledgeable, and some of them do care. Doctors are greedy. Doctors are un-*

trustworthy. Doctors are trustworthy. Doctors don't really tell you the truth.)

---

3. What are your beliefs about why you got cancer?

(For example: *I got cancer because I smoked cigarettes. Because I ate bad food for many years of my life. Because I lived near a toxic manufacturing plant as a child. Because I lived near power lines for ten years. Because I inherited bad genes from my mother or father. Because I am being tested by God. Because I am being punished by God.*)

---

4. What are your beliefs about chemotherapy (or radiation, or surgery)?

(For example: *Chemotherapy will save my life. Chemotherapy will not save my life but will help me live longer. Chemotherapy is poison. Chemotherapy will destroy my immune system. Chemotherapy will make me sick. Chemotherapy is a great gift. Chemotherapy will help me.*)

_____

_____

_____

_____

_____

5. What are your beliefs and expectations about what will happen to you?

(For example: *I will probably die. I may suffer for a while, but I will probably be okay. I don't really know what will happen to me.*)

_____

_____

_____

_____

_____

6. What are your beliefs about God?

(For example: *I don't believe there is a God. I believe that God is nature. I believe there is a supreme being called God who is kind and good. I believe that God is all-loving. I believe that God judges and punishes us for our sins.*)

_____

_____

_____

7. What are your beliefs about spirituality?

(For example: *I believe there is a spiritual dimension to life that is real. Spirituality is important to me. I don't believe there is a spiritual dimension to life; what you see is all there is. Spirituality is not important.*)

8. What are your beliefs about death and life after death?

(For example: *I believe that life ends when you die, and that nothing exists beyond death. I believe that we all have a soul that lives on after the body, but I don't know what happens to it after death. I believe in heaven and hell, and that you will be judged and sent to one place or the other. I believe in reincarnation.*)

Here is a story that illustrates how someone's unconscious beliefs about a particular drug greatly influenced her decision whether to have more treatment for breast cancer.

Joyce Holt was a forty-three-year-old registered nurse with extensive medical experience. When she was diagnosed with Stage II breast cancer she suddenly found herself transformed from caregiver to patient. After her initial surgery Joyce was faced with important decisions about adjuvant treatment. She had consultations at several leading cancer centers around the country, and all of them strongly recommended four cycles of chemotherapy with Adriamycin (doxorubicin) and Cytoxan (cyclophosphamide) to be given over twelve weeks, followed by five years of oral hormone therapy with the estrogen-blocking drug Nolvadex (tamoxifen). Joyce readily agreed to the four cycles of chemotherapy, but she felt highly resistant to taking tamoxifen.

My intention here is not to argue the merits of tamoxifen. However, it is important to note that tamoxifen is a drug that has been tested successfully in many thousands of women over several decades, and its risks and benefits have been clearly defined. The drug is associated with relatively small but real risks of blood clots, uterine cancer, hot flashes, weight gain, and other potential side effects. But these side effects must be weighed against its very real and substantial benefits in terms of proven reduction in the recurrence of breast cancer.

Every year, thousands of women face the decision of whether to take tamoxifen or other hormonally active drugs as adjuvant treatment for breast cancer. The numbers are even increasing, because these drugs are now also being used to *prevent* breast cancer in women who are at high risk of developing the disease. Many women readily agree to the recommendation to take tamoxifen because of its measurable, documented, and unmistakably significant benefits—which, in the vast majority of cases, far outweigh its potential risks.

Many other women, however, struggle deeply with the decision. Why? It is usually not because they are unaware of the data or statistics, which clearly spell out the potential benefits of the drug. Rather, when a patient struggles with a decision like this, it is because of her *beliefs* about what taking the drug will really mean in her life.

Joyce Holt was such a patient. A highly intelligent, highly educated professional nurse, she was fully conversant with all of the arguments about tamoxifen's risks and benefits. Yet, even though she had readily agreed to undergo initial treatment with Adriamycin and Cytoxan—drugs that in many ways are much more toxic than tamoxifen—she felt uncomfortable at the prospect of taking tamoxifen. The more strongly it was recommended by various physicians, the more resistant she became.

When I spoke with her about this, she was uncharacteristically emotional and defensive about her feelings. "I just don't want to take it," she said emphatically. "I know about the data and all that, and I know it might be a mistake. But I just don't want to do it."

I quickly realized that something deeper was going on here. There was no question in my mind that this otherwise calm and clearheaded woman was having an emotional reaction to conscious—or unconscious—fears and beliefs. I also realized that trying to "talk her into" taking tamoxifen, regardless of how strongly I felt it would be good for her, was doomed to failure because she was not approaching this particular decision from a rational place. She had already made up her mind. Furthermore, I was sure that if I pushed her to take tamoxifen I would destroy the trust and rapport we had carefully and tenderly built in our relationship over the prior months of treatment. If I tried to influence her decision by intimidating her, or filling her mind with more fear—specifically with ominous references to how her cancer could come back if she didn't take tamoxifen—I knew I would drive a wedge between us and make it harder for her to trust and count on me.

Whether Joyce's fears and beliefs about tamoxifen were accurate was not the point. This was someone I cared about, and I could see she was in pain. She was also making a decision that I honestly believed was not in her best interests. I realized, though, that she was a bright and intelligent woman who was capable of making the best choice for herself *if* she really had all the information she needed. Although she had facts and figures about the risks and benefits of tamoxifen, she didn't have information *about her own conscious or unconscious fears and beliefs* that were so obviously influencing her decision. What was ultimately important to me was that she make her decision, whatever that might be, from a place of real strength, confidence, knowledge, and wisdom—rather than from fear, uncertainty, and potentially inaccurate and disempowering beliefs.

I asked Joyce if she would be interested in exploring exactly what was going on inside her mind and heart, either consciously or unconsciously, that was so strongly influencing her decision to refuse tamoxifen. I reassured her that I would accept whatever decision she chose, and not try to pressure her. However, I did want to help her find real clarity and peace of mind about her decision. After she felt reassured, she agreed.

I then asked her to write down, in a general way, her principal beliefs about tamoxifen. These were her responses:

My beliefs about tamoxifen are . . .
1. It has many side effects.
2. It is an unnatural and unhealthy substance.
3. It will make me have hot flashes.
4. It will decrease my sex drive.
5. It will increase my risk of uterine cancer.
6. It will disrupt the hormonal equilibrium of my body, which I
   believe goes against the laws of nature and is not good for me.

Joyce and I then discussed her beliefs in detail. I didn't do so with the intention of arguing with her or convincing her she was wrong, or right. What she had written, after all, was certainly understandable from her perspective. I simply asked her how and why she believed these particular things about tamoxifen, how certain she felt that she would experience the side effects she listed, and why. In general, tamoxifen is a drug with relatively low toxicity. As a medical professional, Joyce was aware of that. But beliefs are not necessarily determined by known facts, and when I asked her these questions in a nonjudgmental way, she acknowledged that she really wasn't *sure* she would experience every one of the side effects she listed, but she was *afraid* she would. Even though she also knew that she could stop taking tamoxifen at any time if she did experience any of the unwanted side effects, she was still adamant about not even trying it.

Without contradicting what Joyce said or had written, I asked her to think for a few moments and list some of her thoughts about what it might cost her to hold on to her particular beliefs about tamoxifen, particularly if it meant that she would ultimately decide not to take it as prescribed. This was not asserting that she was wrong, but simply focusing on the results her beliefs could bring about. It was a matter of asking her a question and letting her provide the answers.

What could holding on to my beliefs about tamoxifen cost me?
1. A possible recurrence.
2. A lot of grief as a result of a recurrence.
3. Irreplaceable time with my husband.
4. Increased risk of heart disease and osteoporosis.
5. It could cost me my life if I were to have a recurrence.

Finally, I asked her to write down what she could possibly gain from taking tamoxifen.

What could I possibly gain by taking tamoxifen?
1. I could improve my chances of not having a recurrence and living a long and healthy life.
2. I could significantly improve my chances of avoiding heart disease and osteoporosis.
3. I could gain the knowledge that I was getting the benefit of everything medical science has to offer me right now.
4. I could gain the benefit of making my husband feel reassured.

It is fascinating to realize the extent to which Joyce's responses go directly to the heart of her personal hopes and fears. These are concerns that would never have come up if I had simply presented the statistics about adjuvant therapy with tamoxifen. If I had said, "Here are the numbers, now you decide," her core issues would have remained unacknowledged and unresolved—and the deepest possible healing would not have taken place, regardless of whether she took tamoxifen.

Once Joyce's negative fears and beliefs were clearly revealed to herself, and their possible costs were weighed against the possible benefits of treatment, it was easy for her to make the prudent decision of going ahead with the therapy. While I do believe that this was the wisest choice for her, the *way* she made her decision was just as important to me, as was the sense of clarity and empowerment she had afterward. It was now truly *her choice,* not mine or anyone else's. Furthermore, since her mind and her heart were now aligned with the decision, I felt certain that she would have no unnecessary toxicities that can arise when treatment choices are made from fear-based, unconscious beliefs, or when they are made with doubts and ambivalence. I also felt certain that she would now get the most benefit possible from her treatment, because she had come to the decision on her own, with real understanding and insight about what was most important to her.

MEANINGS

If beliefs are the "truths" we attach to ideas and experiences in the real world, meanings are the *significance* we give to those ideas and experiences. The mind assigns meaning to virtually everything it focuses upon, and the degree of significance can range from the unimportant and trivial to the highly spiritual and profound. In fact, whenever *anything* happens within our awareness, our mind assigns it a meaning. Just as with our thoughts and beliefs, this process is usually unconscious and instantaneous. To a greater degree than most people ever suspect, the meaning we assign to events fundamentally affects our entire experience of life in that moment.

If your boss calls you unexpectedly one day, the meaning you consciously or unconsciously assign to the call determines whether you are filled with fear, curiosity, elation, or dread. If you think the call means you are about to be fired, you might feel fear and tension. But if you think you are about to be given a raise, you might feel elation. And if you have no idea what the call means, your mind will start searching for a meaning. *What is this call about? Did I do something wrong?*

Similarly, if your spouse does not show up to meet you at the time you agreed upon, the meaning you give to his or her absence will determine how you feel. If your mind thinks the reason your spouse is late is because he was in a car accident and he was hurt, you will have one kind of experience internally. On the other hand, if your mind says something like, "She is always late. I can never count on her to keep her word. She doesn't respect me!" you will have an entirely different experience.

The point here is that in both of these situations, *as with every situation that we can or will ever experience in life,* it is not the event that determines our experience, but the meaning and significance we give it. I realize this is a radical assertion, but there is no question in my mind that it is true—and it is especially true when dealing with cancer. I have seen over and over again how the meaning cancer patients give to their illness can dramatically affect how they respond to their diagnosis, choose treatment, and deal with possible side effects. What is often overlooked in this process is how these meanings can have very negative—as well as positive—effects.

Most people are comfortable with the meaning they ascribe to their situation in life, but others may find themselves chronically unhappy or unable to change habitual self-sabotaging patterns in their lives. Often some personal conviction—deeply held but incompletely understood—stops them from moving forward. For a physician, helping patients to identify and understand the meanings they find in illnesses should be an important element of the treatment process.

The contrasting experiences of two patients with virtually identical diagnoses provides a dramatic illustration of this. But before recounting the story, let me pause to make an important observation. Again and again in my work as an oncologist I've seen the importance of God and religion in the lives of a large percentage of patients. Although religion may not play a major role in everyone's life, it is extremely important to a great many people in our society. During a crisis like cancer, it often, and understandably, becomes even more important. The frequency with which God is mentioned in this book is not an attempt to proselytize, judge, or even comment upon the value or significance of religion. Nor is it necessarily a reflection of my own personal beliefs. It is simply a reflection of what oncologists often encounter in dealing with real patients in the real world.

At the age of fifty-four, Ken Mitchell was found to have extensive lung and liver metastases of a high-grade malignant melanoma. He was a devoted family man, with a profound religious faith. His diagnosis plunged him into a deep depression, and nothing seemed to help him feel better emotionally. Despite everyone's attempts to reach out to him, he remained angry, bitter, and resentful. After many soul-searching conversations, I asked Ken if he would tell me his thoughts about the meaning of his ill-ness and why he believed he got cancer. "I'm a sinner, Dr. Geffen," he confided in me. "God gave me this illness to punish me for my sins."

Michael Hart, also fifty-four, was diagnosed with the same cancer as Ken. He too was very devoted to his family and to his religion. After his diagnosis, Michael did not fall into despair. Instead, he focused even more intently than before on the people in his life he cared most about. He refused to feel sorry for himself or to become depressed, and never sank into self-pity or resentment. In the midst of his overwhelmingly challenging situation, he was calm, cheerful, and optimistic—and every-one who met him was uplifted simply by being in his presence. I asked him how he did it, and what his thoughts were about the meaning of his illness, and why he believed he got cancer.

"I don't really know why I got cancer, Doc," he explained. "But I do know this—this experience is making me a better, stronger person. And it is bringing me closer to my Creator, to myself, and to the people I love—closer than I ever could have imagined. So no matter what hap-pens, it's okay. I know I've been given this challenge for a purpose that can and will serve me and those I love. As a matter of fact, how are you doing, Doc? Don't forget, I'm praying for *you* every single day."

What was the difference between Ken and Michael? Their medical situ-ations were as similar as the importance of family and religion in their lives. But because of the different *meaning* they gave to their illnesses, they were living in two completely different worlds. This had a direct bearing on their experiences during treatment and strongly influenced everyone around them as well.

These distinctions are merely a glimpse of the understanding and clarity that this level of the Seven Levels of Healing gives to patients and family members. My goal is to help patients and family members discover and explore the beliefs, values, and meanings they would consciously choose to have at this most critical time in their lives—beliefs, values, and meanings that are empowering, uplifting, and health-promoting, rather than the unconscious beliefs, values, and meanings that they may carry with them from their past, which may not be supporting them at all.

Focus

Another important component of the activity of our mind can contribute significantly to how we feel and respond to any experience, including the experience of cancer. I refer to this component as *focus*. Our experience of events is influenced not only by our thoughts, beliefs, and ascribed meanings but by *what we focus on*. This is a basic tenet of biofeedback, which trains people how to consciously redirect their focus away from unpleasant thoughts or emotions and toward pleasant and relaxing ones. By changing your focus, you can change how you feel.

There are many examples of this, and the effects can be both positive and negative. For example, ignoring the warning signs of cancer by focusing on something else can lead to a crucial delay in diagnosis. Conversely, focusing only on possible adverse side effects of cancer treatment can make the experience significantly more difficult and actually leads some people to forgo potentially life-saving therapies.

There is no question that patients who are able to shift their focus in positive ways not only have a less stressful experience with challenges such as cancer but also often have better outcomes. In fact, this is repeatedly seen in medicine among people with strong religious faith. Without attempting to answer the question of whether people are indeed able to draw upon a higher power, or the extent to which a strong spiritual or religious faith may make a difference in a particular patient's clinical course, it is very clear that faith allows many patients to radically change their focus in the face of great, or even overwhelming, challenges. The following story illustrates how clear and powerful this can be when it occurs.

Jack Montgomery was a delightful seventy-eight-year-old gentleman from Georgia who had been admitted to the hospital with fever, a productive cough, and abdominal pain of several days' duration. CT scans of his chest and abdomen were highly suggestive of a primary lung cancer with extensive liver metastases. I was called to see him for a consultation on a Saturday, as he and his family awaited the results of a liver biopsy to determine the nature of his apparent malignancy.

For fifty years Jack had worked as a carpenter and also as a gardener. He loved to grow his own food, and his face and skin were thickened and engraved with lines that looked like tire treads from spending so many years in the hot Georgia sun. He was most proud when his son and daughter grew up, got married, and had children, whom he loved dearly. Like most men of his time, Jack smoked cigarettes. In fact, he had smoked one or two packs of cigarettes a day for nearly fifty years.

As we got to know each other, Jack tried to put up a brave face in light of his impending diagnosis. At moments, however, he would let down his guard enough to allow me to see the intense fear and sadness in his heart as he thought about the idea of having cancer and possibly dying. Most of all, he was overwhelmed with grief at the thought of leaving his beloved family.

When I arrived at the hospital the following Monday morning, I went immediately to the pathology department and reviewed Jack's slides. The diagnosis of extensive-stage small cell carcinoma of the lung was unequivocal. With a heavy heart, I made my way up to Jack's room, wishing there was a way to avoid giving him and his family the information for which they were waiting.

As I entered Jack's room, I found his family surrounding his bed. There were his wife, his son and daughter, his son-in-law and daughter-in-law, and his brother. We greeted one another and made small talk for a few minutes, trying to ease the obvious fear and tension in the air. Finally, I could delay the discussion no further.

"Mr. Montgomery," I began, "I have some results of your liver biopsy now, if you would like to discuss them."

I looked at him lying in bed and waited for his acknowledgment before going further. Jack closed his eyes, as if bracing himself, and gently nodded. He then opened his eyes again and looked at me.

"Unfortunately," I continued, as gently as I could, "the biopsy has confirmed that the mass in your lung is a lung cancer, and it has spread into your liver."

Silence came over the room as the family tried to absorb this. I searched for something further to say. If I told Jack his disease was almost certainly incurable, all hope would have been destroyed in a heartbeat. He might have felt deeply abandoned, and any belief in the possibility of meaningful survival, let alone unexpected cures, would be greatly diminished in his mind and heart. On the other hand, it is cruel and unfair to overstate what one can reasonably expect to achieve with conventional medicine. There is a fine line between telling the truth and not destroying a patient's hope and spirit.

Facing many such moments over the years, I have developed a personal style that seems to work well for both my patients and myself. I always try to find something positive and hopeful to say about the situation, no matter how grim it may be. In this case, the specific subtype of his lung cancer gave me a very real potential opening.

"Mr. Montgomery," I said, "the kind of lung cancer that you have is the small cell type. This type tends to be readily treatable. We can definitely treat you with chemotherapy, and it is also very possible that chemotherapy will be of benefit, perhaps even very significant benefit."

"But is it curable, Dr. Geffen? Can you cure me?"

"I have to tell you that it is very, very difficult to cure this kind of lung cancer with the treatments that are available right now. I'm not saying it can't be cured, because there is always a great mystery in what ultimately happens to any of us in life. And my own conviction and experience in these kinds of situations is that, in truth, *anything* can happen, including being cured, even when that doesn't seem likely or possible. But it is also important for you to understand that this kind of disease is usually extremely difficult, if not impossible, to cure, particularly when it has already spread so extensively. Nonetheless, we can definitely treat it, if you wish, and try to get it under control at least for a while. If the treatments are successful, then it will help you feel a lot better. And it may help you live longer, too."

After a long silence, his wife finally spoke. She was sitting in a chair in the corner of the room, literally trembling, fighting back tears.

"Dr. Geffen," she asked, "how long are we talking about if my husband takes chemotherapy? And how long will he live if he doesn't take chemotherapy?"

For an oncologist, these are some of the most difficult questions that can be asked by terrified patients and family members. They are also some of the most common. Typically, the physician responds by citing published survival statistics. For a man like Jack Montgomery, the median survival is in the range of six to nine months, which might or might not be prolonged by treatment. However, blurting out numbers in a situation like this is, I believe, insensitive and cruel. I also believe it is misleading. Every human being is absolutely unique, and no one can predict with any certainty how long any one of us is going to live. Every oncologist has seen patients with advanced cancer who died much sooner than anyone expected. And there are also many patients who lived far, far longer than the median survival statistics would predict.

Patients and family members are looking for a specific time frame in this situation. They want some certainty about what to expect. Unfortunately, the sense of certainty that patients get when they are told they have six to nine months to live often turns out to be completely wrong. Or it becomes a self-fulfilling prophecy.

When I try to answer these questions without giving specific numbers, many times patients feel somewhat frustrated. I believe the answer I commonly give is much gentler to their hearts, even if their minds are not entirely satisfied.

"Well, Mrs. Montgomery," I began, "the question that you are asking me is very reasonable, very real, and very understandable. I am asked that question almost every day by patients and their families. Unfortunately, it is very difficult to answer with any certainty. There are various published statistics that suggest what the average survival of patients in this kind of situation is, but I hesitate to draw on those statistics or give them too much credence. Your husband is not a statistic. He is a unique, very special, and precious individual, and no one can truly predict his destiny in this situation. Some lung cancer patients live only a few weeks, with or without chemotherapy. Others, particularly those who have successful chemotherapy treatment, can live for many months. Occasionally, some will live even longer still. It's very difficult to predict in any individual case."

I then paused once again as this painful but honest information was slowly assimilated by Jack and his family.

After some time, he looked up at me from his bed and said, "Well, Dr. Geffen, what should I do?"

This is yet another difficult question. In the field of oncology, in many situations the best option for a given patient is straightforward. Many other times, however, it is not clear at all, and this was the case in Jack Montgomery's situation. His type of malignancy can be very sensitive to chemotherapy, and I have seen extraordinary responses on many occasions, even in elderly patients with advanced disease. If he tolerated chemotherapy well, and if his tumor was responsive, he might indeed gain a great deal from having treatment. On the other hand, Jack was elderly, not in the best overall shape, and furthermore, had very advanced cancer. His liver function was already showing signs of compromise. He also had severe underlying emphysema and a weak heart. Treating patients with chemotherapy in these kinds of circumstances is much harder and more dangerous. Although Jack was looking to me for guidance, it was difficult to know what was best for him.

"Mr. Montgomery," I began, "let me tell you how other people in your situation have approached this. Some patients feel that if there is some reasonable hope of benefit from treatment, they want to go ahead with it. Those patients understand that chemotherapy can be difficult at times, even when the patient is young, and at your age it can be even harder. Nevertheless, some patients are willing to accept this, because they want to do everything they can to fight and prolong their lives. They are simply not ready to let go.

"Other people take a different approach. These are patients who say, 'Well, regardless of my age, I feel that I've lived a good life. If this chemotherapy is not likely to cure me, then I'm not sure I want to spend the time I have left on this earth undergoing treatment, running back and forth to the doctor's office, and spending time away from my family.' Those patients feel that they are ready to think about letting go and not going through the struggle of battling cancer.

"I want to emphasize to you, Mr. Montgomery, that in my mind either one of these approaches is perfectly reasonable and acceptable. If you want to have treatment and if you want to fight, then I am ready to roll up my sleeves and fight with you. On the other hand, if you feel that you're not up for that kind of struggle at this point, then that too is reasonable. Ultimately, this is a personal choice that you and your family will want to make together."

We then had a detailed conversation about the range of chemotherapy treatments that might be appropriate for him, covering the expected benefits as well as the possible side effects. When we had gone over all these issues, there seemed to be nothing left to say. Jack and his family were facing one of the most difficult decisions of their lives. Without anyone saying so directly, it was clear from the tone and direction of their questions that different family members felt very differently—but very strongly—about the best way to proceed.

Then, something extraordinary happened. Jack reached out and asked if he could take my hand in his. He grasped my hand tightly and held it to his chest. Closing his eyes, Jack began to speak in his thick Georgian drawl. He began to pray.

"Lord Jesus, I'm lying here in this moment and calling out to you for help and guidance. Lord Jesus, I don't know which way to go. I pray for your guidance.

"But Lord," he continued, "before I ask you for your help, I want to praise you and honor you and thank you from the depths of my heart for all of your blessings in my life. Lord, I *thank you* for all you have given to me and my family for so many years. I *thank you* and *praise you* for your love and your guidance and protection. Thank you for guiding us, and for lifting us up. Lord, we love you and honor you and thank you. *Thank you,* Jesus. Thank you, thank you."

As Jack prayed, tears started welling up in my eyes, and a surge of love filled my heart like a big wave. I was afraid that this wave would rise and rise and spill over and I would start weeping, because I was so moved by his pure, raw, and absolutely breathtaking declaration of love and gratitude to God.

I glanced around the room and saw everyone standing silently, their hands clasped together. Everyone's head was bowed in reverent prayer, and I realized that—in truth—church, or temple, or whatever you want to call it, is created *instantly* when human beings simply turn their hearts and minds toward God. There, at 9:03 A.M. on a Monday morning in room 468 of Indian River Memorial Hospital, we were all in a sacred space. And Jack Montgomery's prayer had brought us there.

"Lord," he went on, "now I need your help. I am facing a very difficult decision, Lord. It's the hardest one I've ever faced in my life, and I don't know which way to go. Lord, I want you to guide me and guide my family so we can know which road to take. Lord, please above all give your blessings to my family. And Lord, please bless this doctor, who also loves you.

"Lord, guide me and show me what is your will. If it's my time to leave this earth, then so be it. Then take me, Lord. Forgive me for my sins and my trespasses and take me home to you. If you want me to fight this disease, then show me how, Lord, and give me the strength and courage to fight. Whatever you wish, Lord, that is the wish of my heart. I want nothing else. Please love and bless my beloved family, Lord. In Jesus' name we honor and praise you. Thank you. Amen."

During his prayer, which was so profound and heartfelt, the space in the room had become completely transformed. The presence of love and grace filled every heart and every corner of that room. The fear and discord had been instantly transformed into unity and gratitude. The members of Jack's family were holding one another, blowing their noses, and offering one another Kleenex. In those few short moments the unmistakable love, courage, and faith of this man and his family were established beyond question.

It was extraordinary to see how powerfully and elegantly Jack had responded to hearing from his physician that he had a very advanced form of lung cancer that had spread into his liver and was very difficult, if not impossible, to cure. Yet Jack completely transformed the fear and distress of this moment by simply *shifting his focus*, turning to his spiritual faith. He believed he would be guided by a higher power, and he put his focus there. In doing so, he transformed not only his own experience but *everyone else's as well*. His prayer and the power of his faith and focus created an absolutely sublime and healing experience for everyone in the room. I only wished that every human being could face terrifying circumstances with such calm, clear equanimity and joy in one's heart. I also believed that through this process, Jack had opened himself and his family to the possibility of a deeper healing of the mind, heart, and spirit—as well as the body—of everyone involved.

I reached down and gave Jack a big hug. He grabbed me tightly, as if we had known each other forever. "Thank you, Doctor," he said. "I would like to ask if I can have a day to think about everything and make my decision."

"Of course. Please take all the time you need."

As I was preparing to leave, I noticed how much I wanted to stay in the room. It was an amazing realization. Here I was, the doctor of this beautiful man who had just been diagnosed with an aggressive form of metastatic lung cancer, and *I* felt healed by his prayers. *How fortunate I am*, I thought, *to have had this experience this morning*. I also thought how blessed this man and his family were to have such a clear and strong spiritual faith. I felt I couldn't leave without acknowledging at least some of this, in some way.

"Mr. Montgomery," I said, "I want you to know how moved and grateful I am to have had this experience with you this morning. I wish that so many other of my patients could have the experience that we've just had. I feel honored to know you, and thank you for including me in your prayers."

With tears still running down her cheeks, Jack's wife looked at me and said, "Dr. Geffen, our faith has always guided and sustained us, and it always will. It is the most precious thing we have."

Finally, I pulled myself away from the extraordinary presence of love surrounding this family and, holding back tears of my own, went out in the hall and took a few deep breaths before moving on in my rounds.

My next patient that morning was in many ways strikingly similar, yet radically different. Harvey Bruce was a seventy-six-year-old man who had been undergoing treatment for a chronic blood disorder, which had recently transformed into full-blown acute leukemia.

Both Harvey and his wife, Ruth, were bitter, angry, and depressed, and visiting with them was always a challenge. Over the six months I had known them, I had tried to engage them on a personal and empathetic level, but to no avail. I had always been rebuffed with more questions about Harvey's blood counts, a journal article his wife had found, or possible new treatments.

Before I was even through the door, Ruth was demanding to know her husband's morning white blood cell count, whether his hemoglobin was up or down, and what his platelet count was. She was consistently dissatisfied with the nursing care, demanding that Harvey be turned more frequently or that his vital signs not be taken so often. The food was always either too hot or too cold, too mushy or too firm, and she couldn't understand why in the world her husband should have to go through any of this. She also demanded that I not fully disclose how dreadful his prognosis truly was. She kept repeating that he would not be able to handle the truth. "I know him better than all of you," she said over and over. "I know that he can't handle it. He'll start crying and crying. . . ."

I calmly looked at her and said gently, "Mrs. Bruce, what's so wrong and terrible about the possibility that your husband might cry if he learns that he has leukemia, and that he might be dying?"

A long, pregnant pause followed, and then the truth was revealed. With tears welling up in her own eyes, she said, "I can't bear it. I just can't stand to see him cry."

In her resistance to her own pain and grief, Ruth was making herself, her husband, and every one around them miserable. The contrast with Jack Montgomery's room, only a few yards away, was too clear to ignore. Here were two men in their late seventies, both diagnosed with a serious advanced malignancy, and their *focus* completely determined their experience. How I wished that Ruth could have the courage, and the willingness, to allow her own pain and heartbreak to come out. How I wished that she could feel the grace and blessing that Jack Montgomery's wife and her family had experienced through Jack's prayers, as he surrendered and asked for guidance from a higher power, and listened with humility and serenity to whatever answer he would hear in his heart. With this awareness, I sent as much love and compassion as I could to Ruth and her beloved husband. For the hundredth time we went over all of the available options and again acknowledged how limited they were.

As I left Harvey's room and moved on in my rounds, I understood once again how profoundly our thoughts and beliefs, the meanings we give to events, and the focus we bring to them affect every aspect of our lives. Blindly spending millions of dollars on many aspects of cancer treatment seems absurd when a simple act of faith and trust can alleviate so much pain and suffering. I then prayed silently in my own heart for the strength and courage to continue in this effort to realize a vision of medicine that honors and cares not only for the body but for the mind, heart, and spirit as well.

9

LEVEL SIX:

LIFE ASSESSMENT

YOU MUST GIVE BIRTH TO YOUR IMAGES. THEY
ARE THE FUTURE WAITING TO BE BORN.
—RAINER MARIA RILKE

L evel Six of this program is an invitation to explore, discover, understand, and reconnect with the deepest longings, intentions, and purposes of your life. Without question, it is one of the most important and transformative steps anyone can take on the journey through cancer.

Why is this so? The answer begins with an obvious but rarely acknowledged truth. Each of us hopes to get what we want in life and to avoid what we don't want. We all want pleasure, and we all want to avoid pain. We all want happiness and want to minimize suffering. Underlying the desire for happiness and pleasure is a fundamental wish for the experience of love, joy, and peace that is, ultimately, our true nature. We can say, therefore, that the foundation of all human behavior is, ultimately, the desire to know one's self.

In our everyday lives these ideas are rarely acknowledged. We are all so busy, who has the time? Without really thinking about it, we continue to plunge ahead each day, doing the things we hope and believe will bring us pleasure and make us happy—or help us to avoid suffering and pain.

What makes human beings so unique, and human endeavors so diverse, however, is that each of us has a different idea about what brings us happiness or what brings us pain. That's why some people exercise, or drink alcohol, or pursue a career, or go hiking in the mountains, or go dancing in nightclubs, and others don't. It's why some individuals become businesspeople, some teachers, some parents, and others monks or priests. Regardless, underlying all of these activities is the same impulse to seek happiness and pleasure, to avoid pain and suffering, and ultimately to experience love and joy. It is the same impulse that compels people to seek medical help when they are diagnosed with a serious illness.

Virtually every cancer patient I have seen is, at least initially, experiencing some kind of physical, mental, emotional, or spiritual pain. In many patients, the distress is most acute at the moment of their diagnosis. As we have discussed, few words in our culture create a bigger avalanche of pain, confusion, and fear than the words "I'm sorry, but you have cancer."

Remarkably, the mental, emotional, and spiritual pain that most cancer patients experience far exceeds their physical pain. This has become even more true in recent years, as advances in screening and diagnosis have led increasingly to the detection of cancer long before the onset of any physical symptoms.

Some cancers present with an unremitting cough, blood in the urine, or an ache in the upper abdomen. Many more are detected by an abnormal blood test, an abnormal mammogram, a small and completely painless lump, or a swollen lymph node. Quite often, patients believed they were in perfect health. *They had no idea they had cancer.*

Regardless of the type of cancer or the stage at the time of diagnosis, the degree of mental, emotional, and spiritual pain is often the same. In a huge number of cases, it is actually the pain and fear *associated* with cancer, rather than any specific physical symptoms, that cause people to seek medical help.

Certainly patients come to physicians because they want to "get rid of" their cancer as quickly and as easily as possible. But on a deeper level, they also want help in changing how they *feel.* Often they are confused. Often they feel overwhelmed. Almost always, they are deeply afraid.

Doctors must understand that patients want them not only to get rid of their disease and take away their physical pain but to *take away their fear as well*. When physicians realize that their role is not only to address clinical symptoms but also to help patients and family members feel better at every level of their being, an important step will be taken toward fulfilling the ultimate, as well as the relative, purpose of medicine.

What is the best way to fulfill both of these purposes? In this book we have explored a number of the key elements, and in this chapter we will explore another important one. Level Six of the Seven Levels of Healing describes a process for identifying the meaning and purpose of your life, clarifying specific goals for the coming year, and considering how you wish to be remembered after you are gone. These are essential, invaluable distinctions for patients and family members.

LIFE ASSESSMENT:
DISCOVERING YOUR REASONS FOR LIVING

Amid all the effort and activity that takes place in helping cancer patients to prolong their lives, two questions are almost never asked of them. The first is "Do you really want to live?" and the second is "If so, *why?*"

Most people respond to these questions as if the answer were self-evident: *Of course I want to live.* This is a basic, human, and understandable response. Throughout nature, after all, life resists death. But when asked exactly *why* they want to live, many patients don't know how to respond. This is usually because no one has ever asked them this question before, or they have never asked it of themselves. Some break down in tears as they realize they don't really know the answer. Others are puzzled and become curious. A few become hostile, outraged to be asked such a thing.

The Dalai Lama of Tibet has explored these questions in terms of humanity as a whole and has stated with clarity and elegance: "All beings want to be happy." But finding happiness is often not as simple as it appears.

We all know that people seek happiness in many different ways, yet the desired result frequently remains elusive. We look to our careers, our children, our relationships, or in a thousand other places for fulfillment and happiness. Sometimes it appears to work, at least for a while. At other times the activities we pursue only lead us to more pain. Despite this almost universal experience, few people take the time to assess whether the way they are living their lives *will ever* really bring them the happiness they seek. Tragically, in their efforts to find happiness in external things and conditions, they lose sight of their deeper needs and priorities and their true meaning and purpose.

When people are diagnosed with cancer, these deeper issues can instantly and dramatically rise to the surface. Basic changes invariably begin to occur in how patients perceive their lives. Everything that had been taken for granted is now no longer certain—including how much longer they may expect to live. In this context, many things that were previously regarded as significant or even essential may, in one moment, not look that way anymore at all.

Prior to getting cancer, most of our hopes and fears in life are focused in the external world. A cancer diagnosis immediately shifts attention inward. An important reason for this is that cancer instantly and forever shatters the illusion of immortality. The collective, unspoken dream that we have all the time in the world is now gone. In its place often comes an entirely new set of questions: *What do I really care about? What is the real meaning and purpose of my life? What are my most important goals? And also, How do I want to be remembered after I am gone from this life?*

As this process of inquiry begins, patients have an opportunity to discover—or rediscover—what is most important to them. It is a chance to identify their true purpose in life and begin moving immediately in the direction of fulfilling it.

There are three very important reasons why finding clear and coherent answers to these questions is so important on the journey through cancer:

1. Cancer often brings about difficult and challenging times. This is especially true of advanced or aggressive cancers, particularly those that cannot be easily cured with surgery. When you know exactly why you want to live, you have a clear and personally compelling motivation for fighting on. You are able to focus on *reasons for living*, rather than on whatever might not be going well at the moment.

Friedrich Nietzsche wrote, "He who has an important enough *why* can bear almost any *how*." We have all heard stories of patients who were given only a few weeks to live but defied their doctors' predictions and survived to be present at a wedding, graduation, or anniversary celebration months later. Some patients live years longer than expected. While many factors influence the outcome of stories like these, it is clear that the patients benefited from well-defined and compelling reasons for living.

2. On the journey through cancer you will have diminished resources of time and energy, at least temporarily. As we have seen, cancer challenges patients and family members on many levels. Dealing with the myriad logistical elements of cancer care consumes valuable resources of time, money, emotional energy, and physical strength. This may persist through treatment, and sometimes even beyond. As a result, cancer patients simply cannot afford unfulfilling or destructive thoughts, activities, and relationships. Many people find that cancer is the catalyst for long-avoided changes. Some people finally stop smoking or drinking, change their diet, and start exercising. Others might reconsider or completely change a job or career. Still others might change or even end a relationship, or begin a new one. And for some patients, the experience of cancer will cause them to begin to examine and explore some of their deepest beliefs and ideas about why they are alive.

3. Some people will discover that they don't really want to fight their disease. Patients may feel, for whatever reason, that they are unwilling to undergo surgery, radiation, or chemotherapy, or even alternative or complementary approaches to healing. After reflecting on their situation, some people feel that they have lived a good life and are ready to let go. Others may come to the same conclusion but by a very different route. They may feel that life has been a difficult or even an exhausting experience. They have suffered, and struggled, perhaps for a long time, and they don't wish to make any further efforts to keep living.

Unfortunately, in our society this perspective is rarely supported. All too often, patients endure arduous medical procedures and treatments because they are simply not clear about what they truly want to do. Rarely are they helped to explore these issues in the most open, supportive, and conscious way.

There are other instances in which patients are indeed clear about what they want to do, but they can't *give themselves permission* to let go. They're forbidden to do so by their religious beliefs or their cultural training. Or the medical environment in which they find themselves may not support such a decision. Except for the most elderly, the most frail, and the most infirm, our culture gives very, very few people permission to say, "I want to die." Great shame is attached to feeling this way, let alone saying it outright. From moral as well as medical-legal perspectives, it is usually considered to be hugely insensitive, if not outright criminal, even to suggest that it might be in someone's best interest to end his or her struggle to keep the physical body alive. I want to clarify that in pointing this out, I am not advocating physician-assisted suicide or euthanasia. In my experience as a physician, and especially as an oncologist, I have seen very few patients who could not be made comfortable with appropriate care and adequate doses of medications. I am speaking here only of supporting a patient's right to decline treatment for any disease, even if the refusal seems unreasonable to us, and even if it hastens his or her death.

Perhaps most tragic of all are people with advanced cancer who are truly prepared to die, have given themselves permission and are at peace with their choice, *and* have the support of their physician—but can't let go because of pressure from family members. The family is unable and unwilling to face their own unresolved pain, grief, guilt, or anger, so the patient must suffer through tears, pleas, and guilt.

Gloria Parker was a sixty-eight-year-old woman with advanced ovarian cancer that kept progressing after a number of different treatments. When she came to my office for a scheduled follow-up visit, she was exhausted.

In fact, she was dying, but her family would not accept it. Over the weekend her four children had flown in from different parts of the country. They all had ideas of what was wrong with her, what was wrong with her medical care, and what should be done to "turn this situation around." One of her daughters, a strict vegetarian, wanted her to immediately start a macrobiotic diet. A second daughter was convinced that her mother was "starving to death," and demanded to know why I wouldn't give her high-dose intravenous vitamins, which she was sure would save her life. One of her sons wanted to fly her immediately to the Memorial Sloan-Kettering Cancer Center in New York City, certain that "they will have something to offer that you don't." Another son wanted to take her to a clinic in Tijuana, Mexico, that he'd heard had "great success" in curing cancer with herbs and coffee enemas. Meanwhile, Gloria's husband was out in the parking lot, crying.

Gloria herself was getting weaker and weaker, and was starting to feel short of breath. She was gravely ill, and a decision had to be made about what to do. As we started to discuss the options, she told me that she understood what was happening and that she did not want to do anything more to prolong her life. She told me very clearly and serenely that she was "ready to go." I asked her if she wanted to go home to die, or if she would prefer to go into the hospital. She said, "Please, put me in the hospital, because my family is driving me crazy. They won't let me die in peace. I'm ready to go, but they won't let me."

THE LIFE-ASSESSMENT PROCESS

We have covered many important issues in the preceding pages. To help patients address these issues, I ask them to begin by responding in writing to some basic questions:

- What is the meaning and purpose of your life?
- What are your most important goals for the next year?
- How do you want to be remembered after you are gone?

In the balance of this chapter, we'll look at these questions one by one.

1. What is the meaning and purpose of your life?

As we have discussed, a diagnosis of cancer often irrevocably shatters the illusion of immortality that so many of us harbor. For many cancer patients and their loved ones, this marks one of the most important turning points in their lives. As the illusion of immortality shatters, an opening can occur—a unique opportunity in which to explore some of the deepest and most important questions of life.

In the life-assessment process, patients' responses to the question *What is the meaning and purpose of your life?* are often referred to as "mission statements." They actually include three distinct but closely related components: the *purpose* of your life, your *mission* in life, and the *vision* you may hold for your life. These three concepts—purpose, mission, and vision—are often confused in people's minds. But the distinctions between them can be critical, particularly for someone on the journey through cancer.

If I may use myself as an example, I would say, most succinctly, that the *purpose* of my life is *to be a whole, authentic, fully alive, and integrated human being; to know and celebrate my true Self—the timeless, eternal essence of God, of spirit, and of all beings; and to be a powerful presence of love, joy, wisdom, compassion, awareness, and truth for myself and others.* These are the values that inspire me most deeply and call to my heart, again and again and again. These are the qualities that I aspire to understand and embody in my life. And these are the ideals that bring me the greatest experience of love, joy, and fulfillment in life.

It has been humorously said, "At the end of your life, God will not ask you, 'Why didn't you spend more time at the office?' "—and there is real wisdom in this. I am convinced that at the end of *my* life the questions that will matter most to me are: *Did I come to know my true Self? Did I live and embody the highest truths and values I discovered? Did I share the gifts that were given to me? Did I live my life as fully as possible? And, above all, did I love—myself as well as others—as fully and completely as possible?*

You may notice that my purpose in life includes no mention of my work as a physician, writer, and speaker, or my specialty as an oncologist. My *mission,* however, is to create a new paradigm of multidimensional medicine: one that promotes awareness, healing, and transformation at the deepest levels of the body, mind, heart, and spirit of all beings. It is clear to me that the ultimate purpose of this new paradigm of medicine is *to assist all beings to experience unbounded love, joy, and peace, and to know that this is the essence of who we all truly are.* This is the gift I want to bring forth and share with the world. This is the mission I want to accomplish while I am alive on this earth.

Finally, my *vision* is the worldly expression of my mission. My own personal vision is to see this new paradigm of multidimensional medicine made available to everyone in the world. My vision, therefore, is the tangible and full realization of my mission.

Cancer patients and their family members—like many other people—are often not clear about the important distinctions between their purpose, mission, and vision. Achieving clarity about these issues can be life-transforming, and this was certainly true for Beverly Martin, the woman with breast cancer we met in Chapter 2.

When Beverly underwent a modified radical mastectomy and axillary lymph node dissection, the tumor was found to have spread to thirteen of her nineteen axillary lymph nodes. Following her surgery, Beverly was advised by several leading medical centers to undergo conventional-dose adjuvant chemotherapy, followed by high-dose chemotherapy and stem cell rescue, which at the time was often recommended for women with so many positive lymph nodes. This would not have been easy for anyone to accept, but it was even harder for Beverly, an otherwise healthy and vibrant woman who had "barely taken a pill" in her entire life. She'd had no prior illnesses or surgeries, and before the discovery of her breast cancer all of her encounters with the health care system were completely routine and unremarkable.

Her experiences following her breast cancer diagnosis had been quite traumatic. It was at this stage of her journey through cancer that Beverly and I had our first talk on the phone. Our conversation that day prompted her initial appoitment with me at my cancer center in Florida.

I have a vivid memory of her first visit. Beverly had a quiet but striking intensity. Within a few minutes of meeting her, I was convinced that she wanted to do everything possible to overcome her fears and conquer her disease. As I began to talk with her and her husband, Jeff, it also became clear that she brought this same intensity to all areas of her life.

Underlying her determination was the honest, very human fear that I'd heard in our first telephone conversation. Beverly's husband was also struggling with that fear. They were both successful people and were used to being in control of their lives. In fact, in most situations they were used to helping others. Now *they* were the ones who needed help, and everything seemed to be coming unhinged.

Our initial visit covered a wide range of topics, including the serious nature of her breast cancer. Beverly understood the risks of her situation and was determined to do everything she could to help herself. Although she certainly did not wish to abandon conventional medicine, she was also interested in pursuing any complementary and alternative modalities that might be of benefit to her. We discussed a variety of options, and she asked me what I would do in her situation. I answered her question honestly and gave her some extra advice to think about before she made any final decisions, as she and her husband went off for a brief vacation.

About a week later, Beverly called and told me that she and Jeff had decided to take my advice and go through conventional chemotherapy, followed by radiation. She had also decided that she would consider having further treatment with high-dose chemotherapy and stem cell transplant, but not until the first part of her treatment was done.

Beverly also said that she wanted to do everything else she could to help herself heal at all levels. Would it be possible for her and Jeff to move to Vero Beach so she could have her treatment at my center? She wanted to go through the entire Seven Levels of Healing program, and Jeff was very supportive of the idea. What did I think?

I told her I thought it was a terrific idea, and that I would be honored to have her as a patient.

Several days later, Beverly and Jeff arrived and were ready to get started. We reviewed all of the medical aspects of her case and discussed the details of her proposed chemotherapy treatments. The numerous logistical questions about all the aspects of her medical care were addressed and answered, and arrangements were made for her to receive her first chemotherapy treatment in two days.

After going through all of the technical issues, I asked Beverly and Jeff if they *both* wanted to participate in the entire Seven Levels of Healing program. Beverly was enthusiastic, but Jeff was less so, although he did offer his full support to Beverly's participation. He also agreed to take part to the extent that he felt comfortable and interested.

I have found it is best if patients and their spouses engage in this entire program together, with equal interest and focus. However, this is not always possible, nor is it absolutely required. Even if the patient alone participates, everyone benefits.

Toward the end of our first visit, I asked Beverly if she was ready to start the program. She said, "You bet!"

I then asked if she would be willing to take a few minutes to write out an answer to one of the questions in our "homework packet." This is part of the materials used by patients and family members as they go through the program. She again quickly agreed, and I took a sheet of paper from the packet and handed it to her. At the top of the page were spaces for her name, the date, and for her to indicate which version of the document this would be, since her responses might change over time. Below was a single statement: *The meaning and purpose of my life is* . . . followed by a number of blank lines in which to write her answer.

I watched as Beverly silently read, with Jeff looking over her shoulder. "Dr. Geffen," she said after a few moments, "I have no idea how to answer this. It would take me all day! I have never really thought about this before."

"That's completely understandable and okay," I replied. "Don't feel like you have to write a PhD thesis, or that you have to express yourself perfectly. We'll be revisiting this question periodically during the program, and your answer may change with time. But for now, all that matters is that we get started and see what comes up. Are you willing to do that?"

"All right," Beverly said, closing her eyes.

"Take a few deep breaths," I said, "and begin to look inside yourself, maybe deeper now than ever before. Exhale slowly, and relax. Begin to go into your heart, and ask yourself, 'What am I here to do?' 'What do I really want to accomplish while I am alive?' 'What is the real meaning and purpose of my life?' "

I watched Beverly's face as she began to ask herself these questions. I've had the privilege of facilitating this process with patients and family members many times, but seeing it happen is always captivating. People are often frustrated at first, as Beverly was. They're concerned about finding the "right" answer, when there's really no such thing as a "wrong" one.

After a few moments, I asked Beverly if she was ready to write an answer to the question. She opened her eyes and firmly nodded, and I saw that she was indeed ready. "The most important thing," I reminded her, "is to write freely and spontaneously, without editing too much or trying to make it absolutely perfect. Later we can go back and see if it makes sense to you."

Beverly picked up the pen and began writing. A few minutes later she handed me the page, on which were written the following three sentences:

> *My mission is to validate battered women by providing support and information to them in court and in crisis intervention teams established within our country. This mission is not limited to New Jersey, and it has no time constraints. As long as there is inequality between people, my mission is incomplete.*

Beverly watched anxiously as I read her mission statement.

"Thank you for sharing this with me, Beverly," I said. "Would you be willing to read it out loud, so Jeff can hear it, too?"

After a moment of hesitation, Beverly said, "Sure."

For many people, reading their mission statement is an act of unaccustomed and perhaps uncomfortable self-revelation. It is also very often a moment of great revelation for the spouse.

After Beverly finished reading her statement, I thanked her again for sharing it. Then I said, "This mission statement tells me so much about you. Would you like me to tell you what I learned?"

"Oh, yes," she replied. I then described for her the person I saw reflected in her mission statement. In just the first two sentences it was clear that Beverly was a person who was deeply concerned and moved by the problems experienced by abused women. She was a person who was motivated to action. She was someone who not only cared about the plight of others but who also wanted to *do* something about it. Furthermore, she was willing to think big. Her mission was not limited to her home state, and was, in her words, subject to "no time constraints." As with the treatment of her breast cancer, she was willing to do whatever it took to accomplish her goals.

I was somewhat concerned, however, by the third sentence of her mission statement: "As long as there is inequality between people, my mission is incomplete."

There was no question that Beverly was committed to alleviating injustice and inequality in the world, and she was also willing to commit herself over the long term to helping resolve these issues on earth. Unfortunately, her commitment was expressed in a way that seemed to eliminate any chance that it would ever be fulfilled. Although I consider myself a naturally optimistic person, it seems to me that there very likely will be *some* inequality between people on earth for a very long time to come. Based on what Beverly had written, there was no way she could ever achieve the sense of accomplishment and fulfillment that she so clearly desired, and deserved.

"Beverly," I said, "would you like some feedback from me about your mission statement?"

"Yes, absolutely," she replied. "Please tell me what you think."

I related some of the positive impressions I had gained from reading her statement. "Yet," I continued, "I am a bit concerned about your last sentence. Now, I do believe that the world is evolving, and I hope things will improve in the coming years. However, it seems to me that despite everyone's best efforts and intentions, there might be at least *some* inequality between people for a really long time. If so, isn't it possible that you could work your entire life and never fulfill your mission?"

"Yes," she said quietly, "but it doesn't matter, because I have to fight this battle no matter what. I have to keep trying."

"Beverly, I know that's true for you, and I completely understand. In fact, your determination about this is very inspiring, and I want to help you find the strength to accomplish all of your goals. But I'm just as committed to helping you find inner fulfillment as a human being, regardless of whether this external struggle is lost or won."

"What do you mean?" she asked.

"Well, what we do in life is extremely important to most of us and can be very fulfilling and rewarding. However, sometimes we make an effort for many years and our worldly goals are not achieved. Or sometimes they are achieved, and we still don't find the happiness and fulfillment we seek. I believe it is very important—particularly when you are dealing with a situation like cancer—that you commit yourself to finding and experiencing the deepest levels of love, joy, and fulfillment you really want, each and every day, independent of the things you want to do in the world. To a great extent, none of us can really control what happens outside ourselves, so we've got to find the happiness we seek *inside* ourselves—even as we continue to fight the battles that we have chosen to fight, and to work on changing the things that we believe are important to change. This is true with cancer, too. It is *especially* true with cancer. You can do everything right, even perfectly, and it may not turn out the way you want. So along the way, each and every day, it's important that you find and experience the love and joy you truly want."

"How do I do that, Dr. Geffen?" Beverly asked. "What else should I do now?"

"For now, Beverly, what you have done is absolutely beautiful, and certainly enough for today. You've taken a huge step forward, and I want to give you time to let this process unfold naturally. On your next visit, we'll talk some more. In the meantime, when you think about our meeting today, ask yourself how you might begin to experience a deeper sense of fulfillment, here and now, as you and Jeff go through this journey together."

Beverly and Jeff thanked me, and they left with a stack of information about her treatment. They also had a plan of action for exploring the deeper dimensions of healing her body, mind, heart, and spirit. This included getting a better understanding of her upcoming chemotherapy treatments and joining one of our support groups. It also included a plan to begin thinking of and nourishing her body as if it were a garden rather than a machine. She would be evaluating her food and exercise, joining a yoga class, and getting a massage at least once a week, particularly just before her chemotherapy treatments. Jeff agreed to schedule a massage for himself and to accompany Beverly to the support group. They agreed to spend some time together each day, alone—with no TV,

radio, newspaper, or any other distractions—just simply being together
and sharing what was going on for each of them. I asked Beverly to purchase a journal and spend at least ten minutes each day quietly writing
down whatever thoughts, feelings, and questions might come to her. She
would also be signing up for a meditation class the next day.

Over the next week, Beverly and Jeff were in the cancer center every
day, participating in various components of the Seven Levels of Healing
program. She received her first cycle of chemotherapy without any problems and had many conversations with our staff, other patients and their
family members, and our support group leader. During these discussions,
the question occasionally arose: "Why do you want to help other women?
Why do you want to do so much for others?"

Her answers always led to the same place. "Because it makes me
happy to do things for other people," she said. "It brings me joy. It also
helps me to grow and to understand myself better."

Beverly and I had a formal follow-up visit a week after our first meeting. After reviewing her medical status and her progress with the seven
levels of the program, we turned again to her personal mission statement.

"Well, Beverly," I said, "are you ready to go to the next level with your
mission statement?"

"Sure," she replied. "What do I have to do?"

"It's simple. We're just going to go through the same process as before. Only now you've gotten over some of your fears about cancer and
about chemotherapy. You also have some more experience in getting
quiet and going inside of yourself. As a result, you might be able to hear
what your heart is trying to say to you now in a different way than before.
Are you ready?"

"Yes."

"Okay," I began. "Once again, close your eyes and take a few deep
breaths. Let yourself begin to relax, and go inside. Go deep into your
heart, deep into yourself, and ask, *'What is the real meaning and purpose of
my life?'*"

As she closed her eyes and looked silently into her heart, I reminded
Beverly that the key was to allow whatever thoughts, feelings, and ideas
were inside of her to emerge without any stress or strain. She needed only

to listen intently to her own inner voice and express freely and sponta-neously whatever she heard. There was no need to get it "perfect."

A few minutes later she composed the following second draft of her mission statement:

> *It is my mission to heal and benefit from this healing experience spiritually, to learn and grow emotionally, and to mature with a new understanding of myself. It is with this new enlightened self that I will gain joy and peace in my heart by giving to others, in service to those who need support.*

In just one week, the change from the first mission statement was un-mistakable and dramatic. Beverly was now committed to growing and healing, emotionally and spiritually, regardless of her circumstances. She was also getting closer to actually seeing the distinction between her true *purpose* in life and her *mission* and *vision* of helping women who were suf-fering from abuse. She now had a mission statement that gave her, both consciously and unconsciously, a much greater chance of experiencing love, joy, and fulfillment on an ongoing basis, with much less dependence on outside circumstances. The language of her mission statement still re-vealed her longing to serve, support, and care for other human beings. This was not surprising since it was such a strong part of Beverly's character.

When I asked her about the changes in what she'd written, Beverly was bubbling over with excitement. She no longer felt she had to save the world in order to be happy and fulfilled. She didn't feel any less concern for the plight of abused women, but somehow a huge burden had been lifted from her shoulders. She was no longer willing to let events in the external world determine whether she was happy and fulfilled.

A week later, on her third follow-up visit, we went through the mis-sion statement process again. After closing her eyes and going deeply into her heart, Beverly wrote her third and final draft.

> *The purpose of my life is to experience abundant love, joy, and peace in my heart, and to experience physical, mental, emotional, and spiritual health and freedom, and to share this with others.*

Reading this, I sensed that Beverly had now really connected to her true purpose, which was to experience abundant love, joy, and peace in her heart, rather than trying to save the world. She also wanted to experience physical, mental, emotional, and spiritual health and freedom, and she knew she could move in this direction every day of her life. She was no longer asking for perfection, and her fulfillment as a person no longer had anything to do with the conditions of the world. She realized that love, joy, and freedom can exist even in the presence of imperfection and challenge. And in the midst of all of this, the same deep and compelling impulses to share and give to others were once again expressed.

"How do you feel about this mission statement?" I asked Beverly.

She looked at me with her eyes wide, glowing, and excited. "I feel great about it, Dr. Geffen," she said. "It's so simple and so clear. And I can live this and experience it every single day. It all lies within myself, within *me*. There is such a tremendous feeling of strength and freedom in realizing this. Thank you for helping me to see this, and to understand."

2. What are your most important goals for the next year?

The next phase of the process of self-discovery in Level Six has to do with clearly defining and prioritizing your most important goals. Few people ever take the time to write down their specific goals or establish meaningful time frames for achieving them, just as they rarely take the time to identify and understand their true life purpose. These issues can become very important on the journey through cancer, for a variety of reasons. In order to illustrate this, let's look at the following example.

Kate Seymour was a sixty-two-year-old woman from Michigan who was diagnosed with low-grade non-Hodgkin's lymphoma three years before I met her. At the time of her diagnosis she had fairly extensive Stage IV disease and underwent intensive treatment with chemotherapy. The treatment was quite difficult for her, but she got through it and achieved a complete remission of her disease, which lasted for two years. About a year later her lymphoma recurred, and she subsequently underwent evaluation and treatment at several different medical centers around the country. Each time she was treated her enlarged lymph nodes would shrink, but then they would start to grow again. This scenario is not uncommon with low-grade non-Hodgkin's lymphomas. Many patients can be successfully treated on and off like this for a number of years, especially now that a variety of new treatments have become available.

Kate's husband, Ron, was totally devoted to her. Like Kate, he was also devoted to their twenty-eight-year-old daughter, who had Down's syndrome and lived in a residential home in New York State. From the time of Kate's initial cancer diagnosis Ron had accompanied her on all her medical evaluations and treatments, and did everything he could to help care for her and manage the affairs of their family.

The past year had been especially difficult for both of them: for Kate because of all the treatments she had undergone, and for Ron because of all the work he had to do to get everything organized and stay on track. They were both extremely tired from the ordeal they had been through.

Kate and Ron came to see me because she strongly believed that there must be "more that I can do to help myself other than just keep taking chemotherapy." Like Beverly and so many other people with cancer, she didn't want to abandon conventional medicine. She just wanted to do *more*. The problem was that she didn't know what more to do, and she didn't know where to find clear, coherent, and reliable advice.

At our first meeting we went through an extensive standard medical evaluation for Kate. Over the previous month a number of lymph nodes in her abdomen had started to enlarge, and these were now causing her to experience abdominal pain and swelling. It was evident she needed additional treatment, and she was ready and willing to follow my recommendations.

But again, she wanted *more* than just chemotherapy. She wanted to explore the entire Seven Levels of Healing program, which she had heard about from friends.

After Kate's medical plan was established, I asked her and Ron, as I had done with Beverly and her husband, if they both wanted to participate in the program. I was happy when Ron agreed.

I then guided them through the mission statement process. After they were finished writing, I asked them if they would read their mission statements to each other, and they agreed.

Here is Kate's mission statement:

The meaning and purpose of my life is to have a loving, close-knit family that is cemented together with a strong faith in God, in whose footsteps I hope to follow. First and foremost is my strong relationship with Ron, and then my children and grandchildren, which give meaning and purpose to my life.

Ron's eyes filled with tears as he heard Kate read her mission statement. I have to say that this is an almost universal phenomenon. When people share their deepest thoughts and feelings about what is most important to them in life in this way—especially with those whom they love very much—an outpouring of love occurs *almost every single time,* and it is something extraordinary to behold. Facilitating this process for individuals and families is one of the things I most love about my work.

Here is Ron's mission statement:

The meaning and purpose of my life is to be a steadfast and consistent support and provider for my wife and family; to make a productive and positive contribution to the society and environment in which I live; to be a devoted and dependable follower of God's word; to try to live each day to the fullest and minimize regrets; to be self-reliant but not proud; to recognize and accept help when offered and needed; and to appreciate all that has been given me.

As one might have expected, when Kate heard Ron read his mission statement, she couldn't help but cry.

Kate and Ron were inspired by the mission statement process and wanted to keep going. So I handed them the next page in the homework packet. At the top were spaces for name, date, and which version of their answers the page would contain. Below this information was the statement: *My top twenty goals for the next year are . . .*

When they read this, they exclaimed, "Oh my goodness! What a concept!"

"Kate and Ron," I said, "I'm going to ask you to think about your top twenty goals for the next year, and in a few minutes I'll ask you to write them down. But first, there are a few ground rules that are important to understand that will help you get the most out of this process.

"First of all, when I ask you to begin writing down your goals, I want you to write down whatever comes into your mind, *without editing it*. This is really very important. Your mind may have a tendency to say things like, 'Oh, this is unreasonable,' or 'I can't do that,' or 'This is *impossible.*' If you notice that happening, try to ignore it, and write down whatever you were thinking anyway. The main thing at this point is to not edit or filter your goals in any way. Just write down whatever comes to your mind, no matter how crazy or ridiculous you may think it is. We can talk about your goals later, but for now, I just want you to get them out and written down on paper.

"The next thing is, I want you to *keep on writing* whatever comes to your mind until you get to the end of the page. If your mind goes blank and you don't know what to write, allow yourself to think of some things that you would really love to do or experience. Ask yourself, 'What would make me feel really good to do or experience in the next year?' And then just write it down—once again, whether or not you think it is reasonable, crazy, or even possible. Okay?"

They both nodded their agreement, but then Kate asked me, "Why do you want to know these things?"

"That's a great question," I replied, "and I'll answer it for you precisely. You and Ron want my input about how to best fight this lymphoma, feel better, and live as long as possible, right?"

"Yes, exactly," they both said, almost in unison.

"Well, in order to give you the best possible advice, I need to know what your goals are. To begin with, I'd like to know what your goals are for the next year. I want to know what you are fighting for, what you want to accomplish, and what you want to experience—*specifically*—in the next year. It's important to know these things because it might influence what kind of treatment we use for your lymphoma, or when we do it, or how we might want or need to schedule some breaks in your treatment. If I don't know what your goals are, then how can I help you fulfill them?"

"Wow," Ron replied. "That is amazing. No one ever asked us anything like this before."

"But Dr. Geffen," Kate asked, "are you suggesting that I will only live for another year?"

"Absolutely not," I replied. "I'm not suggesting that at all. I can't tell you how long you are going to live. In fact, no one can, really. We've just met each other, and I still don't know how well you are going to respond to your next treatments. You might live a very long time, or less than a very long time. No one can really know for sure right now. But I want to have an idea of what your priorities are for the next year, so we have a place to start, and plan, and have some real goals to work toward and look forward to.

"Now, I'm not saying that you will necessarily meet or fulfill every single one of your goals in the next year, but at least we can take a look and see what they are. If you are meeting some of your goals along the way—and especially if they are some of the most important ones—you are much more likely to feel better than if none of your most important goals is being met. Would you agree?"

After thinking about my question, they nodded.

"Also," I went on, "having a list of your specific goals, which we will be reviewing periodically throughout your treatment, will help keep you focused on what is most important for you to be doing. It will help keep you from getting sidetracked or distracted by things that are bound to come up along the way but which aren't really *that* important. Does this make sense?"

"Yes," they replied.

"Great. Because there is actually another great thing this list can give you."

"What's that?" they asked.

"Well, if you encounter any really rough times along the way, this list can be helpful in reminding you *why* you have chosen to keep fighting your disease. Sometimes, if things get tough, you can forget why you're doing this. It is very human, and natural, and common. But if that happens, each of you will be able to pull out your list and remember exactly what you are fighting for. Does that make sense to you?"

"Yes," they said. "Let's get started."

I then asked them to close their eyes for a few minutes and settle into their hearts. I asked them to take a few deep breaths and to start visualizing all the things they wanted to do in the coming year. I reminded them not to edit anything, just to see and feel all the things that inspired them, things that they would like to do and experience, no matter how mundane or even obvious those things might be. Then I asked them to open their eyes and start writing.

After several minutes of writing Kate and Ron looked up from their pages and indicated to me that they were done. I then asked each of them to read their list out loud.

Here is Kate's list of goals:

1. Become healthy, strong, and energetic
2. Not worry or be fearful—and to have a positive attitude
3. Take one day at a time
4. Find joy in every day
5. Have a family reunion in Colorado at a nice ranch
6. Take a trip to Antigua with Ron
7. Visit my children and grandchildren
8. Take time each day to read the Bible
9. Go on a fishing trip
10. Have a calmer relationship with my mother
11. Stop looking like a cancer patient
12. Find tranquility of spirit
13. Be more involved with Carol [her daughter] and Pathfinder Village [a residential home for people with Down's syndrome]
14. Play golf again
15. Be more at peace with life
16. Take more trips exploring the Northeast
17. Plan a reunion with Sally [her best friend from childhood]
18. Feel strong enough to hike
19. Take an interest in cooking and having friends for dinner
20. Have more courage in the face of adversity

After Kate finished reading her list, I asked Ron how he felt hearing Kate's goals for the year.

"It's a big list," he said. "It's very ambitious. I didn't know she wanted to do all those things."

"That makes sense. But how does it make you *feel* to hear all those things she wants to do?" I asked again.

"Well, it makes me feel excited, and happy. It's a lot to look forward to. But it also makes me a bit worried."

"Why?" I asked.

"Well, is she going to be strong enough to do all those things? Also, I don't know if *I* have the strength to do all those things, or to get them all organized."

These were important and legitimate things for Ron to wonder about, and I commended him for being so open and honest. I also wanted to address his concerns to put his mind at ease.

"Ron, we don't know if Kate will be strong enough to do everything on her list. We're going to look at the list in more detail a bit later, and she will decide what are the most important items for her to try and accomplish. So you don't necessarily have to worry about trying to get everything done.

"And you also don't have to feel responsible for fulfilling Kate's list. I know that you might naturally *feel* responsible, and I know that you will want to help her in any way that you can, but you are not actually responsible for that."

I then turned to Kate. "Is that true, Kate? Do you feel that Ron is responsible for fulfilling everything on your list in the next year?"

"Oh, no," she replied, turning to her husband. "Ron, I love it that you always want to help me. But I don't want you to feel like you always have to do *everything*. I can help, too. And if I'm too tired, well, I'll just change the list, or we can get some other help. Okay?"

Ron looked reassured.

"Great," I said. "Now, Ron, are you ready to read your list to Kate?"

He began reading. Here is Ron's list of goals:

1. Support my wife and see her through this period of hardship
2. Find time to learn how to paint better
3. Become closer to my children and grandkids
4. Find more time to fish
5. Develop more patience
6. Curtail feelings of anger
7. Develop a keener understanding of life
8. Better understand what is most important in life

9. Maintain a sense of humor

10. Give more of myself to others

11. Play more golf

12. Handle frustrations, disappointments, and stress better

13. Be less selfish and introverted

14. Try to be a compassionate and good person

15. Maintain good health

16. Cheerfully step forward and give when asked

17. Try to do some volunteer work

18.

19.

20.

When Ron finished, I asked Kate how she felt hearing Ron's goals for the next year. She was very moved, and said so. She also said she was happy that some of his goals were to take care of himself and do things that he wanted to do. "Ron has sacrificed so much for me," she said. "I want him to do more for himself, too."

I noticed that Ron hadn't completed the last three goals on his list, and I asked him why.

"Well," he said. "I didn't want to fill them all in for myself. I wanted to leave room to find out what Kate's goals were, so I could help her fulfill some of them."

I was amazed at how completely devoted this man was to his wife. His love and concern for her were so apparent, and Kate was moved to tears when she heard Ron say why he had left his last three goals blank.

I asked Kate and Ron to look at their lists and to renumber their goals with a red pen in order of priority. I then asked them both to rewrite their new lists on a clean goal sheet and read them out loud for each other once again.

One of the interesting things that came out of that process was a recognition by both Kate and Ron that the majority of their goals were very possibly attainable within the next year. Some of the goals were simple, others were more complex or challenging. But they realized that if they were committed, and if Kate's strength held up, there was a good chance they could accomplish most of them.

When I asked how they felt about having such a clear picture of what they wanted to accomplish, they both said they felt great. They had a new sense of clarity and focus, and a renewed sense of determination of what they wanted to aim for. It was beautiful to see. They agreed to spend more time talking in the coming days to refine the priorities of their goals, and to find how they could work together to make sure that they both felt that their goals were being pursued. For Ron, seeing Kate's goals written down gave him clarity on how he could really help her the most, which was so obviously his wish. Now he had an absolutely clear blueprint, written by her, of exactly what she wanted to accomplish in the next year, along with her commitment to communicating with him about how best to get there. For Kate, she now had a list of things that were important for Ron, written by him, which she could use to support him in taking care of himself as well.

Toward the end of our session, I had to ask Kate one last question. "I'm really curious about one thing," I said. "I noticed you said you wanted to take a trip to Antigua. Of all the places in the world, why do you want to go to Antigua?"

"Oh," Kate said, starting to blush. "Antigua is where Ron and I met, forty-one years ago. And that is where we went on our honeymoon. I have so many beautiful memories of being there. We haven't been there for so many years, and I thought, 'Wouldn't it be wonderful to go back again?'"

I looked at Ron, and he was smiling. No doubt he was recalling some of those same memories. "I haven't thought of that place for so long," he said. "But what a beautiful idea. If we can do it, let's go!"

Now I too was smiling. We talked about it some more, and agreed to make it a high priority for the coming year.

3. How do you want to be remembered?

A third part of the life-assessment process has to do with acknowledging the fact that at some time in the future we are all destined to die. This is true regardless of our circumstances in life. In the years I have spent working as an oncologist, I have found that it can be extremely powerful, inspiring, and revealing for cancer patients and their family members to take some time to think about how they want to be remembered after they are gone. Obviously this can be a sensitive subject for some people who are on the journey through cancer, because for them the reality of leaving may be closer than they might wish to acknowledge. Most cancer patients and their family members are also quite sensitive and attentive to any subtle nuances in their oncologists' words, tone of voice, facial expressions, and gestures. They often read much more into things that are said—or not said—in those interactions than is intended. As a result, I realize that asking a question such as *How do you want to be remembered?* in an inappropriate or insensitive way—and without a clearly established context—might give the impression that I think the patient might be dying soon.

However, when done properly and with sensitivity, helping patients and family members explore this question in a loving and supportive way can yield insights that are moving, profound, and important.

This was true for Kate and Ron, who returned for a follow-up visit a week after our initial meeting. Kate had started a new chemotherapy regimen several days earlier. Her first treatment had gone well and overall she felt quite stable. After I had carefully examined her, reviewed her lab results for the day, and addressed some additional questions about her treatment plan, they indicated to me that they were both eager to continue with the life-assessment process.

Kate and Ron shared with me that they had been spending time over the past week thinking about the meaning and purpose of their lives and talking more about their goals. This was bringing them closer in ways they had not anticipated, and they wanted to go further in understanding each other, and themselves.

We then reviewed their experience over the previous week and talked about some of the valuable insights they had gained from writing and sharing their personal mission statement and goals with each other.

"The next step of this process," I said, "is something I have also found to be very powerful and helpful for people. It raises a question that some of us may not want to look at, but it is a question that can lead to great insights into ourselves, and especially into the way we live our lives. Now, before we explore this, I want to ask you a different question. I'm curious about something, and maybe you can help me out.

"In the history of the world," I asked Kate and Ron, "since humans have been walking on Earth, how many people would you guess have lived, not counting the people who are alive right now?"

Kate and Ron gave me puzzled looks.

"Well," I said, "let's take a look. Right now, there are about six billion people alive on Earth. And we know that there are a *lot* more people alive today than ever before. True?"

"That seems right," they answered.

"Okay," I continued, "anthropologists estimate that since the beginning of human history there have been about ten billion people who have been alive on Earth, including everyone who is alive right now. Does that seem like a reasonable estimate?"

"I guess so," Kate and Ron said in unison.

"Okay. Now, of the ten billion people who ever lived, not counting the six billion who are alive today, how many does that leave?"

"About four billion people," Ron responded.

"That's right," I said. "And now, let me ask you another question. Of those four billion people who were alive before everyone who is alive now, what percentage of those people died?"

Kate and Ron then burst out laughing, and Kate said, "Well, one hundred percent, of course!"

"That's exactly right," I said. "And if one hundred percent of the people who were ever alive in history before now died, what percentage of the people who are alive today do you think are likely to die at some point in the future?"

Again they laughed, and said, *"One hundred percent."*

"I would agree," I said. "Now, I guess it's possible that somebody, somewhere, has figured out how to never die, but I haven't run into that person yet! So, since one hundred percent of everyone who is alive today is likely to die at some point in the future, what do you think the likelihood is that at some point in the future *you and I* are also going to die?"

"Well, it's pretty certain," Kate said. "In fact, we're all going to die someday."

"Exactly," I said. "At least, it certainly looks that way right now. Anyway, I have another question. Since it seems likely that all of us are going to die at some point in the future, did you ever stop to think for a moment about how you'd like to be remembered after you are gone?"

They said they had never really stopped to think about it.

"Well," I continued, "most people don't really think about it. And sometimes, it's a shame. Because if they did, they might live their lives a bit differently."

"What do you mean?" they asked.

"I've talked to many people about this over the years," I said, "and I've always found it fascinating to explore with them how they want to be remembered after they're gone. I've also been very privileged, as you know, to have been able to serve as a guide for many people who are battling cancer, sometimes very aggressive cancer. It has been especially rewarding to explore these ideas with individuals who really recognize that they will not live forever. In these cases—quite often, but certainly not always—when people think about how they want to be remembered, they realize that they had better start doing some things differently, right now, or they may not be remembered in the way they truly want. And quite often, seeing this so clearly actually spurs them to make the changes they had really wanted to make in their lives all along.

"Another important benefit of this exploration," I went on, "is that it allows people an opportunity to think about the values and standards of behavior that they hold important in life. Knowing how you want to be remembered after you are gone can serve as sort of an inner-directed 'code of conduct,' which can help guide your decisions and actions while you are alive. This can be very helpful for anyone, especially anyone involved in the journey through cancer.

"Would you like to see how this works?" I asked.

"Yes," they replied. "We're ready."

I handed Kate and Ron a new piece of paper from the homework packet. Like the mission statement form, and the top twenty goals form, this page also had space at the top for their names, the date, and version number. Below that was the statement *How and what I want to be remembered for in my life.*

Kate and Ron sat up straight in their chairs and prepared to begin the process.

"Okay," I said. "Let's begin by closing our eyes once again and taking a few deep breaths. I'd like you to begin to relax, as you've done before. I'd like you to start thinking about your life, and about the fact that—cancer or no cancer—someday you will be gone from this earth. When your time to go comes, and you have left, what are some of the things you would like people to say about you? How do you want to be remembered? What contributions do you want to have made? What kind of person do you want to have been? When your family, your children, your friends, and your colleagues think about you and speak about you after you're gone, what kind of person do you want them to say you were? Just go inside your heart right now and listen to what your inner voice is saying. And when you feel ready, open your eyes, and start writing down whatever you feel about how and what you want to be remembered for in your life."

After a moment Kate and Ron each opened their eyes and started writing. After several minutes they looked up at me again and indicated they were done.

"Great," I said. "Who would like to go first and read what they wrote?"

Ron volunteered. Here is what he read, as Kate and I listened.

How and what I want to be remembered for in my life

RON SEYMOUR WAS:

1. Someone who was trustworthy
2. A good husband
3. A good father
4. Somebody who could laugh at his own shortcomings
5. Someone who demonstrated compassion
6. Someone who was able to respect those who disagreed with him
7. Someone who could both work and play hard
8. A man who was true to his word
9. Someone who was a willing and generous giver of his time
10. A caring man

As Ron was reading, Kate's eyes filled with love and admiration. "What do you think about what Ron wrote?" I asked.

"Well," she replied, "it is so moving for me to hear it, because what he wrote is *how he really is.* It's amazing. He really *is* all those things."

"How does it make you feel to hear that, Ron?" I asked.

"It feels very good," he replied. "I try to be that kind of person, but sometimes it's hard to know if I am succeeding." Then he became very quiet, almost withdrawn, and said, "I try very hard, but actually I often don't feel that I really am succeeding."

"Kate," I asked, "do you think Ron is succeeding?"

"Oh, yes," she replied.

"Would you tell him directly?" I asked.

"Yes," she said, turning to Ron. "Ron, I want you to know how much I appreciate everything you do for me. And I want you to know how wonderful I think you are as a husband, as a father to our kids, and as a man."

Ron's eyes welled with tears. "Thank you," he said. "But you never told me that before."

This was followed by a long silence as Kate thought about and really heard what he had said. Then she said softly, "I'm so sorry, Ron. I didn't know you wanted me to tell you. You always seem so self-sufficient, and you never ask for anything. So I thought you just knew."

"No," Ron replied. "I didn't know for sure. Sometimes I just want to be told. It feels good to hear you say it. Thank you."

A rich silence followed this interaction. After some time Kate said she felt ready to read her list. Here it is:

How and what I want to be remembered for in my life

Kate Seymour was

1. Someone who cared deeply for family
2. A loving wife
3. A caring mother and friend
4. A faithful servant of God
5. Someone who was nonjudgmental
6. Someone who had courage in the face of adversity

7. Someone who was sensitive to others' needs
8. A good listener
9. Someone who had a good sense of humor

After Kate finished reading, she and I both turned to Ron for his reaction. He was quiet, and I could tell he was deeply moved. I asked Kate if she would read her list again, and she agreed.

Once again Ron remained quiet, as if it was hard for him to speak. He seemed a bit stunned. I looked at Kate's list and immediately noticed something that, intuitively, I felt was significant for Ron.

"Ron," I said gently, "are you aware that Kate said she wanted to be remembered first as someone who cared deeply for family, as a loving wife, and *then* as a caring mother and friend?"

"Yes," Ron replied quietly.

Something inside me felt inspired to look again at Kate's mission statement, which I had in hand. Immediately, my hunch was confirmed.

"Kate, would you be willing to read your mission statement out loud again?"

"You mean right now?" she asked.

"Yes," I replied.

"Sure," Kate said, and she again read aloud:

> *The meaning and purpose of my life is to have a loving, close-knit family that is cemented together with a strong faith in God, in whose footsteps I hope to follow. First and foremost is my strong relationship with Ron, and then my children and grandchildren, which give meaning and purpose to my life.*

After she finished reading, I said, "Kate, would you read the second sentence one more time?"

"Okay," she replied, then read: " 'First and foremost is my strong relationship with Ron, and then my children and grandchildren, which give meaning and purpose to my life.' "

"Thank you, Kate," I said. "I have one more favor to ask. Would you be willing to read just the first part of that sentence one more time?"

"Sure," she said. " 'First and foremost is my strong relationship with Ron.' "

I looked at Ron, whose eyes were again filled with tears.

"Ron, how does it make you feel to hear what Kate has said? That she wants to be remembered as someone who cared deeply for family and as a loving wife, and *then* as a caring mother and friend?"

"It is amazing," Ron said.

"Why?" I asked.

"Because I never knew," he replied. "We've been married for forty-one years, and I always thought I came second, after the kids."

"Kate," I said, "is that true? In your mind, and in your heart, does Ron come second?"

"Oh, no," she said, turning to Ron. "I just thought you always knew, just like I thought you knew how much I appreciated you."

The look on both of their faces at that moment is impossible to describe. Love, sadness, joy, revelation, forgiveness, and gratitude were all mixed together. Something very deep, significant, and profound had occurred in the minds and hearts of these two courageous people. In their forty-one years together, it was—on some level—only in the past few minutes that they'd really seen and understood how much they loved each other, and how important they were to each other.

They hugged and then looked into each other's eyes, which were filled with tears, tenderness, and love.

Very gently, I broke the silence. "Kate and Ron, I'd like to ask you one final question. What is it worth to you to know what you have discovered about each other and about your relationship today?"

They both looked at me and said, simultaneously, "It is worth everything."

LETTING GO WHEN THE TIME IS RIGHT

As we discussed earlier in this chapter, the journey through cancer sometimes brings people to very different conclusions about where they are in life, and how they might wish to proceed. Most truly wish to do all they can to keep living and to improve their situation. Some, however, come to a point in their journey where they realize that they do not have the will or the desire to fight their disease—for whatever reason. When this occurs, I believe it is an important duty for us all to honor whatever choice an individual might make and to love them unconditionally.

When a person decides not to undertake a battle with his or her illness, a different kind of opportunity arises that can be sacred and profound. It is an opportunity to ask, *If I am going to die, what can I do right now to feel complete with my life? What do I need to do, or say to those who have touched my life, so that I can die without any regrets or any fears? What do I need to do so that I can die with a full heart and a peaceful mind?*

Some people may need a great deal of assistance at such a critical time in their lives. Others might need help with only a few things. And still others may already feel complete, except for one issue that could touch any one of us. That issue is the simple fear of death itself.

The following story shows how this part of the journey through cancer unfolded for one patient.

Mrs. Golashevsky was a lovely seventy-three-year-old Polish woman I was asked to see one day in the hospital to evaluate her newly diagnosed colon cancer. Before entering her room I stopped to read her chart and learned some important things about her.

She lived alone in a small apartment and had not seen a doctor for many years. She and her husband had escaped from Poland after World War II to come to the United States. He had died two years earlier, and they had no children. After her husband's death she started visiting the local Polish American Club near her apartment, where she went regularly to eat. She had no other known relatives and only a few friends. One of those friends was a young Polish woman named Rachel Kosala, who worked as a social worker and had brought Mrs. Golashevsky to the hospital two days before.

Several months previously, Mrs. Golashevsky had started to feel tired and began to lose weight. She seemed more withdrawn than before and came to the club less often. A few friends noticed these changes and asked her if she was okay, but she would always say, "Yes, I'm fine. Thank you." More recently, she'd started to look quite pale. Again her friends asked if she was okay, and she said, "Thank you, really, I'm fine."

A week before I met her, she had stopped coming to the club alto-gether. This was highly unusual, and her friends became alarmed. They tried calling her at home, but got no answer. No one had ever been to her apartment before, and they didn't dare go uninvited. So they called Rachel and told her what was going on.

Rachel had taken the initiative to go to Mrs. Golashevsky's apart-ment. She found her lying in bed, weak and pale, barely able to move. The apartment was a mess, and it was clear that Mrs. Golashevsky had not been eating for days. Rachel called 911 and accompanied Mrs. Golashevsky to the hospital, where she was found to have a colon cancer that was nearly obstructing her bowel and was slowly oozing blood.

The next morning Mrs. Golashevsky underwent surgery to remove the tumor. Unfortunately, at the time of surgery her entire abdominal cavity was found to be full of cancer. Malignant cells had spread every-where, and virtually every organ surface was covered with thick tumor nodules.

Mrs. Golashevsky had tolerated her surgery remarkably well. She was awake, alert, and sitting up in bed, and she appeared to be recovering without difficulty. However, the serious problem of her very advanced cancer remained. This was the reason I had been called to see her.

I knocked softly on the door and heard a voice say, "Come in," before I entered the room. Upon entering, I saw a sweet and gentle-looking pe-tite lady with curly gray hair. She was sitting up in bed with several pil-lows behind her. A nasogastric tube emerged from her left nostril and was hooked up to a suction apparatus on the wall. She looked very tired and very sad. Sitting on a chair close to the bed was a younger woman, about thirty-five years old.

"Good morning, Mrs. Golashevsky," I said, smiling at her. "I'm Dr. Geffen. Dr. Cooper, your surgeon, asked me to come and see you today. I'm pleased to meet you."

I offered Mrs. Golashevsky my hand, and we shook hands gently. Her hand was very small and warm. She looked at the other woman, who said something to her in Polish.

Mrs. Golashevsky then looked at me, and said, "Thank you," with a thick Polish accent.

We looked across the bed at each other, and even though she was only a few feet away, it seemed as if we were separated by a thousand miles. I realized that she had lived through events that I could only try to imagine—and now she was undergoing yet another tremendous challenge. She seemed so tired and lonely. I tried to silently embrace and reassure her with my eyes and my thoughts: *It's okay, Mrs. Golashevsky. You don't have to be scared. I won't hurt you. I'm here to love and care for you, and to help in any way that I can.*

I turned to the other woman in the chair, and introduced myself again. "Hi, Dr. Geffen," she said. "My name is Rachel Kosala. I'm a friend of Mrs. Golashevsky's, from the Polish American Club. Thank you for coming. She's a bit nervous right now, but I'm sure you can understand."

"Of course," I replied.

At that point I wanted to sit down and talk with them some more. Glancing around the room, I noticed that there were no other chairs. So I asked Mrs. Golashevsky if I could sit down beside her on the bed. She was staring at me intently, sizing me up. I smiled at her and waited to see if I would pass the test. Luckily I did. She slowly nodded and motioned to where she wanted me to sit.

I carefully sat down at the appointed place.

"How are you feeling today?" I began.

Before answering me, Mrs. Golashevsky turned to Rachel and spoke to her in Polish, and Rachel responded. Listening to them, I felt as if I had been transported to another time and place. I enjoyed the sound of their language. It reminded me of when I was a child, hearing Russian, Polish, Yiddish, and Hebrew spoken in my grandparents' home.

Finally, Mrs. Golashevsky looked at me and replied to my question. "I feel okay," she said in her thick accent.

"Do you have any pain?" I asked.

"No, thank God," she said.

"Do you feel nauseated?" I asked.

"No."

"Are you comfortable in your room?"

"Yes."

"Have you had any vomiting?"

"No."

"Any other problems?"

"No."

After asking a few more questions like these I felt reassured that she was not having any acute problems that needed to be addressed right away. I also felt that she was beginning to develop some trust in me, so I decided to try to go to the next level in our discussion.

"Mrs. Golashevsky," I asked gently, "do you understand why you are here in the hospital?"

She paused for a long time before answering, "Yes."

"Why?" I asked.

She exchanged a few words with Rachel before answering, "Because I have cancer."

"That's correct," I replied. "And do you understand why I am here to see you today?"

Once again she and Rachel spoke in Polish before she answered.

"Yes. Because you are a cancer doctor."

There was another long pause. Then Mrs. Golashevsky spontaneously asked, "Can you help me, Doctor? I am so afraid."

"What are you afraid of?" I asked.

This time, she paused for a very, very long time.

"I am afraid that I am going to die."

I also paused, before asking, "What is it that makes you feel you are going to die?"

Mrs. Golashevsky again turned to Rachel, and they spoke together in Polish before she turned to me and said, "Because the cancer has spread throughout my abdomen. Dr. Cooper said it couldn't be cured with surgery. He said I needed to see you. When I asked him if you could cure me, he said he didn't know—but he didn't think so. So I am afraid I am going to die."

I took a deep breath and started to think about how to respond in the most sensitive and appropriate way. This was a tough situation. Colon cancer that has spread so extensively is generally incurable with any known means, particularly in someone as frail and weak as Mrs. Golashevsky. Fortunately, though, many patients can have the quality of their life improved with chemotherapy treatments that are relatively mild and easy to tolerate. Some may even have their lives extended as well.

I explained all of this to Mrs. Golashevsky and asked if she was interested in talking further about some chemotherapy treatments that might help her.

I was surprised when she said no. And then she began to sob uncontrollably.

I held her hand and tried to soothe her. After a minute or two she stopped crying, and I asked, "Why are you crying, Mrs. Golashevsky?"

"Because I am afraid to die."

"Then why don't you want treatment for your cancer? It might help you to live longer."

"I don't want any treatment for my cancer. I am all alone. My husband is gone, and I have no children. Why should I go through this? I have lived a good life and have been blessed in many ways. But I am ready to go now. There is nothing to keep me here any longer."

I was impressed by her clarity, and by her honesty with herself and me. This is not such a common thing to see.

"Okay, Mrs. Golashevsky," I said. "I understand how you feel, and I can accept it if you are sure that is what you want. But I don't understand, then, why you were crying so."

"Because I am afraid to die," she said again.

"Please tell me," I said, "why you are so afraid to die?"

Once again she started to cry. This time she gave a long answer to my question in Polish, right through her tears.

Rachel translated for me: "Even though Mrs. Golashevsky feels she has had many blessings in her life, she has also suffered a great deal. She lived through so many deaths, and so many horrible things, especially during the war. She has terrifying images of death in her mind. She is terrified that when she dies she will suffer again. And she has seen so much suffering. How could she not be terrified?"

I looked at Mrs. Golashevsky. She was trembling with fear.

"Please tell her," I said to Rachel, "that she is not going to die right now. And when her time to die does come, she won't have to suffer. Tell her I will make sure she is comfortable."

Rachel translated and Mrs. Golashevsky seemed to understand. She calmed down, and we resumed talking about her current situation. At first everything went well, but soon she started to cry uncontrollably again.

I soon realized that I had to do something significant to shift her focus and her emotional state. The depth of her fear and her negative associations of death and dying were overwhelming her and dragging her deeper and deeper into despair. She kept on crying and sobbing, and was not responding to anything that Rachel or I said to her. But I knew I had to do something, *now*. I silently asked for some kind of inner guidance: *How could I help her? What could I possibly say or do that would be of help? How could I ease her pain and relieve her overwhelming fear?*

Then, in a flash, I remembered a beautiful story that I had once heard, and I thought, *This is it. This will work.*

I took a deep breath and looked at Mrs. Golashevsky, still crying and shaking before me.

"Mrs. Golashevsky," I said, "may I please ask you a question?"

She didn't hear me, so I repeated myself again, louder this time.

Mrs. Golashevsky continued crying, saying, "No, no, no."

I looked at Rachel, and pleaded with my eyes for her help.

"Kashya!" she shouted. "Kashya, listen! Dr. Geffen wants to ask you a question!"

Mrs. Golashevsky stopped crying for a moment and looked at me, still shivering in fear.

"What?" she asked.

"Mrs. Golashevsky, please tell me something. It is very important. I need to know. When you were a very little girl, *did you go to school*?"

I watched the question enter Mrs. Golashevsky's consciousness, and I saw it start to work its magic. At first she looked confused, with an expression on her face that seemed to say, *Of course I went to school. Why in the world are you asking me that? What on earth does that have to do with anything that is happening right now?*

This is exactly what I had hoped would happen. She was no longer thinking of her horrible fears about death.

"Yes," she finally replied.

"Good," I answered. "Now I need to know something else. This is also very important. When you were a little girl, *did you like going to school*?"

I continued to watch her carefully as she thought about my question.

I could see from the expression on her face that she was beginning to call up new images in her mind, images of when she was a little girl, before the war.

Slowly, as the expression on her face continued to change, I could tell we were on the right track. After a moment or two, she started to smile tentatively.

"Great," I said. "Now, this is really important. I really need to know, so I will ask you again. When you were a little girl, *did you like going to school*?"

Now Mrs. Golashevsky broke into a smile and, nodding, said, "Oh, yes. Very much."

Rachel and I both breathed a big sigh of relief. It was clear that her focus had now changed significantly. The tension in the room lifted, and Mrs. Golashevsky stopped shaking and trembling altogether.

I decided to go further.

"Great. Now, Mrs. Golashevsky, I have another question. When you were a little girl, did you ever get a new pair of shoes?"

Once again Mrs. Golashevsky looked puzzled by my question. But then her eyes seemed to light up, and she nodded.

"Did you ever get a new pair of shoes that you *really loved a lot*?"

"Yes," she answered.

"Can you remember what they looked like?"

"Oh, yes," she said.

"How old were you then?" I asked.

After a few moments she said, "Ten years old."

Mrs. Golashevsky's eyes were now starting to actually sparkle. We could see she was *there,* reliving the memory of being ten years old and getting her new pair of shoes.

"What color were they?" I asked.

"They were black," she said, "and very shiny. My father bought them for me. They were my birthday present. He worked so hard to get them."

"Do you remember the first time you wore them?" I asked.

"Yes, I remember it very well. It was the first day of school."

"Great," I said. "Do you remember how it felt wearing them to school for the first time?"

"Oh, yes. I loved them, and felt so proud wearing them."

"Let me ask you another question. Were your shoes a bit tight and stiff the first time you wore them?"

"Yes."

"Did they hurt to walk around in when they were new?" I asked.

"Actually, yes," she replied.

"I can imagine that very well. Very often that is how shoes feel when they are new, when you wear them for the first time. Now, Mrs. Golashevsky, I want to ask you another question. On that first day when you wore your new shoes to school, did you wear them all day?"

She closed her eyes and remembered the day. "Yes," she said.

"And can you remember walking home in your new shoes?"

"Yes."

"And can you remember how your feet felt when you finally got home from school that day?"

"Yes."

"How did they feel?"

"They hurt. *A lot.* By the time I got home my feet were really hurting."

"Exactly," I said. "Now I want to ask you one last question, Mrs. Golashevsky. Do you remember when you finally got home and you took your shoes off? Do you remember that moment? Do you remember how it felt?"

She closed her eyes once again and went back in time to that moment as a ten-year-old girl, taking off her stiff and tight-fitting shoes. Then she started to smile and opened her eyes to look at me.

"Yes," she said, "I remember."

"How did it feel?" I asked.

"Ahhh," she said, "it felt so good. It felt *wonderful.*"

"That's right, Mrs. Golashevsky," I said. "I can imagine how good it felt. And guess what?" I asked.

"What?" she replied.

"Dying is just like that. Dying is like taking off a pair of tight-fitting shoes. It doesn't hurt at all. It is completely safe. And there is nothing to be afraid of."

Mrs. Golashevsky smiled back at me, and her eyes sparkled and filled with tears. She got it. She understood. She nodded and said in Polish, "I see. I see."

Soon we finished up our visit for the day. We had covered a lot of ground, and she needed to rest. I said good-bye and promised to return the next morning. We talked more each day while she remained in the hospital. During this time she continued to say no whenever I asked her if she wanted to consider receiving any further treatment. After about a week she left the hospital and returned to her apartment, feeling much stronger.

A few days later she came to my office to talk further about her situation. Rachel, who brought her in, had many new questions. Mrs. Golashevsky's abdomen was starting to fill up with fluid, and we talked about things that could be done to help relieve this. However, Mrs. Golashevsky was still not interested in treatment. She wasn't having any pain or discomfort and didn't want the fluid drained off. And she definitely didn't want chemotherapy.

What she really wanted was to see me every week and talk.

And so we did. Each week she would come in for a visit, and I would examine her carefully and review how she was feeling. During these visits we talked about everything, including her childhood, and so many of the things she had lived through. We would also occasionally talk about that beautiful pair of tight-fitting shoes that she loved so much, which had now developed a new and even deeper meaning for her. Little by little, even though her body was slowly dying, inside she seemed more alive. And little by little, each time we talked, her fear of death diminished.

After a while Mrs. Golashevsky decided that she would allow me to drain off the fluid in her abdomen, which had started to make her uncomfortable. This provided her great and instant relief. She was amazed at how dramatic the effects were. But she still refused to consider undergoing treatment with chemotherapy to try to extend her life.

The fluid soon reaccumulated in her abdomen, and she needed to have the procedure performed weekly. Initially, she didn't mind at all. It got her out of the house and kept her going.

During this time we openly discussed the fact that her cancer was inevitably going to take her life. I asked Mrs. Golashevsky if she wanted to be at home when her time came to die, or if she would prefer to be in the hospital. By now she was no longer terrified of dying and was quite clear about her wishes. "I want to be at home," she said without hesitation. "And I want Rachel to be there with me." I asked Rachel if she agreed, and she said, "Yes, of course." So Mrs. Golashevsky was enrolled into the hospice program, and all the appropriate arrangements were made so she could be at home, safely and comfortably, until the end.

A week later the swelling in her abdomen increased dramatically— much more than on previous occasions. She started to have severe pain and felt much weaker than before. Moving around now required great effort. Her interest in eating, or in doing anything at all, faded and disappeared. But she insisted that Rachel bring her to see me one last time.

She arrived in a wheelchair, a blanket wrapped around her legs, looking thin and frail. Her eyes were tired but also filled with determination to see me. While examining her I felt heartsick, because there was no question that her cancer had now reached a very advanced stage. When I explained this to her and Rachel, Mrs. Golashevsky softly asked, "Am I going to die now, Dr. Geffen?"

"Probably not today, Mrs. Golashevsky, but probably sometime soon," I replied. We reviewed everything one last time, and she confirmed her feeling that she had made the right choice for her. She also confirmed that she didn't want any more treatments of any kind, and that she was now truly ready to let go. She had insisted on coming in today only because she wanted to hear from me directly what she intuitively knew was happening. And she wanted to say good-bye, in person.

We hugged each other, then sat quietly together for a few minutes. We spoke again about her life, and how we had met in the hospital all those weeks before. We talked about all she had been through, including her impending death, which no longer terrified her. And we talked once more about her childhood and that pair of beautiful shoes she loved so much.

Finally, it was time to go. I promised her again that I would make sure she was comfortable all the way until the end, and that she would have no pain. We laughed, cried, hugged once more, and said good-bye one last time.

As she and Rachel left, my heart was sad, but also filled with love and appreciation for her. What a beautiful, courageous soul Mrs. Golashevsky was. I knew I was blessed to have met her.

Two weeks later I received a letter from Rachel.

> *Dear Dr. Geffen,*
>
> *Last Tuesday morning, at 2:30 A.M., Mrs. Golashevsky took off her shoes, as I held her hand. Thank you for everything.*
>
> *With love,*
>
> *Rachel*

10

LEVEL SEVEN:

THE NATURE OF SPIRIT

SILENCE IS THE ABSOLUTE POISE OR BALANCE
OF BODY, MIND AND SPIRIT. THE MAN WHO
PERCEIVES HIS SELFHOOD IS EVER CALM AND
UNSHAKEN BY THE STORMS OF EXISTENCE.
—OHIYESA (1858–1939)

I AM THE SELF THAT RESIDES IN
THE HEART OF ALL BEINGS.
—BHAGAVAD GITA

WHATEVER BE THE MEANS ADOPTED,
YOU MUST AT LAST RETURN TO THE SELF.
SO WHY NOT ABIDE IN THE SELF HERE AND NOW?
—BHAGAVAN SRI RAMANA MAHARSHI (1879–1950)

Who are you?

It's a deceptively simple question. Are you your body? Are you your mind? Are you the feelings in your heart? If you *have* a body, mind, and heart, can you also *be* those things? And if you are not those things, then what are you?

So far, we've given our attention to the physical, mental, and emotional aspects of ourselves. Now, in this seventh level, we will open our eyes to a whole new dimension of being—the dimension of spirit. This dimension is different in a number of important ways. It is also vitally important in the journey through cancer.

Most of us, out of necessity, live our lives on the surface of things. We're like the navigators of ships; our greatest concern is to get from the point of departure to our destination, often as quickly as possible. Needless to say, the waters can get choppy—and rarely more so than after a diagnosis of cancer.

At such a time, our primary concern is certainly the immediate clinical issues—the high winds and waves, if you will. But it is a mistake to focus on these issues exclusively. The journey through cancer is a time when it is vitally important to look beneath the surface, into the vast depths that are untouched by even the greatest and most turbulent waves.

This exploration is not simply a digression or distraction from the "real world." Although it can be, admittedly, difficult to find, the profound serenity that underlies our everyday experience is, in a sense, the *real* real world.

When your attention is directed toward the dimension of spirit, even for just a few minutes each day, your entire experience of life can be transformed. Just a glimpse of this reality can change everything. It is as if someone who had been born and raised in an enclosed room is one day shown a window on the world. All it takes is one glance, one breath of fresh air, one glimpse of the larger environment, and their understanding of reality is expanded exponentially. From that moment on, life will never be the same.

By discovering or reconnecting with the realm of spirit, many people with cancer have this very experience. Their illness has isolated them, both physically and emotionally, from the world at large. Cancer and its treatments can be so overwhelming that the possibility of another reality may seem inconceivable. But another reality does exist.

The window to this reality opens when you sit quietly, allow the mind to calm down, and begin to look within your own self. There you will find a world that can never be fully reached through thought, effort, or activity of any kind—a gentle, silent awareness and presence of love, joy, and peace that lies within the heart of every human being. This reality is always present. It is that aspect of ourselves that is timeless, dimensionless, and untouched by any circumstance—including illness, disease, cancer, and even death.

When patients and their family members are in touch with this aspect of themselves, their experience of the journey through cancer can change in extraordinary ways. The process is greatly enhanced when some time is taken each day to shift awareness away from the all-consuming drama of the physical body and the demands of daily life, as well as the emotional storms that accompany them. By entering the dimension of being that is untouched by events in the mental, emotional, and physical realms, the peaks and valleys of the journey are softened. A genuine sense of peace and serenity can appear—even in the midst of the fiercest storms—that is of tremendous benefit to everyone.

By nurturing an ongoing awareness of the deepest level of self, patients gain direct access to the most profound source of the love, joy, and peace we all seek. Though at times it may be difficult to grasp, the realm of spirit is actually the source of everything that cancer patients and their families really want. This includes not only love, joy, and peace, but physical healing as well. Although consciously allowing your awareness to abide in the realm of spirit on a regular basis is not a guarantee that physical healing will occur, I deeply believe that it improves the chances, perhaps significantly.

Incorporating a spiritual dimension into the practice of medicine brings joy and fulfillment not only to patients but to doctors, nurses, and all other members of the health care team as well. Something profoundly healing and uplifting occurs in acknowledging the aspect of our work that reaches beyond the physical realm. When we take the time to honor and care for the spiritual dimension of life that we all share—no matter what role we happen to be playing in the journey—everyone gains.

This is an extremely important point, because a new vision of medicine that embraces all the dimensions of who we are as human beings must include awareness of the consciousness and intentions of the caregivers. Such a vision of multidimensional medicine has barely begun to enter the awareness of the mainstream medical world. Nonetheless, it has been an honored and cherished reality for millennia in many of the world's ancient healing traditions. This vision speaks to a great truth that doctors, caregivers, and health practitioners of all types are well advised to remember: we can't give what we don't have. We cannot help people heal as deeply as we want, or as deeply as they want, unless *we ourselves* are healed. Understanding and embracing the nature of spirit is an essential step for everyone seeking a deep and long-lasting experience of wholeness and healing in their lives, whether for themselves or others.

ENTERING THE REALM OF SPIRIT

Finding our spiritual essence is an intimate process of self-discovery. Most often, it takes place through time spent in silence, in meditation and prayer, in nature, and in communion with family, friends, loved ones, and other patients.

Drugs and radiation may kill cancer cells, but they don't make a human being healthy or joyful. That power comes from the intangible realm of spirit. In addition—and my words are chosen carefully here—if so-called spontaneous recoveries or remissions do occur, they must ultimately come along this pathway. They will enter your body through your soul—yet, remarkably, even the soul is not the deepest truth of who you are.

From my perspective, the soul is the first ripple of individuality on a vast ocean of pure awareness that underlies everything in existence. That ripple eventually grows into a solid wave, until the physical body comes into being. If we wish to find the true origin of the physical body, we must go all the way to the ultimate source. Stopping at the wave is not going all the way home.

"You are not the wave," said Ramana Maharshi, one of India's greatest and most revered sages. "You are the ocean."

Indeed, as we will explore further, who we all truly are is the vast and timeless ocean of awareness out of which every being, and in fact all of creation, arises and eventually falls away. By recognizing your deeper identity as the ocean rather than the wave—regardless of how healthy, diseased, powerful, or powerless the wave may appear—you can find freedom not only from cancer but even from birth and death. This is the ultimate message of this book.

ASKING THE ULTIMATE QUESTIONS

In our daily lives, we view ourselves as separate beings, or as separate waves, existing independently from one another. Our common perception is that we are limited in time and space by our physical bodies, our personal histories, our worldly identities, and our unique memories, hopes, fears, and desires. In fact, we tend to identify *completely* with these aspects of ourselves.

For both classical Buddhism and the Vedic traditions of India, however, the experience of an independent self is an illusion. Clinging to the idea of an independent self is regarded as the fundamental cause of the suffering, illness, disease, and death that human beings experience over and over again. This attachment, and all the suffering that goes with it, arises from a basic misunderstanding about our true nature.

On a relative level, we do experience ourselves as solid, separate physical beings. But there is a deeper level of reality in which this separation is seen and experienced as a limiting misperception; indeed, an illusion. When the illusion of our separateness is dispelled, the interconnectedness of everything is clearly recognized and understood. The level of reality at which this interconnectedness exists is the "ocean of awareness" referred to earlier. Throughout history, this reality has been given many different names by the great spiritual traditions of the world. In Buddhism, it is called *Shunyata,* or "emptiness." In the Vedic tradition, it is called *Brahman,* or the Self. In the mystical tradition of Judaism, known as Kabbalah, it is called *Ein Sof,* the boundless, unending source of all creation. And some Christians refer to it as the *kingdom of heaven within,* or *Christ consciousness.* This transcendent reality does not exist at some point light-years away. It exists within each of us. At the ultimate level, it is the deepest truth of who we really are.

In Sanskrit, one of the most powerful expressions of this truth is *Aham Brahmasmi,* or "I am That." And That which I am—and which we *all* are—is absolutely still, immaculate, and pure. It is beyond conception, beyond birth and death, and beyond illness of any kind.

Thousands of years ago, the sages of ancient India saw and understood the unity, the oneness, underlying all of creation and recognized that we are not separate from that oneness in any way. Twenty-five

hundred years ago, Buddha also saw and understood the fundamental illusion of the separate self. Since then, mystics and saints from all the
world's religious and spiritual traditions have proclaimed this same truth.
Remarkably, in the twentieth century, Albert Einstein arrived at the
same conclusion, which he described this way:

> *A human being is part of the whole, called by us the universe, a part
> limited in time and space. He experiences himself, his thoughts, and
> feelings as something separated from the rest . . . a kind of optical
> delusion of his consciousness.*

In facing cancer, and in directly confronting the very real possibility of
death, patients and their family members have a pressing need and opportunity to examine this question of who we all really are. Few people
ever do this without the imperative of a serious illness. But cancer can
bring the question into sharp focus, often like nothing else. Finding the
most enlightened answer is the ultimate reward of the journey through
cancer, and the journey through life.

What is the ultimate cause of cancer?

Discussion of ultimate realities offers an opportunity to address this important and mysterious question. As with most fundamental questions,
the answer depends on the point of view of the questioner.

If you perceive your existence in terms of a physical body that is born
and dies, whose consciousness is wholly dependent upon brain activity
and function, your viewpoint is consistent with the current biomolecular
model of medicine. In that worldview, cancer is caused by genetic derangements occurring deep within a cell, most notably involving oncogenes or tumor-suppressor genes. These derangements in turn are caused
by physical events occurring in the external world, such as exposure to
various toxins, chemicals, radiation, or other harmful substances. They
can also be precipitated by hormonal or other biochemical changes within
the body or by inherited genetic predispositions. Or they can occur randomly, as cells divide repeatedly and multiply over time. On the relative

level of existence, these derangements are seen as the fundamental cause of cancer.

Another point of view might find the cause of cancer in God, or even the devil. Perhaps there is an omnipotent being who works in inscrutable ways to punish, reward, or test the faith and endurance of individuals. In this view, the cause of disease is often related to the concepts of right and wrong, good and evil, or virtue and sin.

An atheistic or existential philosophy might see cancer, and life itself, as a completely random event that is entirely without meaning. For individuals who hold this point of view, there is no more meaning in cancer than there is in the flip of a coin.

Finally, there is what I consider a more expanded view, in which the universe is recognized as an emanation of our own consciousness. In this view, nothing exists independently of our own perception, understanding, and ultimately, our intention as well. Despite the experience of our senses, despite appearances to the contrary, in truth we are not separate from anything in the universe at all. Who we ultimately are is indeed the ocean of pure awareness out of which everything arises and falls away again.

In this context, cancer is not an event that happens *to* us in a random or disordered way. Rather, cancer is seen a mysterious phenomenon arising in the body in which we are nonetheless involved, on some level, however remote or esoteric it may seem. In this view, toxins, chemicals, radiation, and oncogenes are understood not as the *cause* of cancer but as the *mechanisms* through which cancer is expressed in the body. As emphasized in "Level Five: The Nature of Mind" (page 151), this is not to suggest that an individual should ever, in any way, be accused of "causing" his or her cancer. Rather, this view offers an invitation to consider the intimate interconnectedness of all beings and all creation, and to acknowledge our ultimate inseparability from all that is occurring in our lives and our world, including our health and illness. Rather than adding guilt, blame, or shame to the mix, this perspective in fact does the opposite: it opens up new and inspiring vistas of possibility for greater wisdom, kindness, and compassion for ourselves and others on the healing journey. This is not a trivial matter since, sooner or later, each of us or a loved one will all face a personal health challenge of some kind—cancer or otherwise—and will need and want to experience wisdom, kindness, and compassion from those around us, particularly those involved in providing our medical care.

The ultimate serenity of spirit that patients and family members discover in Level Seven is intimately linked with this understanding and direct experience of our oneness with all of existence. An additional aspect of this involves the recognition that who we are at the deepest level is also never truly touched by the storms of existence.

When there is a storm at sea, at the very bottom of the ocean there is stillness. No matter how turbulent the waves appear on the surface, the bottom of the ocean remains still, silent, and untouched. In a similar way, we are not the images or events that appear and disappear in our lives. In fact, our awareness itself can be seen as the screen onto which the images and events of life are projected. Regardless of their content—whether they contain fires, earthquakes, hurricanes, or even nuclear explosions—the screen itself is always unaffected. Thus also with the "movie" of cancer. The drama feels and appears very real, but in every moment, at the deepest level of reality, the timeless, dimensionless, inner Self is untouched by it, and indeed, remains whole and complete.

In this discussion it is important to emphasize that I am in no way suggesting that we ignore the outer world of appearances in which we abide—the domain of *doing*—which includes the worlds of sensory experience, everyday life, and comprehensive cancer treatment. I firmly advocate doing everything possible to help people heal and transform physically, mentally, and emotionally. But in Level Seven of the Seven Levels of Healing, another possibility is revealed. That possibility is the invitation to acknowledge and embrace the other domain of existence—the domain of *being*—that exists simultaneously with the domain of doing. This domain of being is the doorway to ultimate freedom and to the ultimate healing journey. This doorway leads to the recognition of our true nature, the true Self, the truth of who we all are—beyond what can be seen and known, beyond name and form, and even beyond time and space. This truth of who we all are is not separate in any way from God, spirit, the cosmos, and all that exists.

How is this related to the cause of cancer? As long as you regard yourself as an individual being who is isolated and separate from others, and from creation itself, you will experience yourself as being subject to the laws of nature, physics, and biology.

You may also experience yourself as an independent soul on a journey through many lives. According to Eastern philosophy, the soul will reincarnate again and again, and will experience events in each life according to its own prior actions. There is no God "out there" who is rewarding you or punishing you. Rather, each of us experiences the results of our own thoughts, feelings, and actions, both positive and negative, which in Sanskrit is called *karma.*

This is not to say that getting cancer is a punishment for behavior in past lives. It just means that the seed of this experience has been planted in some way by ourselves—by our own thoughts, feelings, and actions—at some point in the past. Some of these thoughts, feelings, and actions arise quite mechanically, from social, cultural, and family-of-origin conditioning. Others are genetically programmed and arise from deep within our physiology. Still others, including some of the most potent and emotionally charged of these phenomena, arise from the myriad ways in which we often judge, neglect, or disown parts of ourselves, not to mention others. This process can occur consciously, although just as often, if not more often, it occurs unconsciously. Almost without exception, these judgments arise from a feeling of lack, which stems directly from the fundamental illusion of separateness that afflicts all human beings. These judgments then lead to powerful emotional and energetic dynamics, not to mention behaviors, which can and do impact our health. They also contribute to some of the important learning experiences we will have in life—including cancer.

Cancer, illness, and other life challenges can also be seen as lessons that we ourselves have, on some level, chosen to learn, or dimensions of human experience that we are seeking to understand. The individual soul wants to grow, to learn and expand, and ultimately to discover and experience the fullness of itself. The wave wants to experience itself as a wave, with all its ups and downs, before falling back into the ocean and remembering its deeper identity. Throughout my career, I have repeatedly watched in awe as the journey through cancer became, for so many, a profound catalyst for just this remembering.

As we've discussed, karma is unrelated to punishment or reward. It simply expresses the phenomenon of cause and effect. If one waters a plant, it will grow. If one doesn't, it will die—with no guilt or judgment involved. Similarly, over time, the presence of kindness, compassion, and love for oneself and others—or its absence—will ultimately be felt and manifested in the physical realm, including the body. As we've discussed, since we are not separate from all that exists, there are no events that occur "out there" or happen "to" us without our involvement; indeed without our participation on some level, no matter how remote or intangible that level may appear.

From this perspective, one could say that we participate in creating the events of our lives because, ultimately, we want to learn and grow—and sometimes we learn and grow the most from painful and difficult experiences. We don't create difficult experiences to punish ourselves, but to gain what we need to evolve and move forward on our journeys. Sometimes, the most difficult experiences of our lives prove to be the most evolutionary. If nothing else, they bring us face-to-face with our humanity, and the reality that we are ultimately not in control. If we are fortunate, they also lead us into domains of healing and discovery that can only be reached through the experience of humility, surrender, and trust.

It is impossible for ordinary people to really know *why* something happens to one person and not to another. Only truly enlightened people can comprehend why things happen as they do. Therefore, holding judgments, ideas, or opinions about events or life experiences that happen to us or to others leads nowhere. It can also divert precious time and energy from more important and fruitful concerns. Knowing *why* something happens is not the most important thing. *Why me?* is an especially disempowering question. The better questions are:

What can I do now to learn and grow, and make the most of this experience?

How can I use this experience to discover and fulfill the purpose of my life?

How can I use this journey through cancer to discover who I really am?

11

CONCLUSION

SOMEDAY, AFTER WE HAVE MASTERED THE
WINDS, THE WAVES, THE TIDE AND GRAVITY, WE
SHALL HARNESS FOR GOD THE ENERGIES OF
LOVE. AND THEN, FOR THE SECOND TIME IN THE
HISTORY OF THE WORLD, MAN WILL HAVE
DISCOVERED FIRE.
                              —TEILHARD DE CHARDIN

I remember one of the final conversations I had with my father, just a few short weeks after we took that taxi ride together through Central Park. This time we were in his hospital room, and he was approaching the end of his life.

We were sitting together, in silence. Drinking together, from the river of silence.

Without speaking, we were appreciating all that we had lived and shared in this life.

Without speaking, we were treasuring our last hours and moments together, and acknowledging how much we were going to miss each other.

And without speaking, we were saying our final good-byes.

Then, suddenly, I felt a deep and powerful presence of energy in the room. I looked up and saw my father beaming, grinning from ear to ear. He looked back at me, and his face was filled with a quiet, peaceful radiance. The room was very still, and I was aware of sunlight streaming in the window.

Quietly, I said, "Sid, what's going on?"

"Jeremy," he answered, "I'm so happy. I'm so happy. *I'm so happy.*"

His words startled me, because here was my father, a relatively young man—only sixty-one years old—lying in a hospital bed, dying. His lungs were filled with metastatic gastric cancer, and his belly was filled with gastric cancer and ascites. He was barely able to move without pain, barely able to breathe without oxygen. And yet, here he was, saying he was *so happy.*

"How can this be?" I asked. "Please tell me."

"I'm so happy," he replied, "because now I really understand. It's all so clear. We are not our positions, and we are not our possessions. *All we are is love. All that exists is love. And, all that matters is love.* And in seeing this, I'm so happy."

For me, the kind of awareness that my father had in that moment represents the true power and significance of the Seven Levels of Healing and the vision of multidimensional medicine that we have explored in this book. This is a vision that honors and cares for the body, mind, heart, and spirit of all beings with equal skill, strength, and integrity. It is a vision that honors all paths of healing, from every culture in the world, in a spirit of humility, open-mindedness, and respect. And it is a vision that recognizes the dimension of who we are as humans, beyond all appearances, that is the source of the love, joy, fulfillment, and peace that we all seek.

There is no question in my mind that as our understanding deepens of how all the dimensions of ourselves are interwoven, and how different approaches to medicine can likewise be interwoven into a tapestry of stunning beauty and power, we will discover ways of healing ourselves and one another we could never have imagined before.

And as we proceed further on this amazing journey that we are all taking, we will learn something else. As we continue our adventure through the ever-changing and extraordinary realms of medicine and healing—through the domain of doing into the domain of being, from action into stillness, from speech into silence—we will appreciate even more the great mystery of how the body, mind, heart, and spirit not only are interwoven but indeed are *one and the same.* Here, we will ultimately discover our true nature as human beings and the essence of who we really are. In doing so, I am certain, we will come to understand the true meaning of love, the power of love, and the meaning of life itself.

ACKNOWLEDGMENTS

The Journey Through Cancer has been as much a labor of love and the heart as it has been an effort of the mind and intellect. One of the greatest joys in completing both the initial and revised editions of the book is the opportunity to publicly thank all those individuals who have made such important contributions to my life over so many years.

Thus, I wish to say thank you, from my heart:

To my grandfather David Geffen, who demonstrated honor, wisdom, and integrity in all aspects of his life, and who inspired in me a deep love of learning and contributing to others.

To my father, Sidney Geffen, who showed me the example of a man who always followed his dreams, even in the face of incredible pressure, and who always saw the humor and irony of life.

To my uncle, Merwin Geffen, MD, for his love, guidance, and never-ending support and encouragement.

To my mother, Dita Geffen, who showed me that a mother's love truly never dies, and to my dear sisters, Talia Cohen, Danah Geffen, and Amara Geffen, who have loved and supported me through all the years.

To my agent, Kris Dahl, at ICM, for seeing and understanding the vision of *The Journey Through Cancer,* and for her support and encouragement.

To Ann Patty, for her support in getting the first edition of *The Journey Through Cancer* published.

To Mitch Sisskind, for his invaluable contributions in preparing the original manuscript of *The Journey Through Cancer,* for his friendship and encouragement, and for our heartfelt dialogues about this book and about many deep issues of life.

To Steve Ross, Jaci Updike, Heather Jackson, and Rich Romano, at Random

House, for their initiative and support in publishing and promoting the revised edition of *The Journey Through Cancer*.

To Aimee Snow, for her support and assistance in helping me research and update the revised edition.

To Michael Rudell, Esq., Jason Baruch, Esq., and Neil Rosini, Esq., for their wise, skillful guidance and support throughout the planning and development of *The Journey Through Cancer* and in the years since it was first published.

To Ann Peterson, for her support and encouragement, and for a joyful reunion after so many years.

To Dr. Paul Bass, a phenomenal coach, for his love, faith, confidence, and support, for teaching me so much, and for standing with me through tough times.

To the staff of the Geffen Cancer Center and Research Institute—including Al Boileau, MT, Mary Beth Tessier, Trish Garey, Connie Ozment, LPN, LMT, Brandy Sanders, Jessica Bentley, Doris Eldridge, Gladys Williams, June Goodrich, Shannon Richard, Pam Worthington, Vivian Poulsen, Shirley Ketchpaw, Hidi St. Peter, Sandra Woods, Jennifer Lang, LPN, Darlene Lieffort, CLNI, Richard Hocking, Russell Shoemaker, Charlotte Willis, PhD, LCSW, Phil Flynn, EdD, Donna Terrill, BSN, OCN, CRNI, Jeannine Smith, RN, Maureen Van Name, RN, Natalie Jones, PA, and Kim Klein, ARNP—for their hard work, sacrifice, courage, and faith in helping to fulfill the Center's vision, and for the meticulous and loving care that they consistently gave to all of our patients and their family members.

To Debra Dickerson, CLNI, who was with me at the birth of the Cancer Center and the Seven Levels of Healing program, for her unwavering love, support, hard work, and dedication.

To Rita Rosko, for her wonderful meals, laughter, and hugs, for caring for me with such love and devotion over the years, and for always being there.

To Tracey Fitzgerald, RN, for her unconditional love and friendship, for many treasured times together, and for her contributions to the Foundation and those it served.

To Karen Blackburn and Elaine Amy, for their loyalty, friendship, and support during a time of great transition.

To Julie and S. T. Forgione, Surja Jessup, Sonni Kane, Mary Ann Cooke, Melissa Tripson, and Jack and Sally Ruane, for their extraordinary, longstanding friendship.

To Tony and Sage Robbins, for their very special love, friendship, and inspiration.

To David Simon, MD, and Deepak Chopra, MD, for their friendship, confidence, and support.

To Harry Offut, CPA, Gertrude Terry, Sue Young, Robert Compton, Esq., Eddi Winter, Jana Barile, Jerry Swanson, Gage Gwyn, ARNP, and Lora Grabach, for their important and deeply appreciated contributions in the early years of the Cancer Center.

To Ash Andon and Herman Becker, for their love, faith, confidence, and humor.

To Ross Cotherman, CPA, John Moore, Esq., Charley Perry, Doug Sweeney, Marvin and Jean Messex, Nancy McLarty, George and Norma Gray, Amos and Louise Prescott, Kay Brown, Carol Webb, Bev and Bruce Gordon, Joan DeGregorio, PhD, Will Murphy, Esq., and Reverend Dr. Barbara King, for believing in me and the vision of the Geffen Cancer Center and Research Institute and Foundation, and for all their help and support.

To Bill and Penny George, for their friendship, support, and pioneering leadership in advancing the cause of integrative medicine.

To Tom McCarthy, Bruce and Carolann Fenton, Colleen Pyke, Diane Agnello, Michael Stillwater, Gary Malkin, Susan Osborn, Marcy Shimoff, Junior Allen, Chris Robedee, Mike and Tammy Rhodes, Kathy Zavada, Sara O'Donnell, Brandon Bays, Debra Angeletti, Carole Abrahams, Debra Frasier, Staton Grant, Sarah Kinel Lorraine and Lou Blankenmeier, Amy and Michael Pinneo, Michael Sautman, Allen Keller, MD, Larry Trivieri, Virginia Bell, Peter Amato, Sheila Moses, Penelope Young, Michael Spatuzzi, Paul Winter, Anna Triebel Thome, Lexie Brockway Potamkin, Hector Moré, Esq., Ben Newman, Esq., David Illig, PhD, Jennifer Jacobs, Jody and Wingaite Paine, Mirabai Starr Little, Suzanne Starr, Yashoda Hutner, Ananda Devi, Neeraja Tronca, and Gopal Verhague, for their love, support, and friendship.

To Philip Lee, MD, Frank Valone, MD, Michael Weiner, MD, Alan Venook, MD, Stephen Wasserman, MD, and Alvin Friedman-Kien, MD, for their mentoring and encouragement during my years in academic medicine.

To Jerry Pierone, MD, Nancy Cho, MD, George Duvall, MD, Bill Maples, MD, Mary O'Connor, MD, Debu Tripathy, MD, and Bhoomi Mehrotra, MD, for their friendship, and for the joy and privilege of working together.

To John Suen, MD, for his amazing support, friendship, and encouragement during some of the most extraordinary and challenging years of our lives.

To my other colleagues and friends at Indian River Memorial Hospital, for their friendship and support over the years we worked together.

To my dear friends and allies in Boulder, Colorado—including Shana Stanberry Parker, ScD, Doug Parker, John Steiner, Margo King, Ellin Todd, Judith and Robert Gass, David Friedman, Tom and Sylvia Hast, Adam Engle, Ginny Jordan, Chris Hibbard, PhD, Gunther Weil, PhD, Katharine and Makasha Roske, David and Lila Tressemer, Marc Barasch, Katherine Moritz, Lorell Frysh, David Luce, MD, David Scrimgeour, LAc, Ben Levi, Naomi Rusk, Sina Simantob, Jorian and Topher Wilkins, Rhonda Akin, RN, Sara Schaffer, Tarron Estes, Rosemarie Comacho, and Nan de Grove—for welcoming me so deeply into this wonderful community.

To Gemma Wilcox and Teresa Sparks, my wonderful assistants, for their invaluable help and support.

To Deb Flores, Pam and Chris Hendrickson, Travis Decker, Ulli Haslacher, Eric Weissman, Laura Crites, Uma and Tandu Sivanathan, and Karolyn Gazella, for their friendship, encouragement, and support.

To Rabbi Zalman Schachter-Shalomi and Rabbi Tirzah Firestone, for their love and inspiration.

To Peggy Wrenn, for her incredible, unwavering, and deeply appreciated love, support, friendship, and encouragement.

To Sandy Sela-Smith, PhD, for her years of indescribably kind, wise, loving, and skillful guidance, support, and confidence.

To the doctors, nurses, caregivers, and healers who work so hard and give so much, through long days and even longer nights, caring for the sick and weary, who have taught me so much and whose lives are an example for the world.

And finally . . .

To Neem Karoli Baba, for wrapping me in his blanket when I was so young, and for keeping me there always.

To Ma Jaya Sati Bhagavati, for guiding me, training me, and teaching me to always follow the deepest inner voice of my heart, for showing me the River . . . and teaching me to swim.

And to H. W. L. Poonja, known to so many as Papaji, for his supreme gifts of the Ocean, and of Silence. I bow in gratitude.

SOURCES AND SELECTED REFERENCES

PREFACE

Barnes PM, Powell-Grinner E, McFann K, and Nahin RL. Complementary and alternative medicine use among adults: United States 2002. Advance data from vital and health statistics; no. 343. Hyattsville, MD: National Center for Health Statistics. 2004.

Jemal A, Murray T, Ward E, et al. Cancer statistics, 2005. *CA: A Cancer Journal for Clinicians.* 2005;55(1):10–30.

Tindle HA, Davis RB, Phillips RS, and Eisenberg DM. Trends in use of complementary and alternative medicine by U.S. adults: 1997–2002. *Alternative Therapies in Health and Medicine.* 2005;2(1):42–49.

Wetzel MS, Kaptchuk TJ, Haramati A, and Eisenberg DM. Complementary and alternative medical therapies: implications for medical education. *Annals of Internal Medicine.* 2003;138(3):191–196.

CHAPTER 1: WHAT IS THE PURPOSE OF MEDICINE?

Clifford T. *Tibetan Buddhist Medicine and Psychiatry: The Diamond Healing.* York Beach, ME: Samuel Weiser. 1990.

Devrode G. On a practitioner's "being" as the true healing agent. *Advances in Mind-Body Medicine.* 1999;15:134–136.

Dossey L. Do religion and spirituality matter in health? A response to the recent article in *The Lancet* [special commentary]. *Alternative Therapies in Health and Medicine.* 1999;5(3):16–18.

Godman, David, ed. *Be As You Are: The Teachings of Sri Ramana Maharshi.* London: Arkana Books. 1991.

Kahn DL and Steeves RH. Spiritual well-being: a review of the research literature. *Quality of Life—A Nursing Challenge.* 1993;2(3):60–64.

Lintz KC, Penson RT, Chabner BA, and Lynch TJ. A staff dialogue on caring for an intensely spiritual patient: psychosocial issues faced by patients, their families, and caregivers. *The Oncologist.* 1998;3:439–445.

Passik SD, Dugan W, McDonald MV, et al. Oncologists' recognition of depression in their patients with cancer. *Journal of Clinical Oncology.* 1998;16(4): 1594–1600.

Sloan RP, Bagiella E, and Powell T. Religion, spirituality, and medicine. *The Lancet.* 1999;353(9153):664–667.

Voljc B. On the spirituality of the doctor-patient relationship. *Annals of the New York Academy of Science.* 1997;809:80–82.

CHAPTER 2: BEVERLY IS EVERY ONE OF US

American Cancer Society. *Cancer Facts and Figures 2006.* Atlanta: American Cancer Society. 2006.

Andersen LD, Remington P, Trentham-Dietz A, and Reeves M. Assessing a decade of progress in cancer control. *The Oncologist.* 2002;7:200–204.

Barnes PM, Powell-Grinner E, McFann K, and Nahin RL. Complementary and alternative medicine use among adults: United States 2002. Advance data from vital and health statistics; no. 343. Hyattsville, MD: National Center for Health Statistics. 2004.

Bernstein BJ and Grasso T. Prevalence of complementary and alternative medicine use in cancer patients. *Oncology.* 2001;15:1267–1272.

Brown ML, Riley GF, Schussler N, and Etzioni R. Estimating health care costs related to cancer treatment from SEER-Medicare data. *Medical Care.* 2002;40 (suppl 8):IV-104–IV-117.

Cassileth BR and Deng G. Complementary and alternative therapies for cancer. *The Oncologist.* 2004;9:80–89.

Cohen MH, Johnson JR, Chen YF, et al. FDA drug approval summary: erlotinib (Tarceva) tablets. *The Oncologist.* 2005;10(7):461–466.

Complementary and alternative medicines in cancer therapy. Publication BFHC0462. *Datamonitor.* Published June 30, 2002. http://www.datamonitor. com/all/reports/product_summary.asp?pid=BFHC0462. Accessed September 6, 2005.

Eisenberg DM, Kessler RC, Foster C, et al. Unconventional medicine in the United States: prevalence, costs, and patterns of use. *New England Journal of Medicine.* 1993;328(4):246–252.

Eisenberg DM, Davis RB, Ettner SL, et al. Trends in alternative medicine use in the United States, 1990–1997: results of a follow-up national survey. *Journal of the American Medical Association*. 1998;280(18):1569–1575.

Feuer EJ. Lifetime probability of cancer. *Journal of the National Cancer Institute*. 1997;89(4):279.

Hurwitz H, Fehrenbacher L, Novotny W, et al. Bevacizumab plus irinotecan, fluorouracil, and leucovorin for metastatic colorectal cancer. *New England Journal of Medicine*. 2004;350:2335–2342.

Jacobsen SJ, Katusic SK, Bergstralh MS, et al. Incidence of prostate cancer diagnosis in the eras before and after serum prostate-specific antigen testing. *Journal of the American Medical Association*. 1995;274(18):1445–1449.

Jemal A, Clegg LX, Ward E, et al. Annual report to the nation on the status of cancer, 1975–2001, with a special feature regarding survival. *Cancer*. 2004; 101(1):3–27.

Jemal A, Murray T, Ward E, et al. Cancer statistics, 2005. *CA: A Cancer Journal for Clinicians*. 2005;55(1):10–30.

Kantarjian H, Sawyers C, Hochhaus A, et al. Hematologic and cytogenetic responses to imatinib mesylate in chronic myelogenous leukemia. *New England Journal of Medicine*. 2002;346:645–652.

King SE and Schottenfeld D. The "epidemic" of breast cancer in the U.S.—determining the factors. *Oncology*. 1996;10(4):453–462.

Landis SH, Murray T, Bolden S, and Wingo PA. Cancer statistics, 1999. *CA: A Cancer Journal for Clinicians*. 1999;49(1):8-31.

Mell LK, Mehrotra AK, and Mundt AJ. Intensity-modulated radiation therapy use in the U.S., 2004. *Cancer*. 2005;104(6):1296–1303.

National Cancer Institute. The nation's investment in cancer research: A plan and budget proposal for fiscal year 2006. Bethesda, MD: U.S. National Cancer Institute, National Institutes of Health. 2005.

Nelson WG, De Marzo AM, and Isaacs WB. Prostate cancer. *New England Journal of Medicine*. 2003;349:366–381.

Parker SL, Tong T, Bolden S, and Wingo PA. Cancer statistics, 1996. *CA: A Cancer Journal for Clinicians*. 1996;46(1):5–27.

Pedrazzoli P, Tarenzi E, Tullio C, et al. High dose chemotherapy and hematopoietic progenitor cell transplantation for breast cancer. *Journal of Chemotherapy*. 2004;16 (suppl 4):108–111.

Pharmaceutical Research and Manufacturers of America. 2005 Survey: medicines in development for cancer. *PhRMA*. 2005;1–60.

Richardson MA, Sanders T, Palmer JL, et al. Complementary/alternative medicine use in a comprehensive cancer center and the implications for oncology. *Journal of Clinical Oncology*. 2000;18(13):2505–2514.

Schuette HL, Tucker TC, Brown ML, et al. The costs of cancer care in the United States: implications for action. *Oncology*. 1995;9(suppl 11):19–22.

Slamon DJ, Leyland-Jones B, Shak S, et al. Anti-HER2 monoclonal antibody plus chemotherapy for metastatic breast cancer. *New England Journal of Medicine*. 2001;344(11):783–791.

Stat Bite: Cancer incidence trends in U.S. women. *Journal of the National Cancer Institute*. 1996;88(24):806.

Stat Bite: Cancer incidence trends in U.S. men. *Journal of the National Cancer Institute*. 1997;89(1):14.

Tindle HA, Davis RB, Phillips RS, and Eisenberg DM. Trends in use of complementary and alternative medicine by U.S. adults: 1997–2002. *Alternative Therapies in Health and Medicine*. 2005;2(1):42–49.

VandeCreek L, Rogers E, and Lester J. Use of alternative therapies among breast cancer outpatients compared with the general population. *Alternative Therapies in Health and Medicine*. 1999;5(1):71–76.

CHAPTER 3: THE BASICS: STATE-OF-THE-ART MEDICAL CARE

Agrawal A, Gutteridge E, Gee JMW, et al. Overview of tyrosine kinase inhibitors in clinical breast cancer. *Endocrine-Related Cancer*. 2005;12(s):135–144.

Baselga J, Norton L, Albanell J, et al. Recombinant humanized anti-HER2 antibody (Herceptin) enhances the antitumor activity of paclitaxel and doxorubicin against HER2/*neu* overexpressing human breast cancer xenografts. *Cancer Research*. 1998;58(13):2825–2831.

Berger AM and Clark-Snow RA. Nausea and vomiting. In: DeVita VT, Hellman S, and Rosenberg SA, eds. *Cancer: Principles and Practice of Oncology*. 7th edition. Philadelphia: Lippincott Williams & Wilkins. 2004:2515–2522.

Bonadonna G, Valagussa P, Moliterni A, et al. Adjuvant cyclophosphamide, methotrexate, and fluorouracil in node-positive breast cancer: the results of 20 years of follow-up. *New England Journal of Medicine*. 1995;332(14): 901–906.

Bruera E and Kim HN. Cancer pain. *Journal of the American Medical Association*. 2003;290(18):2476–2479.

Calvo KR, Petricoin EF, and Liotta LA. Genomics and proteomics. In: DeVita VT, Hellman S, and Rosenberg SA, eds. *Cancer: Principles and Practice of Oncology*. 7th edition. Philadelphia: Lippincott Williams & Wilkins. 2004:51–72.

Carbone D and Meyerson M. Genomic and proteomic profiling of lung cancers: lung cancer classification in the age of targeted therapy. *Journal of Clinical Oncology*. 2005;23(14):3219–3226.

Chan KC, Lucas DA, Hise D, et al. Analysis of the human serum proteome. *Clinical Proteomics*. 2004;1(2):101–226.

Cohen MH, Johnson JR, Chen YF, et al. FDA drug approval summary: erlotinib (Tarceva) tablets. *The Oncologist*. 2005;10(7):461–466.

Coiffier B. Rituximab in diffuse large B-cell lymphoma. *Clinical Advances in Hematological Oncology*. 2004;2(3):156–157.

Collins FS, Patrinos A, Jordan E, et al. New goals for the U.S. Human Genome Project: 1998–2003. *Science*. 1998;282:682–689.

Cortes J and Kantarjian H. New targeted approaches in chronic myeloid leukemia. *Journal of Clinical Oncology*. 2005;23(26):6316–6324.

Cunningham D, Humblet Y, Siena S, et al. Cetuximab monotherapy and cetuximab plus irinotecan in irinotecan-refractory metastatic colorectal cancer. *New England Journal of Medicine*. 2004;351(4):337–345.

Davis TA, White CA, Grillo-López AJ, et al. Single-agent monoclonal antibody efficacy in bulky non-Hodgkin's lymphoma: results of a phase II trial of rituximab. *Journal of Clinical Oncology*. 1999;17(6):1851–1857.

Domon B and Broder S. Implications of new proteomics strategies for biology and medicine. *Journal of Proteome Research*. 2004;3(2):253–260.

Dranoff G. Cancer gene therapy: connecting basic research with clinical inquiry. *Journal of Clinical Oncology*. 1998;16(7):2548–2556.

Espinoza-Delgado I. Cancer vaccines. *The Oncologist*. 2002;7(suppl 3):20–23.

Faderl S, Kantarjian HM, and Talpaz M. Chronic myelogenous leukemia: update on biology and treatment. *Oncology*. 1999;13(2):169–184.

Fisher B, Dignam J, Wolmark N, et al. Tamoxifen and chemotherapy for lymph node–negative, estrogen receptor–positive breast cancer. *Journal of the National Cancer Institute*. 1997;89(22):1673–1682.

The Genome Sequencing Consortium. Initial sequencing and analysis of the human genome. *Nature*. 2001;409:860–921.

Hicklin DJ and Ellis LM. Role of vascular endothelial growth factor pathway in tumor growth and angiogenesis. *Journal of Clinical Oncology*. 2005;23(5): 1011–1027.

Jackman AL, Boyle FT, and Harrap KR. Tomudex (ZD1694): from concept to care, a programme in rational drug discovery. *Investigational New Drugs*. 1996;14(3):305–316.

Jaffee EM and Greten TF. Cancer vaccines. *Journal of Clinical Oncology*. 1999; 17(3):1047–1060.

Jemal A, Murray T, Ward E, et al. Cancer statistics, 2005. *CA: A Cancer Journal for Clinicians*. 2005;55(1):10–30.

Kirsch DG and Kaston MD. Tumor-suppressor p53: implications for tumor development and prognosis. *Journal of Clinical Oncology*. 1998;16(9):3158–3168.

Krause DS and Van Etten RA. Tyrosine kinases as targets for cancer therapy. *New England Journal of Medicine*. 2005;353(2):172–187.

Kressner U, Inganas M, Byding S, et al. Prognostic value of p53 genetic changes in colorectal cancer. *Journal of Clinical Oncology*. 1999;17(2):593–599.

Kyle RA and Rajkumar SV. Multiple myeloma. *New England Journal of Medicine*. 2004;351(18):1860–1873.

Lo HW, Day CP, and Hung MC. Cancer-specific gene therapy. *Advances in Genetics*. 2005;54:235–255.

Lum LG. T cell–based immunotherapy for cancer: a virtual reality? *CA: A Cancer Journal for Clinicians*. 1999;49(2):74–100.

Malawer MM, Helman LJ, and O'Sullivan B. Sarcomas of bone. In: DeVita VT, Hellman S, and Rosenberg SA, eds. *Cancer: Principles and Practice of Oncology*. 7th edition. Philadelphia: Lippincott Williams & Wilkins. 2004:1638–1660.

McCormick F. Cancer therapy based on p53. *The Cancer Journal*. 1999;5(3): 139–144.

McLaughlin P, Grillo-López AJ, Link BK, et al. Rituximab chimeric anti-CD20 monoclonal antibody therapy for relapsed indolent lymphoma: half of patients respond to a four-dose treatment program. *Journal of Clinical Oncology*. 1998;16(8):2825–2833.

Meyerhardt JA and Mayer RJ. Systemic therapy for colorectal cancer. *New England Journal of Medicine*. 2005;352(5):476–487.

Mughal TI. Current and future use of hematopoietic growth factors in cancer medicine. *Hematological Oncology*. 2004;22(3):121–134.

Myers EW, Sutton GG, Smith HO, et al. On the sequencing and assembly of the human genome. *Proceedings of the National Academy of Sciences*. 2002;99(7): 4145–4146.

National Human Genome Research Institute, National Institutes of Health. The Human Genome Project. http://www.genome.gov. Accessed September 14, 2005.

Ornstein DK and Petricoin EF. Proteomics to diagnose human tumors and provide prognostic information. *Oncology*. 2004;18(4):521–532.

Pegram MD, Lipton A, Hayes DF, et al. Phase II study of receptor-enhanced chemosensitivity using recombinant humanized anti-p185HER2/*neu* monoclonal antibody plus cisplatin in patients with HER2/*neu*-overexpressing metastatic breast cancer refractory to chemotherapy treatment. *Journal of Clinical Oncology*. 1998;16(8):2659–2671.

Pegram MD, Pietras R, and Bajamonde A. Targeted therapy: wave of the future. *Journal of Clinical Oncology*. 2005;23(8):1776–1781.

Peters KF and Hadley DW. The Human Genome Project. *Cancer Nursing*. 1997;20(1):62–71.

Piccart-Gebhart MJ, Procter M, Leyland-Jones B, et al. Trastuzumab after adjuvant chemotherapy in HER2-positive breast cancer. *New England Journal of Medicine*. 2005;353(16):1659–1672.

Pollack A. Drugs may turn cancer into manageable disease. *New York Times.* June 6, 2004.

Portenoy RK and Lesage P. Trends in cancer pain management. *Cancer Control.* 1999;6(2):136–145.

Ragaz J, Jackson SM, Le N, et al. Adjuvant radiotherapy and chemotherapy in node-positive premenopausal women with breast cancer. *New England Journal of Medicine.* 1997;337(14):956–962.

Reed JC. Dysregulation of apoptosis in cancer. *Journal of Clinical Oncology.* 1999;17(9):2941–2953.

Ribas A, Butterfield LH, and Economou JS. Genetic immunotherapy for cancer. *The Oncologist.* 2000;5:87–98.

Ribas A, Butterfield LH, Glaspy JA, and Economou JS. Current developments in cancer vaccines and cellular immunotherapy. *Journal of Clinical Oncology.* 2003;21(12):2415–2432.

Ries LAG, Eisner MP, Kosary CL, et al., eds. *SEER Cancer Statistics Review, 1975–2002,* National Cancer Institute. Bethesda, MD, http://seer.cancer.gov/csr/1975_2002/, based on November 2004 SEER data submission, posted to the SEER Web site 2005. Accessed September 10, 2005.

Romond EH, Perez EA, Bryant J, et al. Trastuzumab plus adjuvant chemotherapy for operable HER2-positive breast cancer. *New England Journal of Medicine.* 2005;353(16):1673–1684.

Rosen LS. VEGF-targeted therapy: therapeutic potential and recent advances. *The Oncologist.* 2005;10:382–391.

Rosenberg SA. Shedding light on immunotherapy for cancer. *New England Journal of Medicine.* 2004;350(14):1461–1463.

Scappaticci FA. Mechanisms and future directions for angiogenesis-based cancer therapies. *Journal of Clinical Oncology.* 2002;20(18):3906–3927.

Schiffer CA and Stone RM. Acute myeloid leukemia in adults. In: Holland JF, Frei E, Bast RC, et al., eds. *Cancer Medicine.* 6th edition. Baltimore: Williams & Wilkins. 2003:2095-2116.

Schrump DS, Altorki NK, Henschke CL, et al. Non-small cell lung cancer. In: DeVita VT, Hellman S, and Rosenberg SA, eds. *Cancer: Principles and Practice of Oncology.* 7th edition. Philadelphia: Lippincott Williams & Wilkins. 2004:753-809.

Springfield D and Rosen G. Bone tumors. In: Holland JF, Frei E, Bast RC, et al, eds. *Cancer Medicine.* 6th edition. Baltimore: Williams & Wilkins. 2003: 2015-2048.

Stat Bite: Persons living with major cancers in the United States, 1998. *Journal of the National Cancer Institute.* 1998;90(8):565.

Staudt LM. Molecular diagnosis of the hematologic cancers. *New England Journal of Medicine.* 2003;348(18):1777–1785.

Stuhler G and Walden P. *Cancer Immune Therapy: Current and Future Strate-gies.* Weinheim, Germany: Wiley-VCH. 2002.

Tan M. Granisetron: new insights into its use for the treatment of chemotherapy. *Expert Opinion Pharmacotherapy.* 2003;4(9):1563–1571.

Velders MP, Schreiber H, and Kast WM. Active immunization against cancer cells: impediments and advances. *Seminars in Oncology.* 1998;25(6):697–706.

Venter JC, Adams MD, Myers EW, et al. The human genome. *Science.* 2001;291:1304–1353.

Vorburger SA and Hunt KK. Adenoviral gene therapy. *Oncologist.* 2002;7:46–59.

Waterson RH, Lander ES, and Sulston JE. On the sequencing of the human genome. *Proceedings of the National Academy of Sciences.* 2002;99(6): 3712–3716.

Weston AD and Hood L. Systems biology, proteomics, and the future of health care: toward predictive, preventative, and personalized medicine. *Journal of Proteome Research.* 2004;3(2):179–196.

CHAPTER 4: LEVEL ONE: EDUCATION AND INFORMATION

A Century of Oncology: A Photographic History of Cancer Research and Therapy. With commentary by J. Lynne Dodson. Greenwich, CT: Greenwich Press. 1997.

American College of Physicians. Screening for prostate cancer. *Annals of Internal Medicine.* 1997;126(6):480–484.

Armstrong, D. K., Bundy B., Wenzel L, et al. Intraperitoneal cisplatin and pacli-taxel in ovarian cancer. *New England Journal of Medicine.* 2006;354(1):34–43.

Arpino G, Weiss H, Lee AV, et al. Estrogen receptor–positive, progesterone receptor–negative breast cancer: association with growth factor receptor expression and tamoxifen resistance. *Journal of the National Cancer Institute.* 2005;97:1254–1261.

Awada A and Klastersky J. Ovarian cancer: state of the art and future directions. *European Journal of Gynaecologic Oncology.* 2004;25(6):673–676.

Baker L, Wagner TH, Singer S, and Bundorf KM. Use of the internet and e-mail for health care information: results from a national survey. *New England Journal of Medicine.* 2003;289(18):2400–2406.

Bhatnagar V and Kaplan RM. Treatment options for prostate cancer: evaluating the evidence. *American Family Physician.* 2005;71(10):1915–1922.

Berry DA, Cronin KA, Plevritis SK, et al. Effect of screening and adjuvant ther-apy on mortality from breast cancer. *New England Journal of Medicine.* 2005;353(17):1784–1792.

Bick RL, guest ed. Paraneoplastic syndromes. *Hematology/Oncology Clinics of North America.* 1996;10(4).

Biermann JS, Golladay GJ, Greenfield ML, and Baker LH. Evaluation of cancer information on the Internet. *Cancer*. 1999;86(3):381–390.

Blum RH. Adjuvant chemotherapy for lung cancer—a new standard of care. *New England Journal of Medicine*. 2004;350(4):404–405.

Bonadonna G, Valagussa P, Moliterni A, et al. Adjuvant cyclophosphamide, methotrexate, and fluorouracil in node-positive breast cancer: the results of 20 years of follow-up. *New England Journal of Medicine*. 1995;332(14):901–906.

Boon T and Van Baren N. Immunosurveillance against cancer and immunotherapy—synergy or antagonism? *New England Journal of Medicine*. 2003;348(3): 252–254.

Brenner C and Duggan D. *Oncogenomics: Molecular Approaches to Cancer*. Hoboken, NJ: Wiley-Liss. 2004.

Burnet FM. Immunological surveillance in neoplasia. *Transplantation Review*. 1971;7:3–25.

Buzdar AU. The ATAC (Arimidex, Tamoxifen, alone or in combination) trial: an update. *Clinical Breast Cancer*. 2004;5 (suppl 1):S6–S12.

Cannistra SA. Cancer of the ovary. *New England Journal of Medicine*. 2004;351(24):2519–2529.

Catalona WJ, Partin AW, Slawin KM, et al. Use of the percentage of free prostate-specific antigen to enhance differentiation of prostate cancer from benign prostatic disease. *Journal of the American Medical Association*. 1998; 279(19):1542–1547.

Closing in on Cancer: Solving a 5000-Year-Old Mystery. A publication of The National Cancer Institute. U.S. Department of Health and Human Services. NIH Publication no. 98-2955. 1998.

Cody HS. Sentinel lymph node mapping in breast cancer. *Oncology*. 1999;13(1): 25–34.

Coiffier B., Lepage E., Brière J, et al. CHOP chemotherapy plus rituximab compared with CHOP alone in elderly patients with diffuse large-B-cell lymphoma. *New England Journal of Medicine*. 2002;346(4):235–242.

Colditz GA. Estrogen, estrogen plus progestin therapy, and risk of breast cancer. *Clinical Cancer Research*. 2005;11(2 Pt 2):909s–917s.

Colditz GA. Epidemiology and prevention of breast cancer. *Cancer Epidemiology, Biomarkers, and Prevention*. 2005;14(4):768–772.

Connors J. Radioimmunotherapy—hot new treatment for lymphoma. *New England Journal of Medicine*. 2005;352(5):496–499.

Daly PA. Genetic counselling in breast and colorectal cancer. *Annals of Oncology*. 2005;16 (suppl 2):ii163–169.

David YB, Chetrit A, Hirsh-Yechezkel G, et al. Effect of BRCA mutations on the length of survival in epithelial ovarian tumors. *Journal of Clinical Oncology*. 2002;20(2);463–466.

Davies AJ, Rohatiner AZ, Howell S, et al. Tositumomab and iodine I-131 tositumomab for recurrent indolent and transformed B-cell non-Hodgkin's lymphoma. *Journal of Clinical Oncology.* 2004;22:1469–1479.

DeVita VT, Hellman S, and Rosenberg SA, eds. *Cancer: Principles and Practice of Oncology.* 7th edition. Philadelphia: Lippincott Williams & Wilkins. 2004.

Dillman RO. Radiolabeled anti-CD20 monoclonal antibodies for the treatment of B-cell lymphoma. *Journal of Clinical Oncology.* 2002;20(16):3545–3557.

Dunn GP, Bruce AT, Ikeda H, et al. Cancer immunoediting: from immunosurveillance to tumor escape. *Nature Immunology.* 2002;3(11):991–998.

Dunn GP and Old LJ. The immunobiology of cancer immunosurveillance and immunoediting. *Immunity.* 2004;21:137–148.

Eifel PJ, Berek JS, and Markman MA. Gynecologic cancers. In: DeVita VT, Hellman S, and Rosenberg SA, eds. *Cancer: Principles and Practice of Oncology.* 7th edition. Philadelphia: Lippincott Williams & Wilkins. 2004:1295–1398.

Elmore JG, Armstrong K, Lehman CD, and Fletcher SW. Screening for breast cancer. *Journal of the American Medical Association.* 2005;293(10):1245–1256.

Finek J, Holubec L, Topolcan O, et al. Clinical relevance of tumor markers for the control of chemotherapy. *Anticancer Research.* 2005;25(3A):1655–1658.

Fisher B, Bauer M, Margolese R, et al. Five-year results of a randomized clinical trial comparing total mastectomy and segmental mastectomy with or without radiation in the treatment of breast cancer. *New England Journal of Medicine.* 1985;312:665–673.

Fisher B, Dignam J, Wolmark N, et al. Tamoxifen and chemotherapy for lymph node–negative, estrogen receptor–positive breast cancer. *Journal of the National Cancer Institute.* 1997;89(22):1673–1682.

Fox S. Health information online. *Pew Internet and American Life Project Online Report.* May 17, 2005. www.pewinternet.org/PPF/r/156/report_display.asp. Accessed October 24, 2005.

Garcia-Martinez C, Costelli P, Lopez-Soriano FJ, and Argiles JM. Is TNF really involved in cachexia? *Cancer Investigation.* 1997;15(1):47–54.

Glode LM. Challenges and opportunities of the Internet for medical oncology. *Journal of Clinical Oncology.* 1996;14(7):2181–2186.

Gradishar WJ, Tjulandin S, Davidson N, et al. Phase III trial of nanoparticle albumin-bound paclitaxel compared with polyethylated castor oil–based paclitaxel in women with breast cancer. *Journal of Clinical Oncology.* 2005;23(31):7794–7803.

Grove A. Taking on prostate cancer. *Fortune.* May 13, 1996.

Grube BJ and Giuliano AE. The current role of sentinel node biopsy in the treatment of breast cancer. *Advances in Surgery.* 2004;38:121–166.

Hamilton AB. Psychological aspects of ovarian cancer. *Cancer Investigation.* 1999;17(5):335–341.

Harris KA. The informational needs of patients with cancer and their families. *Cancer Practice*. 1998;6(1):39–46.

Harris NL, Jaffe ES, Diebold J, et al. World Health Organization classification of neoplastic diseases of the hematopoietic and lymphoid tissues: report of the clinical advisory committee meeting—Airlie House, Virginia, November 1997. *Journal of Clinical Oncology*. 1999;17(12):3835–3849.

Holland JF, Frei E, Bast RC, et al., eds. *Cancer Medicine*. 6th edition. Baltimore: Williams and Wilkins. 2003.

Hudis CA and Dang CT. Adjuvant therapy for breast cancer: practical lessons from the early breast cancer trialists' collaborative group. *Breast Disease*. 2004;21:3–13.

Inui A. Cancer anorexia-cachexia syndrome: current issues in research and management. *CA: A Cancer Journal for Clinicians*. 2002;52(2):72–91.

Jemal A, Murray T, Ward E, et al. Cancer statistics, 2005. *CA: A Cancer Journal for Clinicians*. 2005;55(1):10–30.

Kaklamani VG and Gradishar WJ. Adjuvant therapy of breast cancer. *Cancer Investigation*. 2005;23(6):548–560.

Kalidas M and Brown P. Aromatase inhibitors for the treatment and prevention of breast cancer. *Clinical Breast Cancer*. 2005;6(1):27–37.

Kaminski MS, Tuck M, Estes J, et al. 131 I–tositumomab therapy as initial treatment for follicular lymphoma. *New England Journal of Medicine*. 2005;352(5):441–449.

Kempin SJ. Hemostatic defects in cancer patients. *Cancer Investigation*. 1997;15(1):23–36.

Kolonel LN, Nomura AM, and Cooney RV. Dietary fat and prostate cancer: current status. *Journal of the National Cancer Institute*. 1999;91(5):414–428.

Landis SH, Murray T, Bolden S, and Wingo PA. Cancer statistics, 1999. *CA: A Cancer Journal for Clinicians*. 1999;49(1):8–31.

Lichtenstein P, Holm NV, Verkasalo PK, et al. Environmental and heritable factors in the causation of cancer—analyses of cohorts of twins from Sweden, Denmark, and Finland. *New England Journal of Medicine*. 2000;343:78–85.

Lyman GH, Giuliano AE, Somerfield MR, et al. American Society of Clinical Oncology guideline recommendations for sentinel lymph node biopsy in early-stage breast cancer. *Journal of Clinical Oncology*. 2005;23(30):7703–7720.

Maloney DG. Immunotherapy for non-Hodgkin's lymphoma: monoclonal antibodies and vaccines. *Journal of Clinical Oncology*. 2005;23(26):6421–6428.

McGuire WP, Hoskins WJ, Brady MF, et al. Cyclophosphamide and cisplatin compared with paclitaxel and cisplatin in patients with stage III and stage IV ovarian cancer. *New England Journal of Medicine*. 1996;334(1):1–6.

Melnick AM, Adelson K, and Licht JD. The theoretical basis of transcriptional therapy of cancer: can it be put into practice? *Journal of Clinical Oncology.* 2005;23(17):3957–3970.

Meyerhardt JA and Mayer RJ. Systemic therapy for colorectal cancer. *New England Journal of Medicine.* 2005;352(5):476–487.

Mouridsen HT and Robert NJ. The role of aromatase inhibitors as adjuvant therapy for early breast cancer in postmenopausal women. *European Journal of Cancer.* 2005;41(12):1678–1689.

Mulshine JL. New developments in lung cancer screening. *Journal of Clinical Oncology.* 2005;23(14):3198–3202.

Narod SA and Offit K. Prevention and management of hereditary breast cancer. *Journal of Clinical Oncology.* 2005;23(8):1656–1663.

Pass HI, Carbone DP, Johnson DH, Minna JD, and Turrisi AT, eds. *Lung Cancer: Principles and Practice.* 3rd Edition. Philadelphia: Lippincott Williams & Wilkins. 2004.

Pergament D, Pergament E, Wonderlick A, and Fiddler M. At the crossroads: the intersection of the Internet and clinical oncology. *Oncology.* 1999;13(4): 577–583.

Pisano ED, Gatsonis C, Hendrick E, et al. Diagnostic performance of digital versus film mammography for breast-cancer screening. *New England Journal of Medicine.* 2005;353(17):1773–1783.

Ries LAG, Eisner MP, Kosary CL, et al. *SEER cancer statistics review, 1975–2002,* National Cancer Institute, Bethesda, MD, http://seer.cancer.gov/csr/1975_2002/, based on November 2004 SEER data submission, posted to the SEER web site 2005. Accessed September 10, 2005.

Rosenthal A and Jacobs I. Ovarian cancer screening. *Seminars in Oncology.* 1998;25(3):315–325.

Skalla KA, Bakitas M, Furstenberg CT, et al. Patients' need for information about cancer therapy. *Oncology Nursing Forum.* 2004;31(2):313–319.

Smith-Warner SA, Spiegelman D, Yuan SS, et al. Alcohol and breast cancer in women: a pooled analysis of cohort studies. *Journal of the American Medical Association.* 1998;279(7):535–540.

Sobue T, Moriyama N, Kaneko M, et al. Screening for lung cancer with low-dose helical computed tomography: anti–lung cancer association project. *Journal of Clinical Oncology.* 2002;20(4):911–920.

Veronesi U, Boyle P, Goldhirsch A, et al. Breast cancer. *The Lancet.* 2005;365(9472): 1727–1741.

Wolk A. Diet, lifestyle and risk of prostate cancer. *Acta Oncologica.* 2005;44(3): 277–281.

Whiteman T and Hassouna HI. Hypercoagulable states. *Hematology Oncology Clinics of North America.* 2000;14(2):355–377.

Winer EP, Hudis C, and Burstein HJ. American society of clinical oncology technology assessment on the use of aromatase inhibitors as adjuvant therapy for postmenopausal women with hormone receptor–positive breast cancer: status report 2004. *Journal of Clinical Oncology*. 2005;23(3):619–629.

Winawer SJ. A quarter century of colorectal cancer screening: progress and prospects. *Journal of Clinical Oncology*. 2001;19(18s):6s–12s.

Witzig TE, White CA, Gordon LI, et al. Safety of yttrium-90 ibritumomab tiuxetan radioimmunotherapy for relapsed low-grade, follicular, or transformed non-Hodgkin's lymphoma. *Journal of Clinical Oncology*. 2003;21(7):1263–1270.

Wu AH, Pike MC, and Stram DO. Meta-analysis: dietary fat intake, serum estrogen levels, and the risk of breast cancer. *Journal of the National Cancer Institute*. 1999;91(6):529–534.

Yip I, Heber D, and Aronson W. Nutrition and prostate cancer. *Urologic Clinics of North America*. 1999;26(2):403–411.

Zhang S, Hunter DJ, Forman MR, et al. Dietary carotenoids and vitamins A, C, and E and risk of breast cancer. *Journal of the National Cancer Institute*. 1999;91(6):547–556.

Chapter 5: LEVEL TWO: CONNECTION WITH OTHERS

Brown KW, Levy AR, Rosberger Z, et al. Psychological distress and cancer survival: a follow-up 10 years after diagnosis. *Psychosomatic Medicine*. 2003;65:636–643.

Brown SL, Nesse RM, Vinokur AD, and Smith DM. Providing social support may be more beneficial than receiving it: results from a prospective study of mortality. *Psychological Science*. 2003;14(4):320–327.

Carlson LE and Bultz BD. Efficacy and medical cost offset of psychosocial interventions in cancer care: making the case for economic analysis. *Psychooncology*. 2004;13(12):837–849.

Classen C, Butler LD, Koopman C, et al. Supportive-expressive group therapy and distress in patients with metastatic breast cancer: a randomized clinical intervention trial. *Archives of General Psychiatry*. 2001;58(5):494–501.

Cohen S, Doyle WJ, Skoner DP, et al. Social ties and susceptibility to the common cold. *Journal of the American Medical Association*. 1997;277(24):1940–1944.

Coreil J and Behal R. Man to man prostate cancer support groups. *Cancer Practice*. 1999;7(3):122–129.

Creagan ET. Attitude and disposition: do they make a difference in cancer survival? *Mayo Clinic Proceedings*. 1997;72–164.

De Boer MF, Ryckman RM, Pruyn JF, and Van den Borne HW. Psychosocial correlates of cancer relapse and survival: a literature review. *Patient Education and Counseling*. 1999;37(3):215–230.

Dreher H. The scientific and moral imperative for broad-based psychosocial interventions for cancer. *Advances: The Journal of Mind-Body Health*. 1997;13(3):
38–49.

Fawzy FI, Cousins N, Fawzy NW, et al. A structured psychiatric intervention for
cancer patients. I. Changes over time in methods of coping and affective disturbance. *Archives of General Psychiatry*. 1990;47:720–725.

Fawzy FI, Fawzy NW, Arndt LA, et al. Critical review of pyschosocial interventions in cancer care. *Archives in General Psychiatry*. 1995;52:100–113.

Fawzy FI, Fawzy NW, Hyun CS, et al. Malignant melanoma: effects of an early
structured psychiatric intervention, coping, and affective state on recurrence and
survival 6 years later. *Archives of General Psychiatry*. 1993;50:681–689.

Fawzy FI, Kemeny ME, Fawzy NW, et al. A structured psychiatric intervention for
cancer patients. II. Changes over time in immunologic measures. *Archives of
General Psychiatry*. 1990;47:729–735.

Fobair P. Cancer support groups and group therapies: part I. Historical and theoretical background and research on effectiveness. *Journal of Psychosocial Oncology*.
1997;15(1):63–81.

Fox BH. The role of psychological factors in cancer incidence and prognosis. *Cancer*. 1995;9(3):245–253.

Garssen B. Psychological factors and cancer development: evidence after 30 years of
research. *Clinical Psychology Review*. 2004;24(3):315–338.

Gavrin JR. World wide web resources for cancer support groups. *Journal of Pain and
Palliative Care Pharmacotherapy*. 2005;19(3):69–73.

Glaser R and Kiecolt-Glaser JK. Stress-induced immune dysfunction: implications
for health. *Nature Reviews Immunology*. 2005;5(3):243–251.

Goodwin PJ. Support groups in breast cancer: when a negative result is positive.
Journal of Clinical Oncology. 2004;22(21):4244–4246.

Goodwin PJ, Leszcz M, Ennis M, et al. The effect of group psychosocial support
on survival in metastatic breast cancer. *New England Journal of Medicine*.
2001;345(24):1719–1726.

Hawkley LC and Cacioppo JT. Loneliness and pathways to disease. *Brain, Behavior
and Immunity*. 2003;17(1):98–105.

Heffner KL, Loving TJ, Robles TF, et al. Examining psychosocial factors related to
cancer incidence and progression: in search of the silver lining. *Brain, Behavior
and Immunity*. 2003;17(suppl 1):S109–S111.

Holland JC and Breitbart W, eds. *Psychooncology*. New York: Oxford University
Press. 1998.

Holland JC and Rowland JH, eds. *Handbook of Psychooncology: Psychological Care of
the Patient with Cancer*. New York: Oxford University Press. 1991.

Horowitz S. The power of more than one: the role of support groups in mind-body
healing. *Alternative and Complementary Therapies*. 1998;4(2):84–88.

Kash KM, Mago R, and Kunkel EJ. Psychosocial oncology: supportive care for the cancer patient. *Seminars in Oncology.* 2005;32(2):211–218.

Kiecolt-Glaser JK, Robles TF, Heffner KL, et al. Psycho-oncology and cancer: psychoneuroimmunology and cancer. *Annals of Oncology.* 2002;13(suppl 4): 165–169.

Kogon MM, Biswas A, Pearl D, et al. Effects of medical and psychotherapeutic treatment on the survival of women with metastatic breast carcinoma. *Cancer.* 1997;80(2):225–230.

Krizek C, Roberts C, Ragan R, et al. Gender and cancer support group participation. *Cancer Practice.* 1999;7(2):86–92.

Leedham B and Ganz PA. Psychosocial concerns and quality of life in breast cancer survivors. *Cancer Investigation.* 1999;17(5):342–348.

Leiberman MA and Goldstein BA. Self-help online: an outcome evaluation of breast cancer bulletin boards. *Journal of Health Psychology.* 2005;10(6):855–862.

LeShan L. An emotional life-history pattern associated with neoplastic disease. *Annals of the New York Academy of Science.* 1966;125(3):780–793.

Lillquist PP and Abramson JS. Separating the apples and oranges in the fruit cocktail: the mixed results of psychosocial interventions on cancer survival. *Social Work in Health Care.* 2002;36(2):65–79.

Lutgendorf SK, Sood AK, Anderson B, et al. Social support, psychological distress, and natural killer cell activity in ovarian cancer. *Journal of Clinical Oncology.* 2005;23(28):7105–7113.

Manne S. Cancer in the marital context: a review of the literature. *Cancer Investigation.* 1998;16(3):188–202.

Maunsell E, Brisson J, and Deschenes L. Social support and survival among women with breast cancer. *Cancer.* 1995;76(4):631–637.

Osborne C, Ostir GV, Du X, et al. The influence of marital status on the stage at diagnosis, treatment, and survival of older women with breast cancer. *Breast Cancer Research and Treatment.* 2005;93(1):41–47.

Penson RT, Talsania SHG, Chabner BA, et al. Help me help you: support groups in cancer therapy. *The Oncologist.* 2004;9:217–225.

Rehse B and Pukrop R. Effects of psychosocial interventions on quality of life in adult cancer patients: meta analysis of 37 published controlled outcome studies. *Patient Education and Counseling.* 2003;50(2):179–186.

Richardson JL, Shelton DR, Krailo M, and Levine AM. The effect of compliance with treatment on survival among patients with hematologic malignancies. *Journal of Clinical Oncology.* 1990;8(2):356–364.

Rosenbaum E, Gautier H, Fobair P, et al. Cancer supportive care, improving the quality of life for cancer patients: a program evaluation report. *Supportive Care in Cancer.* 2004;12(5):293–301.

Sapp AL, Trentham-Dietz A, Newcomb PA, et al. Social networks and quality of life among female long-term colorectal cancer survivors. *Cancer.* 2003;98(8): 1749–1758.

Seeman TE. Health promoting effects of friends and family on health outcomes in older adults. *American Journal of Health Promotion.* 2000;14(6):362–370.

Shrock D, Palmer RF, and Taylor B. Effects of psychosocial intervention on survival among patients with stage I breast and prostate cancer: a matched case-controlled study. *Alternative Therapies in Health and Medicine.* 1999;5(3):49–55.

Simonton SS and Sherman AC. Psychological aspects of mind-body medicine: promises and pitfalls from research with cancer patients. *Alternative Therapies in Health and Medicine.* 1998;4(4):50–67.

Spiegel D. *Living Beyond Limits: New Hope and Help for Facing Life-Threatening Illness.* Boulder, CO: Bull Publishing. 2005.

Spiegel D. Psychosocial interventions in cancer. *Journal of the National Cancer Institute.* 1993;85(15):1198–1205.

Spiegel D. Health caring: psychosocial support for patients with cancer. *Cancer.* 1994;74(suppl 4):1453–1457.

Spiegel D. Psychological distress and disease course for women with breast cancer: one answer, many questions. *Journal of the National Cancer Institute.* 1996; 88(10):629–631.

Spiegel D, Bloom JR, Kraemer HC, and Gottheil E. Effect of psychosocial treatment on survival of patients with metastatic cancer. *The Lancet.* 1989; 2:888–891.

Uchino BN, Cacioppo JT, and Kiecolt-Glaser JK. The relationship between social support and physiological processes: a review with emphasis on underlying mechanisms and implications for health. *Psychological Bulletin.* 1996;119(3): 488–531.

Watson M, Homewood J, Haviland J, et al. Influence of psychological response on breast cancer survival: 10-year follow-up of a population-based cohort. *European Journal of Cancer.* 2005;41(12):1710–1714.

Weis J. Support groups for cancer patients. *Supportive Care in Cancer.* 2003; 11(12):763–768.

Zabalaegui A, Sanchez S, Sanchez PD, et al. Nursing and cancer support groups. *Journal of Advanced Nursing.* 2005;51(4):369–381.

Chapter 6: LEVEL THREE: THE BODY AS GARDEN

Abu-Abid S, Szold A, and Klausner J. Obesity and cancer. *Journal of Medicine.* 2002;33(1-4):73–86.

Alimi D, Rubino C, Pichard-Léandri E, et al. Analgesic effect of auricular acupuncture for cancer pain: a randomized, blinded, controlled trial. *Journal of Clinical Oncology.* 2003;21(22):4120–4126.

The Alpha-Tocopherol, Beta Carotene Cancer Prevention Study Group. The effect of vitamin E and beta carotene on the incidence of lung cancer and other cancers in male smokers. *New England Journal of Medicine.* 1994;330(15):1029–1035.

Alphen JV and Aris A, eds. *Oriental Medicine: An Illustrated Guide to the Asian Arts of Healing.* Boston: Shambhala. 1996.

American Cancer Society. *Cancer Prevention & Early Detection Facts & Figures 2005.* Atlanta: American Cancer Society. 2005.

ASCO Special Article. The physician and unorthodox cancer therapies. *Journal of Clinical Oncology.* 1997;15(1):401–406.

The ATBC Study Group. Incidence of cancer and mortality following alpha-tocopherol and beta-carotene supplementation: a postintervention follow-up. *Journal of the American Medical Association.* 2003;290(4):476–485.

Beinfeld H and Corngold E. *Between Heaven and Earth: A Guide to Chinese Medicine.* New York: Ballantine. 1992.

Beresford SAA, Johnson KC, Ritenbaugh C, et al. Low-Fat Dietary Pattern and Risk of Colorectal Cancer: The Women's Health Initiative Randomized Controlled Dietary Modification Trial. *Journal of the American Medical Association.* 2006; 295(6):643–654.

Bingham SE, Day NE, Luben R, et al. Dietary fiber in food and protection against colorectal cancer in the European Prospective Investigation into Cancer and Nutrition (EPIC): an observational study. *The Lancet.* 2003;361(9368): 1496–1501.

Block KI. Antioxidants and cancer therapy: furthering the debate. *Integrative Cancer Therapies.* 2004;3(4):342–348.

Boik J. *Cancer and Natural Medicine: A Textbook of Basic Science and Clinical Research.* Princeton, MN: Oregon Medical Press. 1996.

Borek C. Dietary antioxidants and human cancer. *Integrative Cancer Therapies.* 2004;3(4):333–341.

Bower JE, Woolery A, Sternlieb B, and Garet D. Yoga for cancer patients and survivors. *Cancer Control.* 2005;12(3):165–171.

Broderick JE, Junghaenel DU, and Schwartz JE. Written emotional expression produces health benefits in fibromyalgia patients. *Psychosomatic Medicine.* 2005;67(2):326–334.

Brown JK, Byers T, Doyle C, et al. Nutrition and physical activity during and after cancer treatment: an American Cancer Society guide for informed choices. *CA: A Cancer Journal for Clinicians.* 2003;53(5):268–291.

Brown LM. Epidemiology of alcohol-associated cancers. *Alcohol.* 2005;35(3): 161–168.

Buckner JC, Malkin MG, Reed E, et al. Phase II study of antineoplastons A10 (NSC 648539) and AS2-1 (NSC 620261) in patients with recurrent glioma. *Mayo Clinic Proceedings.* 1999;74:137–145.

Burden B, Herron-Marx S, and Clifford C. The increasing use of Reiki as a complementary therapy in specialist palliative care. *International Journal of Palliative
Nursing.* 2005;11(5):248–253.

Cassileth BR. *The Alternative Medicine Handbook: The Complete Reference Guide to
Alternative and Complementary Therapies.* New York: W. W. Norton. 1998.

Cassileth BR and Deng G. Complementary and alternative therapies for cancer.
The Oncologist. 2004;9:80–89.

Chao A, Thun MJ, Connell CJ, et al. Meat consumption and risk of colorectal cancer. *Journal of the American Medical Association.* 2005;294(3):351–358.

Chen C and Kong AN. Dietary cancer-chemopreventive compounds: from signal-
ing and gene expression to pharmacological effects. *Trends in Pharmacological
Sciences.* 2005;26(6):318–326.

Clark LC, Combs GF, Turnbull BW, et al. Effects of selenium supplementation for
cancer prevention in patients with carcinoma of the skin: a randomized controlled
trial. *Journal of the American Medical Association.* 1996;276(24):1957–1963.

Clifford, Terry. *Tibetan Buddhist Medicine and Psychiatry: The Diamond Healing.*
York Beach, ME: Samuel Weiser. 1990.

Clinton SK, Giovannucci EL, and Miller EC. Nutrition in the etiology and prevention of cancer. In: Holland JF, Frei E, Bast RC, et al., eds. *Cancer Medicine.* 6th
edition. Baltimore: Williams & Wilkins. 2003:397–412.

Cohen AJ, Menter A, and Hale L. Acupuncture: role in comprehensive cancer
care—a primer for the oncologist and review of the literature. *Integrative Cancer
Therapies.* 2005;4(2):131–143.

Coker KH. Meditation and prostate cancer: integrating a mind/body intervention
with traditional therapies. *Seminars in Urologic Oncology.* 1999;17(2):111–118.

Colditz GA. Selenium and cancer prevention: Promising results indicate further trials
required. *Journal of the American Medical Association.* 1996;276(24):1984–1985.

Cooper R, Morre DJ, and Morre DM. Medicinal benefits of green tea: part II. Review of anticancer properties. *Journal of Alternative and Complementary Medicine.* 2005;11(4):639–652.

Corbin L. Safety and efficacy of massage therapy for patients with cancer. *Cancer
Control.* 2005;12(3):158–164.

Courneya KS and Friedenreich CM. Relationship between exercise patterns across
the cancer experience and current quality of life in colorectal cancer survivors.
Journal of Alternative and Complementary Medicine. 1997;3(3):215–226.

D'Andrea GM. Use of antioxidants during chemotherapy and radiotherapy should
be avoided. *CA: A Cancer Journal for Clinicians.* 2005;55(5):319–321.

Demark-Wahnefried W, Aziz NM, Rowland JH, et al. Riding the crest of the
teachable moment: promoting long-term health after the diagnosis of cancer.
Journal of Clinical Oncology. 2005;23:5814–5830.

Deng G and Cassileth BR. Integrative oncology: complementary therapies for pain, anxiety, and mood disturbance. *CA: A Cancer Journal for Clinicians.* 2005;55(2): 109–116.

Dennis LK, Snetselaar LG, Smith BJ, et al. Problems with the assessment of dietary fat in prostate cancer studies. *American Journal of Epidemiology.* 2004;160(5): 436–444.

Dimeo FC, Tilmann MHM, Bertz H, et al. Aerobic exercise in the rehabilitation of cancer patients after high dose chemotherapy and autologous peripheral stem cell transplantation. *Cancer.* 1997;79(9):1717–1722.

DiPaola RS, Zhang H, Lambert GH, et al. Clinical and biological activity of an estrogenic herbal combination (PC-SPES) in prostate cancer. *New England Journal of Medicine.* 1998;339(12):785.

Donaldson MS. Nutrition and cancer: a review of the evidence for an anti-cancer diet. *Nutrition Journal.* 2004;3:19. http://www.nutritionj.com/content/3/1/19). Accessed October 31, 2005.

Donden Y. *Health Through Balance: An Introduction to Tibetan Medicine.* Ithaca, NY: Snow Lion Publications. 1986.

Dorgan JF, Stanczyk FZ, Longcope C, et al. Relationship of serum dehydro-epiandrosterone (DHEA), DHEA-sulfate, and 5-androstene-3 beta, 17 beta-diol to risk of breast cancer in postmenopausal women. *Cancer Epidemiology, Biomarkers, and Prevention.* 1997;6(3):177–181.

Duffield-Lillico AJ, Dalkin BL, Reid ME, et al. Selenium supplementation, baseline plasma selenium status and incidence of prostate cancer: an analysis of the complete treatment period of the Nutritional Prevention of Cancer Trial. *British Journal of Urology International.* 2003;91(7):608–612.

Duffield-Lillico AJ, Reid ME, Turnbull BW, et al. Baseline characteristics and the effect of selenium supplementation on cancer incidence in a randomized clinical trial: a summary report of the Nutritional Prevention of Cancer Trial. *Cancer Epidemiology, Biomarkers, and Prevention.* 2002;11(7):630–639.

Duffield-Lillico AJ, Slate EH, Reid ME, et al. Selenium supplementation and secondary prevention of nonmelanoma skin cancer in a randomized trial. *Journal of the National Cancer Institute.* 2003;95(19):1477–1481.

Eaton NE, Reeves GK, Appleby PN, and Key TJ. Endogenous sex hormones and prostate cancer: a quantitative review of prospective studies. *British Journal of Cancer.* 1999;80(7):930–934.

Ernst E. Complementary therapies in palliative cancer care. *Cancer.* 2001;91(11): 2181–2185.

Evans RC and Rosner AL. Alternatives in cancer pain treatment: the application of chiropractic care. *Seminars in Oncology Nursing.* 2005;21(3):184–189.

Ezzo J, Vickers A, Richardson MA, et al. Acupuncture-point stimulation for chemotherapy-induced nausea and vomiting. *Journal of Clinical Oncology.* 2005;23(28):7188–7198.

Fenton P. In the realm of the Medicine Buddha. *Shambhala Sun.* January 1998:50–57.

Field T, Ironson G, Scafidi F, et al. Massage therapy is associated with enhancement of the immune system's cytotoxic capacity. *International Journal of Neuroscience.* 1996;84(1–4):205–217.

Field T, Ironson G, Scafidi F, et al. Massage therapy reduces anxiety and enhances EEG pattern of alertness and math computations. *International Journal of Neuroscience.* 1996;86(3–4):197–205.

Finckh E. *Foundations of Tibetan Medicine, According to the Book rGyud bzi.* Volume 1. London: Robinson and Watkins Books. 1978.

Finckh E. *Foundations of Tibetan Medicine, According to the Book rGyud bzi.* Volume 2. Longmead, England: Element Books. 1988.

Frawley D. *Ayurvedic Healing: A Comprehensive Guide.* 2nd edition. Twin Lakes, WI: Lotus Press. 2000.

Fuchs CS, Giovannucci EL, Colditz GA, et al. Dietary fiber and the risk of colorectal cancer and adenoma in women. *New England Journal of Medicine.* 1999;340(3):169–176.

Geffen JR. Traditional medicine in the Himalayas of Nepal. *New York University Physician.* 1985;41(2):58–67.

Gill S and Sinicrope FA. Colorectal cancer prevention: is an ounce of prevention worth a pound of cure? *Seminars in Oncology.* 2005;32(1):24–34.

Giovannucci E, Rimm EB, Liu Y, et al. A prospective study of tomato products, lycopene, and prostate cancer risk. *Journal of the National Cancer Institute.* 2002;94(5):391–398.

Glade MJ. Food, nutrition, and the prevention of cancer: a global perspective. American Institute for Cancer Research/World Cancer Research Fund, American Institute for Cancer Research, 1997. *Nutrition.* 1999;15(6):523–526.

Gotay CC. Behavior and cancer prevention. *Journal of Clinical Oncology.* 2005; 23(2):301–310.

Grindel CG, Whitmer K, and Barsevik A. Quality of life and nutritional support in patients with cancer. *Cancer Practice.* 1996;4(2):81–87.

Hankey A. The scientific value of Ayurveda. *Journal of Alternative and Complementary Medicine.* 2005;11(2):221–225.

Harris AH, Thoresen CE, Humphreys K, and Faul J. Does writing affect asthma? A randomized trial. *Psychosomatic Medicine.* 2005;67(1):130–136.

Hartwell JL. *Plants Used Against Cancer.* Lawrence, MA: Quarterman Publications. 1982.

Hennekens CH, Buring JE, Manson JE, et al. Lack of effect of long-term supplementation with beta carotene on the incidence of malignant neoplasms and cardiovascular disease. *New England Journal of Medicine.* 1996;334(18):1145–1149.

Hensrud DD, Engle DD, and Scheitel SM. Underreporting the use of dietary supplements and non-prescription medications among patients undergoing a periodic health examination. *Mayo Clinic Proceedings.* 1999;74:443–447.

Hernandez-Reif M, Field T, Ironson G, et al. Natural killer cells and lymphocytes increase in women with breast cancer following massage therapy. *International Journal of Neuroscience.* 2005;115(4):495–510.

Hernandez-Reif M, Ironson G, Field T, et al. Breast cancer patients have improved immune and neuroendocrine functions following massage therapy. *Journal of Psychosomatic Research.* 2004; 57(1):45–52.

Holmes MD, Hunter DJ, Colditz GA, et al. Association of dietary intake of fat and fatty acids with risk of breast cancer. *Journal of the American Medical Association.* 1999;281(10):914–920.

Holmes MD, Stampfer MJ, Colditz GA, et al. Dietary factors and the survival of women with breast carcinoma. *Cancer.* 1999;86(5):826–835.

Holt S. Chemoprevention of cancer with green tea. *Alternative and Complementary Therapies.* 1998;4(1):48–52.

Holzbeierlein JM, McIntosh J, and Thrasher JB. The role of soy phytoestrogens in prostate cancer. *Current Opinion in Urology.* 2005;15(1):17–22.

Hou Z, Lambert JD, Chin KV, and Yang CS. Effects of tea polyphenols on signal transduction pathways related to cancer chemoprevention. *Mutation Research.* 2004;555(1-2):3–19.

International Agency for Research on Cancer. *IARC Handbooks of Cancer Prevention.* Volume 8: *Fruits and Vegetables.* Lyon, France. 2003.

Jones JA, Nguyen A, Straub M, et al. Use of DHEA in a patient with advanced prostate cancer: a case report and review. *Urology.* 1997;50(5):784–788.

Kaptchuk TJ. *The Web That Has No Weaver: Understanding Chinese Medicine.* New York: Congdon and Weed. 1983.

Key T, Allen N, Spencer E, and Travis R. The effect of diet on risk of cancer. *The Lancet.* 2002;360(9336):861–868.

Kelly JP, Kaufman DW, Kelley K, et al. Recent trends in use of herbal and other natural products. *Archives of Internal Medicine.* 2005;165(3):281–286.

Kim ES and Hong WK. An apple a day...does it really keep the doctor away? *Journal of the National Cancer Institute.* 2005;97(7):468–470.

Klein EA. Selenium and vitamin E cancer prevention trial. *Annals of the New York Academy of Sciences.* 2004;1031:234–241.

Klein EA. Chemoprevention of prostate cancer. *Critical Reviews in Oncology/ Hematology.* 2005;54(1):1–10.

Kolata G. Which of these foods will stop cancer? *New York Times.* September 27, 2005.

Kosty MP, Fleishman SB, Herndon JE, et al. Cisplatin, vinblastine, and hydrazine sulfate in advanced, non-small-cell lung cancer: a randomized placebo-controlled, double-blind phase III study of the Cancer and Leukemia Group B. *Journal of Clinical Oncology*. 1994;12(6):1113–1120.

Krieg MB. *Green Medicine: The Search for Plants That Heal*. Chicago: Rand McNally. 1964.

Kushi L and Giovannucci E. Dietary fat and cancer. *The American Journal of Medicine*. 2002;113(9):63–70.

Labrie F, Bélanger A, Van LT, et al. DHEA and the intracrine formation of androgens and estrogens in peripheral target tissues: its role during aging. *Steroids*. 1998;63(5–6):322–328.

Labriola D and Livingston R. Possible interactions between dietary antioxidants and chemotherapy. *Oncology*. 1999;13(7):1003–1008.

Lad V. An introduction to Ayurveda. *Alternative Therapies in Health and Medicine*. 1995;1(3):57–63.

Lad V. *Ayurveda: The Science of Self-Healing*. Santa Fe, NM: Lotus Press. 1984.

Ladas EJ, Jaconson JS, Kennedy DD, et al. Antioxidants and cancer therapy: a systematic review. *Journal of Clinical Oncology*. 2004;22:517–528.

Laffery WE, Bellas A, Baden AC, et al. The use of complementary and alternative medical providers by insured cancer patients in Washington state. *Cancer*. 2004;100(7):1522–1530.

Lee CO. Homeopathy in cancer care: part II. Continuing the practice of "like curing like." *Clinical Journal of Oncology Nursing*. 2004;8(3):327–330.

Lee I, Cook N, Gaziano JM, et al. Vitamin E in the primary prevention of cardiovascular disease and cancer. *Journal of the American Medical Association*. 2005;294(1):56–65.

Lerner M. *Choices in Healing: Integrating the Best of Conventional and Complementary Approaches to Cancer*. Cambridge, MA: MIT Press. 1996.

Lichtenstein AH and Russell RM. Essential nutrients: food or supplements? Where should the emphasis be? *Journal of the American Medical Association*. 2005;293(2):172–182.

Liebman B. Keeping abreast of the latest on diet and breast cancer. *Nutrition Action Health Letter*. 2005;32(7):1–8.

Loizzo JJ and Blackhall LJ. Traditional alternatives as complementary sciences: the case of Indo-Tibetan medicine. *Journal of Alternative and Complementary Medicine*. 1998;4(3):311–319.

Lonn E, Bosch J, Yusuf S, et al. Effects of long-term vitamin E supplementation on cardiovascular events and cancer. *Journal of the American Medical Association*. 2005;293(11):1338–1347.

Loprinzi CL, Goldberg RM, Su JQ, et al. Placebo-controlled trial of hydrazine sulfate in patients with newly diagnosed non-small-cell lung cancer. *Journal of Clinical Oncology*. 1994;12(6):1126–1129.

Loprinzi CL, Kuross SA, O'Fallon JR, et al. Randomized placebo-controlled evaluation of hydrazine sulfate in patients with advanced colorectal cancer. *Journal of Clinical Oncology*. 1994;12(6):1121–1125.

Lu W. Acupuncture for side effects of chemoradiation therapy in cancer patients. *Seminars in Oncological Nursing*. 2005;21(3):190–195.

McTiernan A, Ulrich C, Kumai C, et al. Anthropometric and hormone effects of an eight-week exercise-diet intervention in breast cancer patients: results of a pilot study. *Cancer Epidemiology, Biomarkers, and Prevention*. 1998;7(6): 477–481.

Mendoza TR, Wang XS, Cleeland CS, et al. The rapid assessment of fatigue severity in cancer patients. *Cancer*. 1999;85(5):1186–1196.

Michels KB. The role of nutrition in cancer development and prevention. *International Journal of Cancer*. 2005;114(2):163–165.

Michels KB, Fuchs CS, Colditz GA, et al. Fiber intake and incidence of colorectal cancer among 76,947 women and 47,279 men. *Cancer Epidemiology, Biomarkers, and Prevention*. 2005;14(4):842–849.

Miller DR, Anderson GT, Stark JJ, et al. Phase I/II trial of the safety and efficacy of shark cartilage in the treatment of advanced cancer. *Journal of Clinical Oncology*. 1998;16(11):3649–3655.

Moertel CG, Fleming TR, Rubin J, et al. A clinical trial of amygdalin (Laetrile) in the treatment of human cancer. *New England Journal of Medicine*. 1982;306:201–206.

Moertel CG, Ames MM, Kovach JS, et al. A pharmacologic and toxicological study of amygdalin. *Journal of the American Medical Association*. 1981;245:591–594.

Molassiotis A, Fernadez-Ortega P, Pud D, et al. Use of complementary and alternative medicine in cancer patients: a European survey. *Annals of Oncology*. 2005; 16(4):655–663.

Moss RW. *Herbs Against Cancer: History and Controversy*. Brooklyn, NY: Equinox Press. 1998.

Navarro-Peran E, Cabezas-Herrara J, Garcia-Canovas F, et al. The antifolate activity of tea catechins. *Cancer Research*. 2005;65:2059–2064.

Nelson WK. Alternative cancer treatments. *Highlights in Oncology Practice*. 1998;15(4):85–93.

Omenn GS, Goodman GE, Thornquist MD, et al. Effects of a combination of beta carotene and vitamin A on lung cancer and cardiovascular disease. *New England Journal of Medicine*. 1996;334(18):1150–1155.

Patel V. Ayurveda: science of integrative approaches to health and disease. *Internal Journal of Integrative Medicine*. 1999;1(5):7–9.

Paulsen SM. Use of herbal products and dietary supplements by oncology patients— informed decisions? *Highlights in Oncology Practice*. 1998;15(4):94–106.

Pennebaker JW, Kiecolt-Glaser JK, and Glaser R. Disclosures of traumas and immune function: health implications for psychotherapy. *Journal of Consulting and Clinical Psychology.* 1988;56:239–245.

Petire KJ, Booth RJ, et al. Disclosure of trauma and immune response to a hepatitis B vaccination program. *Journal of Consulting and Clinical Psychology.* 1995;63:787–792.

Pinto BM, Maruyama NC, Engebretson TO, and Thebarge RW. Participation in exercise, mood, and coping in survivors of early stage breast cancer. *Journal of Psychosocial Oncology.* 1998;16(2):45–58.

Post-White J, Kinney ME, Savik K, et al. Therapeutic massage and healing touch improve symptoms in cancer. *Integrative Cancer Therapies.* 2003;2(4):332–344.

Prentice, RL, Caan B, Chlebowski RT, et al. Low-Fat Dietary Pattern and Risk of Invasive Breast Cancer: The Women's Health Initiative Randomized Controlled Dietary Modification Trial. *Journal of the American Medical Association.* 2006;295(6):629–642.

Purohit V, Khals J, and Serrano J. Mechanisms of alcohol-associated cancers: introduction and summary of the symposium. *Alcohol.* 2005;35(3):155–160.

Quillan P. The ideal anti-cancer diet. *American Journal of Natural Medicine.* 1998;5(7):21–25.

Ravasco P, Monteiro-Grillo I, Vidal PM, et al. Dietary counseling improves patient outcomes: a prospective, randomized, controlled trail in colorectal cancer patients undergoing radiotherapy. *Journal of Clinical Oncology.* 2005;23:1431–1438.

Reid ME, Duffield-Lillico AJ, Garland L, et al. Selenium supplementation and lung cancer incidence: an update of the Nutritional Prevention of Cancer Trial. *Cancer Epidemiology, Biomarkers, and Prevention.* 2002;11(11):1285–1291.

Rinpoche S. The spiritual heart of Tibetan Medicine: its contribution to the modern world. *Alternative Therapies in Health and Medicine.* 1999;5(3):70–72.

Rock CL. Dietary counseling is beneficial for the patient with cancer. *Journal of Clinical Oncology.* 2005;23(7):1348–1349.

Rock CL and Demark-Wahnefried WD. Nutrition and survival after the diagnosis of breast cancer: a review of the evidence. *Journal of Clinical Oncology.* 2002;20(15):3302–3316.

Rock E and DeMichele A. Nutritional approaches to late toxicities of adjuvant chemotherapy in breast cancer survivors. *Journal of Nutrition.* 2003;133(11 suppl 1):3785S–3793S.

Rosenthal DS and Dean-Clower E. Integrative medicine in hematology/oncology: benefits, ethical considerations, and controversies. *Hematology (American Society of Hematology Educational Program).* 2005;491–497.

Rosser C. Homeopathy in cancer care: Part I. An introduction to "like curing like." *Clinical Journal of Oncology Nursing.* 2004;8(3):324–326.

Sandel SL, Judge JO, Landry N, et al. Dance and movement program improves quality-of-life measures in breast cancer survivors. *Cancer Nursing.* 2005;28(4): 301–309.

Schmitz KH, Holtzman J, Courneya KS, et al. Controlled physical activity trials in cancer survivors: a systematic review and meta-analysis. *Cancer Epidemiology, Biomarkers, and Prevention.* 2005;14(7):1588–1595.

Segar ML, Katch VL, Roth RS, et al. The effects of aerobic exercise on self-esteem and depressive and anxiety symptoms among breast cancer survivors. *Oncology Nursing Forum.* 1998;25(1):107–113.

Serenson I. Integrated Chinese/Western therapies in the treatment of cancer, part 1. *Alternative and Complementary Therapies.* 1997;3(6):441–446.

Serenson I. Integrated Chinese/Western therapies in the treatment of cancer, part 2. *Alternative and Complementary Therapies.* 1998;4(2):134–138.

Singh DK and Lippman SM. Cancer chemoprevention—part 1: retinoids and carotenoids and other classic antioxidants. *Oncology.* 1998;12(11):1643–1658.

Singh DK and Lippman SM. Cancer chemoprevention—part 2: hormones, nonclassic antioxidants, NSAID's, and other agents. *Oncology.* 1998;12(12):1787–1800.

Smith AM. Opening the dialogue: herbal supplementation and chemotherapy. *Clinical Journal of Oncology Nursing.* 2005;9(4):447–450.

Smith MC, Stallings MA, Mariner S, and Burrall M. Benefits of massage therapy in hospitalized patients: a descriptive and qualitative evaluation. *Alternative Therapies in Health and Medicine.* 1999;5(4):64–71.

Smith-Warner SA, Spiegelman D, Adami HO, et al. Types of dietary fat and breast cancer: a pooled analysis of cohort studies. *International Journal of Cancer.* 2001;92(5):767–774.

Smith-Warner SA, Spiegelman D, Yuan SS, et al. Alcohol and breast cancer in women: a pooled analysis of cohort studies. *Journal of the American Medical Association.* 1998;279:535–540.

Smyth JM, Stone AA, Hurewitz A, and Kaell A. Effects of writing about stressful experiences on symptom reduction in patients with asthma or rheumatoid arthritis. *Journal of the American Medical Association.* 1999;281(14):1304–1309.

Sparreboom A, Cox MC, Acharya MR, and Figg WD. Herbal remedies in the United States: potential adverse interactions with anticancer agents. *Journal of Clinical Oncology.* 2004;22(12):2489–2503.

Spiegel D. Healing words: emotional expression and disease outcome. *Journal of the American Medical Association.* 1999;281(14):1328–1329.

Spiegel D and Moore R. Imagery and hypnosis in the treatment of cancer patients. *Oncology.* 1997;11(8):1179–1189.

Stanton AL, Danoff-Burg S, Sworowski LA, et al. Randomized, controlled trial of written emotional expression and benefit finding in breast cancer patients. *Journal of Clinical Oncology.* 2002;20(20):4160–4168.

Sun AS, Ostadal O, Ryznar V, et al. Phase I/II study of stage III and IV non-small cell lung cancer patients taking a specific dietary supplement. *Nutrition and Cancer*. 1999;34(1):62–69.

Taylor PR and Greenwald P. Nutritional interventions in cancer prevention. *Journal of Clinical Oncology*. 2005;23(2):333–345.

Thompson D. Acupuncture works: an NIH panel endorses the ancient needle treatment—at least for some conditions. *Time*. November 17, 1997.

Tokar E. Seeing to the distant mountain: diagnosis in Tibetan Medicine. *Alternative Therapies in Health and Medicine*. 1999;5(2):50–58.

Thune I, Brenn T, Lund E, and Gaard M. Physical activity and the risk of breast cancer. *New England Journal of Medicine*. 1997;336(18):1269–1275.

Upchurch D and Chyu L. Use of complementary and alternative medicine among American women. *Women's Health Issues*. 2005;15(1):5–13.

U.S. Congress, Office of Technology Assessment. *Unconventional Cancer Treatments*. OTA-H-405. Washington, D.C.: U.S. Government Printing Office, September 1990.

U.S. Department of Health and Human Services. Fiscal year 2005 budget request for the NCCAM. Statement by Stephen E. Straus, MD, director, NCCAM. www.hhs.gov/budget/testify/b20040401e.html. Accessed October 11, 2005.

Visovsky C and Dvorak C. Exercise and cancer recovery. *Online Journal of Issues in Nursing*. 2005;10(2). http://nursingworld.org/ojin/hirsh/topic3/tpc3_2.htm. Accessed October 31, 2005.

van Gils CH, Peeters PHM, Bueno-de-Mesquit HB, et al. Consumption of vegetables and fruits and risk of breast cancer. *Journal of the American Medical Association*. 2005;293(2):183–193.

Vickers AJ and Cassileth BR. Unconventional therapies for cancer and cancer-related symptoms. *The Lancet Oncology*. 2001;2(4):226–232.

Vignot S, Spano JP, Lantuejoul S, et al. Chemoprevention of lung cancer. *Recent Results in Cancer Research*. 2005;166:145–165.

Wang XD. Alcohol, vitamin A, and cancer. *Alcohol*. 2005;35(3):251–258.

Willett WC. Cancer prevention: diet and chemopreventive agents. In: DeVita VT, Hellman S and Rosenberg SA, eds. *Cancer: Principles and Practice of Oncology*. 7th edition. Philadelphia: Lippincott Williams & Wilkins. 2004:507–554.

Willett W. Diet and cancer. *The Oncologist*. 2000;5:393–404.

Willett W. Diet and cancer: an evolving picture. *Journal of the American Medical Association*. 2005;293(2):233–234.

Zelnak AB and O'Regan RM. Chemoprevention of breast cancer. *Current Problems in Cancer*. 2004;28(4):201–217.

Chapter 7: LEVEL FOUR: EMOTIONAL HEALING

Bailey RK, Geyen DJ, Scott-Gurnell K, and Hipolito MM. Understanding and treating depression among cancer patients. *International Journal of Gynecological Cancer.* 2005;15(2):203–208.

Carlick A and Biley FC. Thoughts on the therapeutic use of narrative in the promotion of coping in cancer care. *European Journal of Cancer Care.* 2004;13(4): 308–317.

Clark MM, Bostwick JM, and Rummans TA. Group and individual treatment strategies for distress in cancer patients. *Mayo Clinic Proceedings.* 2003;78(12): 1538-1543.

Cordova MJ and Andrykowski MA. Responses to cancer diagnosis and treatment: posttraumatic stress and posttraumatic growth. *Seminars in Clinical Neuropsychiatry.* 2003;8(4):286–296.

Fox BH. The role of psychological factors in cancer incidence and prognosis. *Oncology.* 1995;9(3):245–253.

Garssen B. Psychological factors and cancer development: evidence after 30 years of research. *Clinical Psychology Review.* 2004;24(3):315–338.

Graves KD, Schmidt JE, Bollmer J, et al. Emotional expression and emotional recognition in breast cancer survivors: a controlled comparison. *Psychology and Health.* 2005;20(5):579–595.

Greenberg DB. Barriers to the treatment of depression in cancer patients. *Journal of the National Cancer Institute Monograph.* 2004;32:127-135.

Holland JC and Breitbart W, eds. *Psychooncology.* New York: Oxford University Press. 1998.

Holland JC and Rowland JH, eds. *Handbook of Psychooncology: Psychological Care of the Patient with Cancer.* New York: Oxford University Press. 1991.

Katz A. The sounds of silence: sexuality information for cancer patients. *Journal of Clinical Oncology.* 2005;23(1):238–241.

Kiecolt-Glaser JK and Glaser R. Depression and immune function: central pathways to morbidity and mortality. *Journal of Psychosomatic Research.* 2002;53(4): 873–876.

Kiecolt-Glaser JK, McGuire L, Robles TF, and Glaser R. Emotions, morbidity, and mortality: new perspectives from psychoneuroimmunology. *Annual Reviews of Psychology.* 2002;53:83–107.

Kreitier S. Denial in cancer patients. *Cancer Investigation.* 1999;17(7):514–534.

Massie MJ. Prevalence of depression in patients with cancer. *Journal of the National Cancer Institute.* 2004;(32):127–135.

Passik SD, Dugan W, McDonald MV, et al. Oncologists' recognition of depression in their patients with cancer. *Journal of Clinical Oncology.* 1998;16(4):1594–1600.

Pinto BM and Trunzo JJ. Body esteem and mood among sedentary and active breast cancer survivors. *Mayo Clinical Proceedings.* 2004;79:181–186.

Pirl WF and Roth AJ. Diagnosis and treatment of depression in cancer patients. *Oncology.* 1999;13(9):1293–1301.

Pitceathly C and Maguire P. The psychological impact of cancer on patients' partners and other key relatives: a review. *European Journal of Cancer.* 2003;39(11): 1517–1524.

Ronson A. Psychiatric disorders in oncology: recent therapeutic advances and new conceptual frameworks. *Current Opinion in Oncology.* 2004;16(4):318–323.

Smyth JM, Stone AA, Hurewitz A, and Kaell A. Effects of writing about stressful experiences on symptom reduction in patients with asthma or rheumatoid arthritis. *Journal of the American Medical Association.* 1999;281(14):1304–1309.

Somerset W, Stout SC, Miller AH, and Musselman D. Breast cancer and depression. *Oncology.* 2004;18(8):1021–1034.

Spiegel D. Healing words: emotional expression and disease outcome. *Journal of the American Medical Association.* 1999;281(14):1328–1329.

Theobald DE. Cancer pain, fatigue, distress, and insomnia in cancer patients. *Clinical Cornerstone.* 2004;6(suppl 1D):S15–S21.

CHAPTER 8: LEVEL FIVE: THE NATURE OF MIND

Benson H. *Timeless Healing: The Power and Biology of Belief.* New York: Scribner. 1997.

Bonadonna R. Meditation's impact on chronic illness. *Holistic Nursing Practice.* 2003;17(6):309–319.

Borysenko J. *Minding the Body, Mending the Mind.* New York: Bantam Books. 1988.

Cohen SR, Mount BM, Tomas JJN, and Mount LF. Existential well-being is an important determinant of quality of life. *Cancer.* 1996;77(3):576–586.

Chodron T. *Taming the Monkey Mind.* Torrance, CA: Heian International. 1999.

Dossey L. *Meaning and Medicine: Lessons from a Doctor's Tales of Breakthrough and Healing.* New York: Bantam Books. 1991.

Dossey L. What does illness mean? *Alternative Therapies in Health and Medicine.* 1995;1(3):6–10.

Foster LW and McLellan L. Cognition and the cancer experience. Clinical implications. *Cancer Practice.* 2000;8(1):25–31.

Greenstein M and Breitbart W. Cancer and the experience of meaning: a group psychotherapy program for people with cancer. *American Journal of Psychotherapy.* 2000;54(4):486–500.

Haberman M. The meaning of cancer therapy: bone marrow transplantation as an exemplar of therapy. *Seminars in Oncology Nursing.* 1995;11(1):23–31.

Lipton, B. *The Biology of Belief: Unleashing the Power of Consciousness, Matter and Miracles.* Santa Rosa, CA: Elite Books. 2005.

Little M, Paul K, Jordens CF, and Sayers EJ. Survivorship and discourses of identity. *Psychooncology.* 2002;11(2):170–178.

Moyers B. *Healing and the Mind.* New York: Broadway Books. 2002.

O'Connor AP, Wicker CA, and Germino BB. Understanding the cancer patient's search for meaning. *Cancer Nursing.* 1990;13:167–175.

Richer MC and Ezer H. Understanding beliefs and meanings in the experience of cancer: a concept analysis. *Journal of Advanced Nursing.* 2000;32(5):1108–1115.

Richer MC and Ezer H. Living in it, living with it, and moving on: dimensions of meaning during chemotherapy. *Oncology Nursing Forum.* 2002;29(1):113–119.

Robbins A. *Awaken the Giant Within: How to Take Immediate Control of Your Mental, Emotional, Physical, and Financial Destiny.* Cambridge, MA: Gardners Books. 2003.

Taylor EJ. The search for meaning among persons with cancer. *Quality of Life—A Nursing Challenge.* 1993;2(3):65–70.

Vachon ML. The meaning of illness to a long-term survivor. *Seminars in Oncology Nursing.* 2001;17(4):279–283.

Vickberg SM, Bovbjerg DH, DuHamel KN, et al. Intrusive thoughts and psychological distress among breast cancer survivors: global meaning as a possible protective factor. *Behavioral Medicine.* 2000;25(4):152–160.

CHAPTER 9: LEVEL SIX: LIFE ASSESSMENT

Bauer-Wu S and Farran CJ. Meaning in life and psycho-spiritual functioning: a comparison of breast cancer survivors and healthy women. *Journal of Holistic Nursing.* 2005;23(2):172–190.

Breitbart W, Gibson C, Poppito SR, and Berg A. Psychotherapeutic interventions at the end of life: a focus on meaning and spirituality. *Canadian Journal of Psychiatry.* 2004;49(6):366–372.

Brown JK and Knapp TR. Do people with cancer postpone death to celebrate special occasions? *Cancer Practice.* 1995;3(6):351–355.

Frankl VE. *Man's Search for Meaning.* New York: Pocket Books. 1997.

Hanson LC, Tulsky JA, and Danis M. Can clinical interventions change care at the end of life? *Annals of Internal Medicine.* 1997;126(5):381–388.

His Holiness the Dalai Lama. *The Meaning of Life from a Buddhist Perspective.* (Translated and edited by Jeffery Hopkins.) Boston: Wisdom Publications. 1992.

His Holiness the Dalai Lama and Cutler HC. *The Art of Happiness.* New York: Riverhead Books. 1998.

Jones LB. *The Path: Creating Your Mission Statement for Work and for Life.* New York: NY: Hyperion. 1998.

Kübler-Ross E. *On Death and Dying: What the Dying Have to Teach Doctors, Nurses, Clergy, and Their Own Families.* New York: Scribner. 1997.

LeShan L. *Cancer as a Turning Point: A Handbook for People with Cancer, Their Families, and Health Professionals.* London: Penguin Books. 1989.

Levine S. *A Year to Live: How to Live This Year As if It Were Your Last.* New York: Bell Tower. 1998.

Levine S. *Who Dies? An Investigation of Conscious Living and Conscious Dying.* Dublin: Gill & Macmillan. 2000.

Lo B, Quill T, and Tulsky J. Discussing palliative care with patients. *Annals of Internal Medicine.* 1999;130(9):744–749.

McCarthy KW. *The On Purpose Person: Making Your Life Make Sense.* Colorado Springs, CO: Pinon Press. 2001.

McCue JD. The naturalness of dying. *Journal of the American Medical Association.* 1995;273(13):1039–1043.

McQuellon RP and Cowan MA. Turning toward death together: conversation in mortal time. *American Journal of Hospice Palliative Care.* 2000;17(5):312–318.

Smith TJ and Schnipper LJ. The American Society of Clinical Oncology program to improve end-of-life care. *Journal of Palliative Medicine.* 1998;1(3):221–230.

Singer PA, Martin DK, and Kelner M. Quality end-of-life care: patients' perspectives. *Journal of the American Medical Association.* 1999;281(2):163–168.

Singh KD. *The Grace in Dying: How We Are Transformed Spiritually as We Die.* San Francisco: HarperSanFrancisco. 2000.

Vickers KS, Hathaway JC, Patten CA, et al. Cancer patients' and patient advocates' perspectives on a novel information source: a qualitative study of the art of oncology, when the tumor is not the target. *Journal of Clinical Oncology.* 2005;23(18):4013–4020.

CHAPTER 10: LEVEL SEVEN: THE NATURE OF SPIRIT

Byrom T. *The Heart of Awareness: A Translation of the Ashtavakra Gita.* Boston: Shambhala. 2001.

Copp LA and Copp JD. Illness and the human spirit. *Quality of Life—A Nursing Challenge.* 1993;2(3):50–55.

Cunningham AJ. Integrating spirituality into a group psychological therapy program for cancer patients. *Integrative Cancer Therapies.* 2005;4(2):178–186.

Godman D, ed. *Be as You Are: The Teachings of Sri Ramana Maharshi.* London: Arkana Books. 1991.

Godman D. *Nothing Ever Happened.* Boulder, CO: Avadhuta Foundation. 1998.

The Holy Bible. New International Version. Grand Rapids, MI: Zondervan. 1986.

Huxley A. *The Perennial Philosophy*. New York: HarperCollins Publishers. 2004.

McGrath P and Clarke H. Creating the space for spiritual talk: insights from survivors of haematological malignancies. *Australian Health Review*. 2003;26(3): 116–132.

Meraviglia MG. The effects of spirituality on well-being of people with lung cancer. *Oncology Nursing Forum*. 2004;31(1):89–94.

Miller BS, (trans.). *The Bhagavad-Gita: Krishna's Council in Time of War*. New York: Bantam. 1991.

Nisargadatta M. *I Am That*. Bangalore, India: Chetana Private. 1999.

Poonja Sri HWL and de Jeger P, ed. *The Truth Is*. York Beach, ME: Weiser Books. 2000.

Prabhavananda S and Isherwood C, trans. *Shankara's Crest-Jewel of Discrimination* (Viveka-Chudamani). Hollywood, FL: Vedanta Press. 1978.

Rahula W. *What the Buddha Taught*. New York: Grove Press. 1974.

Schuon, F. *The Transcendent Unity of Religions*. Wheaton, IL: Quest Books. 1993.

Seeman TE, Dubin LF, and Seeman M. Religiosity, spirituality and health. *American Psychology*. 2003;58(1):53–63.

Smith, H. *The Forgotten Truth: The Common Vision of the World's Religions*. New York: HarperCollins Publishers. 1992.

Taylor EJ. Spiritual needs of patients with cancer and family caregivers. *Cancer Nursing*. 2003;26(4):260–266.

Venkatesananda S. *Vasistha's Yoga*. Albany: State University of New York Press. 1993.

Wolf L. *Practical Kabbalah: A Guide to Jewish Wisdom for Everyday Life*. New York: Three Rivers Press. 1999.

APPENDIX I

HELPFUL BOOKS, AUDIO PROGRAMS, AND MUSIC

The world is full of magnificent books and other resources that can be profoundly helpful for anyone dealing with cancer or other serious illnesses. Below is a list of some of the books, audio programs, and CDs that I have found over the years to be of great value for patients, family members, caregivers, and friends. I have taken the liberty of categorizing the books according to the Seven Levels of Healing, because it is a useful way of organizing a potentially overwhelming abundance of resource materials. Please note, however, that many of these books address issues that are dealt with in more than one of the seven levels of the program. In this context, I have placed each book in what I feel is the most relevant category, and have added a supplementary list at the end containing books of general interest.

BOOKS

LEVEL ONE: EDUCATION AND INFORMATION

General Information About Cancer

Abeloff, Martin D., MD, Armitage, James O., MD, Niederhuber, John E., MD, Kastan, M.B., MD, and McKenna, W. Gillies, MD. *Clinical Oncology*. 3rd edition. New York: Churchill Livingstone. 2004.

DeVita, Vincent, Jr., MD, Hellman, Samuel, MD, and Rosenberg, Steven, MD, PhD. *Cancer: Principles and Practice of Oncology*. 7th edition. Philadelphia: Lippincott Williams & Wilkins. 2004.

Dollinger, Malin, MD, Tempero, Margaret, MD, Rosenbaum, Ernest, MD, Mulvihill, Sean J., MD, and Foster, David A., PhD. *Everyone's Guide to Cancer Therapy: How Cancer Is Diagnosed, Treated, and Managed Day to Day*. 4th edition. Kansas City, MO: Andrews McMeel. 2002.

Kufe, Donald W., MD, Pollack, Raphael E., MD, Weichselbaum, Ralph R., MD, Bast, Robert C., MD, and Gansler, Ted, MD. *Holland-Frei Cancer Medicine*. 6th edition. Philadelphia: B. C. Decker. 2003.

Schlessel-Harpham, Wendy, MD. *Diagnosis: Cancer. Your Guide Through the First Few Months*. New York: W. W. Norton. 2003.

Sompayrac, Lauren. *How Cancer Works*. Sudbury, MA: Jones and Bartlett. 2004.

Waldholz, Michael. *Curing Cancer: Solving One of the Greatest Medical Mysteries of Our Time*. New York: Simon & Schuster. 1997.

Weinberg, Robert A. *One Renegade Cell: How Cancer Begins*. New York: Basic Books. 1998.

Weinberg, Robert A. *Racing to the Beginning of the Road: The Search for the Origin of Cancer*. New York: W. H. Freeman. 1996.

Zakarian, Beverly. *The Activist Cancer Patient: How to Take Charge of Your Treatment*. New York: John Wiley & Sons. 1996.

Chemotherapy and Radiation

Baquiran, Delia C., and Gallagher, Jean. *Lippincott's Cancer Chemotherapy Handbook*. Philadelphia: Lippincott Williams & Wilkins. 2001.

Bruning, Nancy P. *Coping with Chemotherapy*. New York: Avery. 2002.

Dodd, Marylin J., RN, PhD. *Managing the Side Effects of Chemotherapy and Radiation*. San Francisco: University of California, San Francisco. 2001.

Drum, David E. *Making the Chemotherapy Decision*. 3rd edition. New York: McGraw-Hill. 2000.

Fischer, David S., Knobf, M. Tish, and Durivage, Henry J. *The Cancer Chemotherapy Handbook*. 6th edition. St. Louis: Mosby. 2003.

Kelvin, Joanne. *100 Q&A About Cancer Symptoms and Cancer Treatment Side Effects*. Sudbury, MA: Jones and Bartlett. 2004.

McCollough, Virginia E. (contributor), and Cukier, Daniel. *Coping with Radiation Therapy: A Ray of Hope*. 3rd edition. New York: McGraw-Hill. 2001.

McKay, Judith, RN, OCN, and Hirano, Nancee, RN, AOCN. *The Chemotherapy & Radiation Therapy Survival Guide: Information, Suggestions, and Support to Help You Get Through Treatment*. Oakland, CA: New Harbinger. 1998.

Skeel, Roland T. *Handbook of Cancer Chemotherapy*. 6th edition. Philadelphia: Lippincott Williams & Wilkins. 2003.

Breast Cancer

Brinker, Nancy. *Winning the Race: Taking Charge of Breast Cancer*. Irving, TX: Tapestry Press. 2001.

Kaelin, Carolyn M., and Coltrera, Francesca. *Living Through Breast Cancer*. New York: McGraw-Hill. 2005.

Lange, Vladimir. *Be a Survivor: Your Guide to Breast Cancer Treatment*. 3rd edition. Los Angeles: Lange Productions. 2005.

Link, John, MD, Waisman, James, MD, and Forsthoff, Cynthia, MD. *The Breast Cancer Survival Manual: A Step-by-Step Guide for the Woman with Newly Diagnosed Breast Cancer*. 3rd edition. New York: Owl Books. 2003.

Love, Susan M., MD. *Dr. Susan Love's Breast Book*. 4th edition. Burlington, VT: Da Capo Lifelong Books. 2005.

Mayer, Musa. *Advanced Breast Cancer: A Guide to Living with Metastatic Disease*. 2nd edition. Sebastopol, CA: Patient Centered Guides. 1998.

Ricks, Delthia. *Breast Cancer Basics and Beyond: Treatments, Resources, Self-help, Good News, Updates*. Alameda, CA: Hunter House. 2005.

Prostate Cancer

Grimm, Peter D., DO, Blasko, John C., MD, and Sylvester, John E., MD. *The Prostate Cancer Treatment Book*. New York: McGraw-Hill. 2003.

Korda, Michael. *Man to Man: Surviving Prostate Cancer*. New York: Random House. 1998.

Marks, Sheldon, MD. *Prostate and Cancer: A Family Guide to Diagnosis, Treatment and Survival*. 3rd edition. Cambridge, MA: Perseus Books. 2003.

Rous, Stephen N., MD. *The Prostate Book: Sound Advice on Symptoms and Treatment*. 3rd edition. New York: W. W. Norton. 2002.

Scardino, Peter, MD. *Dr. Peter Scardino's Prostate Book: The Complete Guide to Overcoming Prostate Cancer, Prostatitis and BPH*. New York: Avery. 2005.

Strumm, Stephen B., MD, and Pogliano, Donna L. *Primer on Prostate Cancer: The Empowered Patient's Guide*. Hollywood, FL: Life Extension Media. 2005.

Walsh, Patrick C., MD. *Dr. Patrick Walsh's Guide to Surviving Prostate Cancer*. New York: Warner Books. 2002.

Lung Cancer

Cox, Barbara G., Carr, David T., Harmon, Eloise, and Lee, Robert E. *Living with Lung Cancer: A Guide for Patients and Their Families*. 4th edition. Gainesville, FL: Triad. 1998.

Henschke, Claudia I., McCarthy, Peggy, and Wernick, Sarah. *Lung Cancer: Myths, Facts, Choices—and Hope*. New York: W. W. Norton. 2003.

Johnston, Lorraine. *Lung Cancer: Making Sense of Diagnosis, Treatment, and Options*. Sebastopol, CA: Patient Centered Guides. 2001.

Ruckdeschel, John C., MD. *Myths & Facts About Lung Cancer*. Melville, NY: PRR. 2002.

Colon Cancer

Couric, Katie (foreword), American Cancer Society, and Levin, Bernard. *American Cancer Society's Complete Guide to Colorectal Cancer*. Atlanta: American Cancer Society. 2005.

Johnston, Lorraine. *Colon & Rectal Cancer: A Comprehensive Guide for Patients &
Families.* Sebastopol, CA: Patient Centered Guides. 2000.

Miskovitz, Paul, MD. *What to Do If You Get Colon Cancer: A Specialist Helps You Take
Charge and Make Informed Choices.* New York: John Wiley & Sons. 1997.

Pazdur, Richard, MD, and Royce, Melanie, MD. *Myths & Facts about Colorectal
Cancer.* 2nd edition. Melville, NY: PRR. 2001.

Ovarian Cancer

Arnold, Nina Davidson. *Living with Ovarian Cancer: A Time for Truth, Hope, and
Love.* Kearney, NE: Morris. 2003.

Miron, Ayala. *Ovarian Cancer Journeys: Survivors Share Their Stories to Help Others.*
Lincoln, NE: iUniverse. 2004.

Piver, M. Steven, MD, and Eltabbakh, Gamal, MD. *Myths & Facts About Ovarian
Cancer.* 3rd edition. Melville, NY: PRR. 2002.

Tilberis, Liz. *No Time to Die: Living with Ovarian Cancer.* New York: HarperPaperbacks. 1999.

Lymphoma

Adler, Elizabeth M. *Living with Lymphoma: A Patient's Guide.* Baltimore: Johns
Hopkins University Press. 2005.

Johnston, Lorraine, and Lamb, Linda. *Non-Hodgkin's Lymphomas: Making Sense
of Diagnosis, Treatment, and Options.* Sebastopol, CA: Patient Centered
Guides. 1999.

Mauch, Peter M., MD, Armitage, James O., MD, Harris, Nancy L., MD, Dalla-
Favera, Riccardo, MD, and Coiffier, Bertrand, MD. *Non-Hodgkin's Lymphomas.*
Philadelphia: Lippincott Williams & Wilkins. 2003.

Parker, James N., MD, and Parker, Philip M., MD (editors). *The Official Patient's
Sourcebook on Adult Hodgkin's Disease: A Revised and Updated Directory for the Internet Age.* San Diego: Icon Health Publications. 2002.

LEVEL TWO: CONNECTION WITH OTHERS

Anderson, Greg. *The Cancer Conqueror: An Incredible Journey to Wellness.* Kansas
City, MO: Andrews McMeel. 2000.

Babcock, Elise. *When Life Becomes Precious: The Essential Guide for Patients,
Loved Ones, and Friends of Those Facing Serious Illnesses.* New York: Bantam
Books. 1997.

Benjamin, Harold H. *Wellness Community Guide to Fighting for Recovery from Cancer.* Los Angeles: Jeremy P. Tarcher. 1995.

LeShan, Lawrence, PhD. *Cancer as a Turning Point: A Handbook for People with
Cancer, Their Families, and Health Professionals.* London: Penguin Books. 1989.

Ornish, Dean, MD. *Love & Survival: The Scientific Basis for the Healing Power of Intimacy*. New York: HarperPaperbacks. 1999.

Rosenbaum, Ernest, MD, and Rosenbaum, Isadora. *Everyone's Guide to Cancer Supportive Care: A Comprehensive Handbook for Patients and Their Families*. Kansas City, MO: Andrews McMeel. 2005.

Schimmel, Selma R., and Fox, Barry. *Cancer Talk: Voices of Hope and Endurance from "The Group Room," the World's Largest Cancer Support Group*. New York: Broadway Books. 1999.

Spiegel, David, MD. *Living Beyond Limits: New Hope and Help for Facing Life-Threatening Illness*. Boulder, CO: Bull Publishing. 2005.

LEVEL THREE: THE BODY AS GARDEN

Complementary and Alternative Cancer Therapies

Boik, John. *Cancer and Natural Medicine: A Textbook of Basic Science and Clinical Research*. Princeton, MN: Oregon Medical Press. 1995.

Cassileth, Barrie R., PhD. *The Alternative Medicine Handbook: The Complete Reference Guide to Alternative and Complementary Therapies*. New York: W. W. Norton. 1999.

Cassileth, Barrie R., PhD, Deng, Gary, PhD, and Vickers, Andrew, PhD. *PDQ Integrative Oncology: Complementary Therapies in Cancer Care*. Hamilton, Ontario: B. C. Decker. 2005.

Cohen, Isaac, OMD, LAc, Tripathy, Debu, MD, and Tagliaferri, Mary, MD, LAc. (editors). *Breast Cancer: Beyond Convention: The World's Foremost Authorities on Complementary and Alternative Medicine Offer Advice on Healing*. New York: Atria Books. 2003.

Goldberg, Burton, Anderson, John W., and Trivieri, Larry. *Alternative Medicine: The Definitive Guide*. 2nd edition. Berkeley, Ca: Ten Speed Press. 2002.

Gordon, James S., MD, and Curtin, Sharon. *Comprehensive Cancer Care: Integrating Alternative, Complementary, and Conventional Therapies*. New York: HarperCollins Publishers. 2001.

Hartwell, Jonathan L. *Plants Used Against Cancer*. Lawrence, MA: Quarterman Publications. 1984.

Jonas, Wayne B., MD, and Levin, Jeffrey S., MD, PhD. *Essentials of Complementary and Alternative Medicine*. Philadelphia: Lippincott Williams & Wilkins. 1999.

Labriola, Dan, ND. *Complementary Cancer Therapies: Combining Traditional and Alternative Approaches for the Best Possible Outcome*. Roseville, CA: Prima Publishing. 2000.

Lerner, Michael, PhD. *Choices in Healing: Integrating the Best of Conventional and Complementary Approaches to Cancer*. Cambridge, MA: MIT Press.1996.

Moss, Ralph W., PhD. *Herbs Against Cancer: History and Controversy.* Brooklyn, NY: Equinox Press. 1998.

O'Toole, Carole, with Hendricks, Carolyn B., MD. *Healing Outside the Margins. The Survivor's Guide to Integrative Cancer Care.* Washington, D.C.: LifeLine Press. 2002.

Simon, David, MD. *Return to Wholeness: Embracing Body, Mind, and Spirit in the Face of Cancer.* New York: John Wiley & Sons. 1999.

Walters, Richard. *Options: The Alternative Cancer Therapy Book For People Who Want to Make Informed Decisions About Alternative Cancer Treatments.* Garden City, NY: Avery. 1993.

Diet and Nutrition

Balch, Phyllis, and Balch, James. *Prescription for Nutritional Healing.* 3rd edition. Garden City, NY: Avery. 2000.

Binzel, Philip E., MD. *Alive and Well: One Doctor's Experience with Nutrition in the Treatment of Cancer Patients.* Westlake Village, CA: American Media. 1994.

Calhoun, Susan. *Nutrition, Cancer and You: What You Need to Know, and Where to Start.* Lenexa, KS: Addax. 2002.

Chace, Daniella, Keane, Maureen, and Lung, John A. *What to Eat If You Have Cancer: A Guide to Adding Nutritional Therapy to Your Treatment Plan.* New York: McGraw-Hill. 1996.

Cousens, Gabriel, MD. *Rainbow Green Live-Food Cuisine.* Berkeley, CA: North Atlantic Books. 2003.

Diamond, Harvey. *Fit for Life: A New Beginning.* New York: Kensington, Twin Streams. 2003.

Katz, Rebecca, Tomassi, Marsha, and Edelson, Mat. *One Bite at a Time: Nourishing Recipes for People with Cancer, Survivors, and Their Caregivers.* Berkeley, CA: Celestial Arts. 2004.

Kushi, Michio, and Jack, Alex. *The Cancer Prevention Diet: Michio Kushi's Macrobiotic Blueprint for the Prevention and Relief of Disease.* New York: Griffin/St. Martin's. 1994.

Pitchford, Paul. *Healing with Whole Foods: Asian Traditions and Modern Nutrition.* 3rd edition. Berkeley, CA: North Atlantic Books. 2003.

Robbins, John. *Diet for a New America: How Your Food Choices Affect Your Health, Happiness and the Future of Life on Earth.* Tiburon, CA: H. J. Kramer. 1998.

Spiller, Gene, PhD, and Bruce, Bonnie, MD, PhD, RD. *Cancer Survivor's Nutrition and Health Guide: Eating Well and Getting Better During and After Cancer Treatment.* Rocklin, CA: Prima Publishing. 1997.

Quillin, Patrick, PhD, RD. *Beating Cancer with Nutrition: Clinically Proven and Easy-to-Follow Strategies to Dramatically Improve Your Quality of Life and Chances for a Complete Remission.* Tulsa, OK: The Nutrition Times Press. 2005.

Herbs and Supplements

Blumenthal, Mark, Brinkmann, Josef, and Wollschlaeger, Bernd. *The ABC Clinical Guide to Herbs*. New York: Thieme Medical Publishers. 2003.

Bown, Deni. *Encyclopedia of Herbs & Their Uses*. New York: DK Adult Publishing. 2001.

Chevallier, Andrew. *Encyclopedia of Herbal Medicine: The Definitive Reference to 550 Herbs and Remedies for Common Ailments*. New York: DK Publishing. 2000.

Foster, Steven, and Tyler, Varro E. *Tyler's Honest Herbal: A Sensible Guide to the Use of Herbs and Related Remedies*. 4th edition. Binghamton, NY: Haworth Press. 1999.

Frawley, David, and Lad, Vasant. *The Yoga of Herbs: An Ayurvedic Guide to Herbal Medicine*. Delhi, India: Motilal Banarsidass. 2004.

Griffith, H. Winter. *Vitamins, Herbs, Minerals & Supplements: The Complete Guide*. Cambridge, MA: Fisher Books. 2000.

Hogan, Victoria. *The All in One Guide to Herbs, Vitamins & Minerals: The Quick and Easy Reference for Everything You Need to Know*. Blaine, WA: Alive Books. 1999.

Murray, Michael T., ND. *The Healing Power of Herbs: The Enlightened Person's Guide to the Wonders of Medicinal Plants*. 2nd edition. New York: Gramercy Publishing. 2004.

Navarra, Tova (editor), Navarra, John G., and Lipkowitz, Myron A. *Encyclopedia of Vitamins, Minerals and Supplements*. 2nd edition. New York: Facts On File. 2004.

Tierra, Michael. *Treating Cancer with Herbs: An Integrative Approach*. Santa Fe, NM: Lotus Press. 2003.

Aromatherapy

Edwards, Victoria H. *The Aromatherapy Companion: Medicinal Uses, Ayurvedic Healing, Body-Care Blends, Perfumes & Scents, Emotional Health & Well Being*. North Adams, MA : Storey Publishing. 1999.

Lawless, Julia. *The Complete Illustrated Guide to Aromatherapy: A Practical Approach to the Use of Essential Oils for Health and Well-Being*. New York: Barnes & Noble. 1999.

Schnaubelt, Kurt. *Advanced Aromatherapy: The Science of Essential Oil Therapy*. Rochester, VT: Healing Arts Press. 1998.

Wildwood, Christine. *The Encyclopedia of Aromatherapy*. Rochester, VT: Inner Traditions International. 1996.

Exercise

Andes, Karen. *The Complete Book of Fitness: Mind, Body, Spirit*. New York: Three Rivers Press. 1999.

Asanaro. *The Secret Art of Seamm Jasani: 58 Movements for Eternal Youth from Ancient Tibet*. Los Angeles, CA: Jeremy P. Tarcher. 2003.

Farhi, Donna. *The Breathing Book: Vitality & Good Health Through Essential Breath Work*. New York: Owl Books. 1996.

Feldenkrais, Moshe. *Awareness Through Movement: Easy-to-Do Health Exercises to Improve Your Posture, Vision, Imagination, and Personal Awareness*. San Francisco: HarperSanFrancisco. 1991.

Hendricks, Gay. *Conscious Breathing: Breathwork for Health, Stress Release, and Personal Mastery*. New York: Bantam Books. 1997.

Hoffman, Lisa, and Freeland, Alison. *The Healing Power of Movement: How to Benefit from Physical Activity During Your Cancer Treatment*. Cambridge, MA: Perseus Publishing. 2002.

Kelder, Peter, and Siegel, Bernie S. *Ancient Secret of the Fountain of Youth*. Book 1. New York: Doubleday. 1998.

Kilham, Christopher S. *The Five Tibetans: Five Dynamic Exercises for Health, Energy and Personal Power*. Rochester, NY: Healing Arts Press. 1994.

Manne, Joy. *Conscious Breathing: How Shamanic Breathwork Can Transform Your Life*. Berkeley, CA: North Atlantic Books. 2004.

Reichler, Gayle, and Burke, Nancy. *Active Wellness: A Personalized 10 Step Program for a Healthy Body, Mind & Spirit*. Alexandria, VA: Time-Life. 1998.

Schwartz, Anna L., and Armstrong, Lance (foreword). *Cancer Fitness: Exercise Programs for Patients and Survivors*. New York: Fireside/Simon & Schuster. 2004.

Zi, Nancy. *The Art of Breathing: Six Simple Lessons to Improve Performance, Health & Well-Being*. 4th edition. Glendale, CA: VIVI. 2000.

Yoga

Desikachar, T. K. V. *The Heart of Yoga: Developing a Personal Practice*. Rochester, VT: Inner Traditions International: 1999.

Farhi, Donna. *Yoga Mind, Body & Spirit: A Return to Wholeness*. New York: Owl Books. 2000.

Feuerstein, Georg. *The Shambhala Guide to Yoga: An Essential Introduction to the Principles and Practice of an Ancient Tradition*. Boston: Shambhala. 1996.

Holtby, Lisa. *Healing Yoga for People Living with Cancer*. Lanham, MD: Taylor Trade Publishing. 2004.

Iyengar, B. K. S., and Menuhin, Yehudi (foreword). *Light on Yoga: The Bible of Modern Yoga*. New York: Schocken Books. 1995.

Pierce, Margaret D., and Pierce, Martin G. *Yoga for Your Life: A Practice Manual of Breath and Movement for Every Body*. New York: Sterling Publishing. 1999.

Sarley, Dinabandhu, and Sarley, Ila. *The Essentials of Yoga*. New York: Dell. 1999.

Satchidananda, Sri Swami. *Integral Yoga Hatha*. Buckingham, VA: Integral Yoga Distribution. 1998.

Sell, Christine, and Friend, John (foreword). *Yoga from the Inside Out: Making Peace With Your Body Through Yoga*. Prescott, AZ: Hohm Press. 2003.

Sivananda Yoga Center and Devananda, Vishnu. *The Sivananda Companion to Yoga: A Complete Guide to the Physical Postures, Breathing Exercises, Diet, Relaxation, and Meditation Techniques of Yoga*. New York: Fireside/Simon & Schuster. 2000.

Relaxation

Benson, Herbert, MD, and Klipper, Miriam Z. *The Relaxation Response*. New York: HarperPaperbacks. 2000.

Blumenfield, Larry (editor), Gawain, Shakti, and Folan, Lilias (contributor). *The Big Book of Relaxation: Simple Techniques to Control the Excess Stress in Your Life*. Roslyn, NY: Relaxation Company. 1994.

Davis, Martha, Eshelman, Elizabeth Robbins, and McKay, Matthew. *Relaxation & Stress Reduction Workbook*. 5th edition. Oakland, CA: New Harbinger. 2000.

George, Mike. *Learn to Relax: A Practical Guide to Easing Tension and Conquering Stress*. San Francisco: Chronicle Books. 1998.

Lacroix, Nitya, and Bown, Deni. *101 Essential Tips: Relaxation*. New York: DK Publishing Merchandise. 1998.

Lazarus, Judith. *Stress Relief & Relaxation Techniques*. New York: McGraw-Hill. 2000.

Levey, Joel, and Levey, Michelle. *Simple Meditation and Relaxation*. Berkeley, CA: Conrai Press. 1999.

Sutcliffe, Jenny. *The Complete Book of Relaxation Techniques*. Allentown, PA: People's Medical Society. 1996.

Massage

Atkinson, Mary, and Floyd, Esme. *The Complete Book of the Massage*. London: Carlton Books. 2004.

Bentley, Eilean. *The Essential Massage Book: The Complete Guide to the Primary Hands-on Therapy*. Sussex, England: Gaia Books. 2005.

Lidell, Lucinda. *The Book of Massage: The Complete Step-by-Step Guide to Eastern and Western Techniques*. 2nd edition. New York: Fireside/Simon & Schuster. 2001.

MacDonald, Gayle. *Medicine Hands: Massage Therapy for People with Cancer*. Portland, OR: Rudra Press. 1999.

Maxwell-Hudson, Clare. *The Complete Book of Massage*. New York: Random House. 1998.

Mitchell, Stewart. *The Complete Illustrated Guide to Massage: A Step-by-Step Approach to the Healing Art of Touch*. New York: Barnes & Noble. 1999.

Mumford, Susan. *Healing Massage: A Practical Guide to Relaxation and Well-Being*. New York: Plume. 1998.

Porter, Sarah. *Massage: For Health, Relaxation and Vitality*. New York: Lorenz Books. 1998.

Journaling

DeSalvo, Louise, PhD. *Writing as a Way of Healing: How Telling Our Stories Transforms Our Lives*. San Francisco: HarperSanFrancisco. 2002.

Forrest, Jan. *Coming Home to Ourselves: Journaling to Wholeness*. West Olive, MI: Heart to Heart. 1999.

Glass, Elaine, Gullo, Shirley M., and Gamiere, Maria. *Journaling Through the Storm: A Journal for Personal Reflections*. Pittsburgh, PA: Oncology Nursing Society. 1998.

Grason, Sandy. *Journolution: Journaling to Awaken Your Inner Voice, Heal Your Life and Manifest Your Dreams*. Novato, CA: New World Library. 2005.

Guarino, Lois. *Writing Your Authentic Self*. New York: Dell. 1999.

Hossler, Bill. *Keys to Open Your Heart: A Journaling Guide for Men and Women*. Fort Wayne, IN: Key Publishing. 2002.

Neimark, Neil F., MD. *The Handbook of Journaling: Tools for the Healing of Mind, Body & Spirit*. 2nd edition. Irvine, CA: R. E. P. Technologies. 2000.

Parnell, Anthony D., MSW. *Healing Through Writing: A Journaling Guide to Emotional and Spiritual Growth*. Lincoln, NE: iUniverse. 2005.

Visualization and Guided Imagery

Achterberg, Jeanne, PhD, Dossey, Barbara, RN, MS, FAAN, and Kolkmeier, Leslie, RN, MEd. *Rituals of Healing: Using Imagery for Health and Wellness*. New York: Bantam New Age Books. 1994.

Brigham, Deirdre Davis. *Imagery for Getting Well: Clinical Applications of Behavioral Medicine*. New York: W. W. Norton. 1996.

Fanning, Patrick. *Visualization for Change: A Step-by-Step Guide to Using the Powers of Your Imagination for Self-improvement, Therapy, Healing, and Pain Control*. 2nd edition. Oakland, CA: New Harbinger. 1994.

Gawain, Shakti. *Creative Visualization*. Novato, CA: New World Library. 2002.

Hammond, Barbara Kline. *Cancer's Gifts: Meditations on Being, Healing, and Forgiving*. Santa Fe, NM: Sunstone Press. 2003.

Naparstek, Belleruth. *Staying Well with Guided Imagery: How to Harness the Power of Your Imagination for Health and Healing*. New York: Warner Books. 1995.

Rossman, Martin L., MD. *Guided Imagery for Self-Healing: An Essential Resource for Anyone Seeking Wellness*. 2nd edition. Tiburon, CA: H. J. Kramer. 2000.

Acupuncture

Firebrace, Peter. *Acupuncture: How It Works, How It Cures*. New York: McGraw-Hill. 1999.

Hecker, Hans-Ulrich, Steveling, Angelika, Peuker, Elmar, Kastner, Jorg, and Liebchen, Kay. *Color Atlas of Acupuncture: Body Points, Ear Points, Trigger Points*. New York: Thieme Medical Publishers. 2001.

Kidson, Ruth. *Acupuncture for Everyone: What It Is, Why It Works, and How It Can Help You.* Rochester, VT: Healing Arts Press. 2001.

Mole, Peter. *Acupuncture: Energy Balancing for Body, Mind and Spirit.* Boston, MA: Element Books. 1997.

Nightingale, Michael. *Acupuncture: An Introductory Guide to the Technique and Its Benefits.* North Pomfret, VT: Trafalgar Square. 1997.

Rothfeld, Glenn S., and LeVert, Suzzanne. *The Acupuncture Response: Balance Energy and Restore Health—a Western Doctor Tells You How.* New York: McGraw-Hill. 2001.

Chiropractic

Burke, Edmund J., and Gravelle, Brent L. *Wellness and Chiropractic.* Longmeadow, MA: Movement Publications. 1997.

Haldeman, Scott. *Principles and Practices of Chiropractic.* New York: McGraw-Hill. 2004.

Koch, William H. *Chiropractic: The Superior Alternative.* New York: Bayeux Arts. 1997.

McGill, Leonard. *The Chiropractor's Health Book: Simple, Natural Exercises for Relieving Headaches, Tension, and Back Pain.* New York: Three Rivers Press. 1997.

Redwood, Daniel. *Contemporary Chiropractic.* New York: Churchill Livingstone. 1997.

Homeopathy

Hammond, Christopher. *The Complete Family Guide to Homeopathy: An Illustrated Encyclopedia of Safe and Effective Remedies.* New York: Element Books/Penguin Studios. 1999.

Jonas, Wayne B., and Jacobs, Jennifer. *Healing with Homeopathy: The Complete Guide.* New York: Warner Books. 1996.

Lansky, Amy L., PhD. *Impossible Cure: The Promise of Homeopathy.* Portola Valley, CA: RL Ranch Press. 2003.

Lockie, Andrew, MD, and Geddes, Nicola, MD. *Complete Guide to Homeopathy: The Principles and Practice of Treatment.* New York: DK Publishing. 2000.

Vithoulkas, George, and Tiller, William A. *Science of Homeopathy.* New York: Grove Atlantic. 1980.

Weiner, Michael. *The Complete Book of Homeopathy.* Garden City, NY: Avery. 1998.

Therapeutic Touch

Airey, Raje. *Healing Hands: A Concise Guide to the Therapeutic Power of Touch.* London: Southwater Publishing. 2004.

Cowens, Deborah, and Monte, Tom. *A Gift for Healing: How You Can Use Therapeutic Touch.* New York: Three Rivers Press. 1996.

Krieger, Dolores. *Accepting Your Power to Heal: The Personal Practice of Therapeutic Touch.* Santa Fe, NM: Bear & Company. 1993.

Krieger, Dolores, PhD, RN. *Therapeutic Touch as Transpersonal Healing.* New York: Lantern Books. 2002.

Kunz, Dora, and Krieger, Dolores, PhD. *The Spiritual Dimension of Therapeutic Touch.* Rochester, VT: Inner Traditions, Bear & Company. 2002.

MacRae, Janet. *Therapeutic Touch: A Practical Guide.* New York: Alfred A. Knopf. 1990.

Reiki Therapy

Horan, Paula. *Empowerment Through Reiki: Path to Personal and Global Transformation.* Delhi, India: Motilal Banarsidass. 2003.

Lubeck, Walter. *The Complete Reiki Handbook: Basic Introduction and Methods of Natural Application, a Complete Guide for Reiki Practice.* Delhi, India: Motilal Banarsidass. 2003.

Parkes, Chris, and Parkes, Penny. *Reiki: The Essential Guide to the Ancient Healing Art.* London: Ebury Press. 2005.

Shuffey, Sandi Leir. *Reiki: A Beginner's Guide.* London: Hodder and Stoughton. 1998.

Stein, Diane. *Essential Reiki: A Complete Guide to an Ancient Healing Art.* Freedom, CA: Crossing Press. 2003.

Upczak, Patrick Rose. *Reiki: A Way of Life.* Nederland, CO: Synchronicity Publishing. 1999.

EASTERN HEALING TRADITIONS

Ayurveda

Frawley, David. *Ayurveda and the Mind: The Healing of Consciousness.* Delhi, India: Motilal Banarsidass. 2000.

Frawley, David. *Ayurvedic Healing: A Comprehensive Guide.* 2nd edition. Twin Lakes, WI: Lotus Press. 2000.

Godagama, Shantha, and Hodgkinson, Liz. *The Handbook of Ayurveda: India's Medical Wisdom Explained.* Berkeley, CA: North Atlantic Books. 2004.

Joshi, Sunil V. *Ayurveda and Panchakarma: The Science of Healing and Rejuvenation.* Twin Lakes, WI: Lotus Light Publications. 1997.

Krishan, Shuhra. *Essential Ayurveda: What It Is and What It Can Do for You.* Novato, CA: New World Library. 2003.

Lad, Vasant. *The Complete Book of Ayurvedic Home Remedies.* New York: Three Rivers Press. 1999.

Lad, Vasant. *The Encyclopedia of Ayurveda.* Albuquerque, NM: Ayurveda Press. 2001.

Mishra, Lakshmi C. *Scientific Basis for Ayurvedic Therapies.* New York: Taylor & Francis/CRC Press. 2003.

Svoboda, Robert. *Ayurveda: Life, Health and Longevity.* Albuquerque, NM: Ayurveda Press. 2004.

Tiwari, Maya. *Ayurveda Secrets of Healing: The Complete Ayurvedic Guide to Healing.* Delhi, India: Motilal Banarsidass. 1998.

Traditional Chinese Medicine

Beinfeld, Harriet, and Corngold, Efrom. *Between Heaven and Earth: A Guide to Chinese Medicine.* New York: Ballantine. 1992.

Kaptchuk, Ted J., OMD. *The Web That Has No Weaver: Understanding Chinese Medicine.* New York: McGraw-Hill. 2003.

Kun, Jia. *Prevention and Treatment of Carcinoma in Traditional Chinese Medicine.* Hong Kong: The Commercial Press. 1985.

Leung, Albert Y. *Chinese Herbal Remedies.* New York: Universe Books. 1989.

Wisemann, Nigel. *Fundamentals of Chinese Medicine: Zhong Yi Xue Ji Chu.* Brookline, MA: Paradigm Publications. 1997.

Wisemann, Nigel. *A Practical Dictionary of Chinese Medicine.* 2nd edition. Brookline, MA: Paradigm Publications. 1997.

Williams, Tom. *Chinese Medicine, Acupuncture, Herbal Remedies, Nutrition, Qigong and Meditation for Total Health.* London: Chrysalis Books. 2002.

Tibetan Medicine

Aschoff, Jürgen C., and Rösing, Ina (editors). *Tibetan Medicine. East Meets West— West Meets East.* Ulm, Germany: Fabri Verlag. 1997.

Avedon, John F. (editor). *The Buddha's Art of Healing: Tibetan Paintings Rediscovered.* New York: Rizzoli Bookstore/Arthur M. Sackler Gallery. 1998.

Chang, Garma C. C. *Teachings of Tibetan Yoga: An Introduction to the Spiritual, Mental, and Physical Exercises of the Tibetan Religion.* Secaucus, NJ: Citadel Press. 1993.

Clark, Barry, Dr. (translator). *The Quintessence Tantras of Tibetan Medicine.* Ithaca, NY: Snow Lion Publications. 1995.

Clifford, Terry. *Tibetan Buddhist Medicine and Psychiatry: The Diamond Healing.* Delhi, India: Motilal Banarsidass. 2003.

Donden, Yeshi, Dr. *Health Through Balance: An Introduction to Tibetan Medicine.* Ithaca, NY: Snow Lion Publications. 1986.

Donden, Yeshi, and Kelsang, Jhampa (translator). *The Ambrosia Heart Tantra: The Secret Oral Teaching on the Eight Branches of the Science of Healing.* Dharamsala, India: Library of Tibetan Works and Archives. 1995.

Dummer, Tom. *Tibetan Medicine, and Other Holistic Health-Care Systems.* New Delhi, India: Paljour Publications. 2001.

Fenton, Peter. *Tibetan Healing: The Modern Legacy of Medicine Buddha.* Wheaton, IL: Quest Books. 1999.

Finckh, Elisabeth. *Foundations of Tibetan Medicine: According to the Book rGyud bzi.* 2 volumes. 2nd edition. London: Element Books. 1994.

Parfionovitch, Yuri (editor). *Tibetan Medical Paintings: Illustrations to the Blue Beryl Treatise of Sangye Gyamtso (1653–1705: Plates and Text).* New York: Henry N. Abrams. 1992.

Rinpoche, Chokyi Nyima. *Medicine and Compassion: A Tibetan Lama's Guidance for Caregivers.* Somerville, MA: Wisdom Publications. 2004.

Rinpoche, Khenchen Thrangu. *Medicine Buddha Teachings.* Ithaca, NY: Snow Lion Publications. 2004.

Samel, Gerti. *Tibetan Medicine: A Practical and Inspiration Guide to Diagnosing, Treating and Healing the Buddhist Way.* Boston: Little, Brown. 2004.

LEVEL FOUR: EMOTIONAL HEALING

Arenson, Gloria. *Five Simple Steps to Emotional Healing: The Last Self-Help Book You Will Ever Need.* New York: Fireside/Simon & Schuster. 2001.

Brach, Tara, PhD. *Radical Acceptance: Embracing Your Life With the Heart of a Buddha.* New York: Bantam Dell. 2003.

Brehony, Kathleen A., PhD. *After the Darkest Hour: How Suffering Begins the Journey to Wisdom.* New York: Henry Holt. 2000.

Borysenko, Joan, PhD. *Guilt Is the Teacher, Love Is the Lesson: A Book to Heal You, Heart and Soul.* New York: HarperCollins Publishers. 1993.

Bradshaw, John. *Healing the Shame That Binds You.* Deerfield Beach, FL: Health Communications. 2005.

Bradshaw, John. *Home Coming: Reclaiming and Championing Your Inner Child.* New York: Random House. 1992.

Greenspan, Miriam. *Healing Through the Dark Emotions: The Wisdom of Grief, Fear, and Despair.* Boston: Shambhala. 2004.

Jampolski, Gerald G., MD. *Love Is Letting Go of Fear.* Berkeley: Ten Speed Press. 2004.

Jampolski, Gerald G., MD. *Out of Darkness into the Light: A Journey of Inner Healing.* New York: Bantam Books. 1990.

Jampolski, Gerald G., MD. *Teach Only Love: The Twelve Principles of Attitudinal Healing.* Hillsboro, OR: Beyond Words Publishing. 2000.

Johnson, Robert. *Owning Your Own Shadow: Understanding the Dark Side of the Psyche.* San Francisco: HarperSanFrancisco. 1993.

Lerner, Harriet. *Fear and Other Uninvited Guests: Tackling the Anxiety, Fear, and Shame That Keep Us from Optimal Living and Loving.* New York: HarperCollins Publishers. 2004.

Schlessel-Harpham, Wendy, MD. *Happiness in a Storm: Facing Illness and Embracing Life as a Healthy Survivor*. New York: W. W. Norton. 2005.

Pennebaker, James W., PhD. *Opening Up: The Healing Power of Expressing Emotions*. New York: Guilford Press. 1997.

Zweig, Connie, PhD, and Wolf, Steve, PhD. *Romancing the Shadow: Illuminating the Dark Side of the Soul*. New York: Wellspring/Ballantine. 1999.

LEVEL FIVE: THE NATURE OF MIND

Allen, James. *As a Man Thinketh*. 3rd edition. San Diego, CA: Laurel Creek Press. 2000.

Benson, Herbert, MD. *Timeless Healing: The Power and Biology of Belief*. New York: Scribner. 1997.

Borysenko, Joan, PhD. *Minding the Body, Mending the Mind*. New York: Bantam Books. 1988.

Chodron, Thubten. *Taming the Monkey Mind*. Torrance, CA: Heian International. 1999.

Dossey, Larry, MD. *Meaning and Medicine: Lessons from a Doctor's Tales of Breakthrough and Healing*. New York: Bantam Books. 1991.

Doyle, Bruce I., III. *Before You Think Another Thought: An Illustrated Guide to Understanding How Your Thoughts and Beliefs Create Your Life*. Charlottesville, VA: Hampton Roads. 1997.

Jampolsky, Gerald G., MD, and Cirincione, Diane V. *Change Your Mind, Change Your Life*. New York: MJF Media. 2002.

Kabat-Zinn, Jon, PhD. *Coming to Our Senses: Healing Ourselves and the World Through Mindfulness*. New York: Hyperion. 2005.

McWilliams, Peter. *You Can't Afford the Luxury of a Negative Thought: A Book for People with Any Life-threatening Illness—Including Life*. Los Angeles: Prelude Press. 2001.

Moyers, Bill. *Healing and the Mind*. Frostburg, MD: Main Street Books. 1995.

Pelletier, Kenneth R. *Mind as Healer; Mind as Slayer: A Holistic Approach to Preventing Stress Disorders*. New York: Dell. 1977.

Robbins, Anthony. *Awaken the Giant Within: How to Take Immediate Control of Your Mental, Emotional, Physical, and Financial Destiny*. New York: Free Press. 1992.

Thondup, Tulku. *The Healing Power of Mind: Simple Meditation Exercises for Health, Well-Being, and Enlightenment*. Boston: Shambhala. 1996.

LEVEL SIX: LIFE ASSESSMENT

Purpose, Mission, and Vision

Adrienne, Carol. *Find Your Purpose, Change Your Life: Getting to the Heart of Your Life's Mission.* New York: HarperPaperbacks. 2001.

Bellamy, D. Richard. *12 Secrets for Manifesting Your Vision, Inspiration, and Purpose: How to Make Your Dreams Come True.* Houston: PHI Publishing. 1999.

Cassidy, Gail A. *Discover Your Passion: An Intuitive Search to Find Your Purpose in Life.* Westfield, NJ: Tomlyn Publications. 2000.

Covey, Stephen R., Merrill, Roger A., and Merrill, Robecca R. *First Things First: To Live, to Love, to Leave a Legacy.* New York: Simon & Schuster. 1996.

Frankl, Victor E. *Man's Search for Meaning.* Boston: Beacon Press. 2000.

Hansen, Mark Victor. *Future Diary.* Newport Beach, CA: Mark Victor Hansen Publishing. 1994.

Jones, Laurie Beth. *The Path: Creating Your Mission Statement for Work and for Life.* New York: Hyperion. 1998.

Levine, Stephen. *A Year to Live: How to Live This Year as if It Were Your Last.* New York: Thorsons. 1997.

McCarthy, Kevin W. *The On-Purpose Person: Making Your Life Make Sense.* Colorado Springs, CO: Pinon Press. 2001.

Millman, Dan. *The Life You Were Born to Live: A Guide to Finding Your Life Purpose.* Tiburon, CA: H. J. Kramer. 1995

Seale, Alan. *Soul Mission, Life Vision: Recognize Your True Gifts and Make Your Mark in the World.* York Beach, ME: Red Wheel/Weiser. 2003.

Letting Go: Death and Dying

Albom, Mitch. *Tuesdays with Morrie: An Old Man, A Young Man, and Life's Greatest Lesson.* New York: Broadway Books. 2002.

Byock, Ira, MD. *Dying Well: Peace and Possibilities at the End of Life.* New York: Riverhead Books. 1998.

Kübler-Ross, Elisabeth, MD. *On Death and Dying: What the Dying Have to Teach Doctors, Nurses, Clergy, and Their Own Families.* Minneapolis: Rebound, by Sagebrush Books. 1999.

Levine, Stephen. *Who Dies? An Investigation of Conscious Living and Conscious Dying.* Dublin: Gill & Macmillan. 2000.

Longaker, Christine. *Facing Death and Finding Hope: A Guide to the Emotional and Spiritual Care of the Dying.* Frostburg, MD: Main Street Books. 1998.

Mullin, Glenn H. *Living in the Face of Death: The Tibetan Tradition.* Ithaca, NY: Snow Lion Publications. 1998.

Singh, Kathleen Dowling. *The Grace in Dying: How We Are Transformed Spiritually as We Die.* San Francisco: HarperSanFrancisco. 1998.

Tadd, Ellen. *Death and Letting Go.* Montague, MA: Montague Press. 2003.

Tobin, Daniel R., MD, with Lindsey, Karen. *Peaceful Dying: The Step-by-Step Guide to Preserving Your Dignity, Your Choice, and Your Inner Peace at the End of Life.* Cambridge, MA: Perseus Books. 1999.

LEVEL SEVEN: THE NATURE OF SPIRIT

Ardagh, Arjuna Nick. *Relaxing into Clear Seeing.* San Rafael, CA: Self Xpress. 1998.

Byrom, Thomas. *The Heart of Awareness: A Translation of the Ashtavakra Gita.* Boston: Shambhala. 2001.

Dossey, Larry, MD. *Healing Beyond the Body: Medicine and the Infinite Reach of the Mind.* Boston: Shambhala. 2003.

Dossey, Larry, MD. *Healing Words: The Power of Prayer and the Practice of Medicine.* New York: HarperCollins Publishers. 1995.

Dossey, Larry, MD. *Prayer Is Good Medicine: How to Reap the Healing Benefits of Prayer.* New York: HarperCollins Publishers. 1997.

Easwaran, Eknath. *Strength in the Storm: Creating Calm in Difficult Times.* Tomales, CA: Nilgiri Press. 2005.

Evans-Wentz, Walter Yeeling (editor). *The Tibetan Book of the Great Liberation.* New York: Oxford University Press. 1983.

Feldman, Christina. *Silence: How to Find Inner Peace in a Busy World.* Berkeley, CA: Rodmell Press, 2003.

Garfield, Jay L. (translation and commentary). *The Fundamental Wisdom of the Middle Way: Nagarjuna's Mulamadhyamakakarika.* New York: Oxford University Press. 1995.

Godman, David. *Nothing Ever Happened.* Boulder, CO: Avadhuta Foundation. 1998.

Godman, David (editor). *Be as You Are: The Teachings of Sri Ramana Maharshi.* London: Arkana Books. 1991.

Goleman, Daniel, PhD, and Tarcher, J. P. *The Meditative Mind.* New York: G. P. Putnam's Sons. 1996.

His Holiness the Dalai Lama. *The Meaning of Life from a Buddhist Perspective.* (Translated and edited by Jeffery Hopkins.) Boston: Wisdom Publications. 1992.

His Holiness the Dalai Lama and Cutler, Howard, MD. *The Art of Happiness: A Handbook for Living.* New York: Riverhead Books. 1998.

Huxley, Aldous. *The Perennial Philosophy.* New York: Perennial Books. 2004.

Kabat-Zinn, Jon, PhD. *Full-Catastrophe Living: Using the Wisdom of Your Body and Mind to Face Stress, Pain, and Illness.* New York: Delta. 1990.

Kabat-Zinn, Jon, PhD. *Wherever You Go, There You Are.* New York: Hyperion. 2004.

Levine, Stephen. *A Gradual Awakening*. Garden City, NY: Anchor Press/Double-day. 1989.

Miller, Barbara Stoler (translator). *The Bhagavad-Gita: Krishna's Counsel in Time of War*. New York: Bantam Books. 1986.

Nisargadatta, Maharaj. *I Am That*. Bangalore, India: Nesma Books. 1997.

Ponlap, Dzogchen. *Wild Awakening: The Heart of Mahamudra and Dzogchen*. Boston: Shambhala. 2003.

Poonja, Sri H.W.L., and de Jeger, Prashanti (editor). *The Truth Is*. San Anselmo, CA: Vidyasagar Publishing. 1999.

Poonja, Sri H. W. L., de Jeger, Prashanti, Vidyavati, and Yudhishtara (compilers and editors). *This: Prose and Poetry of Dancing Emptiness*. San Anselmo, CA: Vidyasagar Publishing. 1997.

Prabhavananda, Swami, and Isherwood, Christopher (translators). *Shankara's Crest-Jewel of Discrimination (Viveka-Chudamani)*. Hollywood, FL: Vedanta Press. 1978.

Rahula, Walpola. *What the Buddha Taught*. 2nd edition. New York: Grove Press. 1974.

Rinpoche, Sogyal. *The Tibetan Book of Living and Dying*. New York: HarperCollins Publishers. 1994.

Schuon, Frithjof. *The Transcendent Unity of Religions*. Wheaton, IL: Quest Books. 1993.

Smith, Huston. *The Forgotten Truth: The Common Vision of the World's Religions*. New York: HarperCollins Publishers. 1992.

Smith, Huston. *The World's Religions*. New York: HarperCollins Publishers. 1991.

Thurman, Robert A. F. (translator). *The Tibetan Book of the Dead*. New York: Bantam Books. 1994.

Venkatesananda, Swami. *Vasistha's Yoga*. Albany: State University of New York Press. 1993.

Zukav, Gary. *The Seat of the Soul*. New York: Fireside/Simon & Schuster. 1990

OTHER HELPFUL BOOKS

Anderson, Gregg. *Healing Wisdom: Wit, Insight and Inspiration for Anyone Facing Illness*. New York: Penguin Books. 1994.

Anderson, Gregg. *The 22 (Non-Negotiable) Laws of Wellness: Feel, Think, and Live Better Than You Ever Thought Possible*. New York: HarperCollins Publishers. 1995.

Bache, Christopher M. *Dark Night, Early Dawn*. Albany: State University of New York Press. 2000.

Barasch, Marc Ian. *The Healing Path: A Soul Approach to Illness*. New York: Penguin Books. 1993.

Brennan, Barbara Ann. *Light Emerging: The Journey of Personal Healing*. New York: Bantam Books. 1993.

Canfield, Jack, and Hansen, Mark Victor. *Chicken Soup for the Soul: 101 Stories to Open the Heart and Rekindle the Spirit*. Deerfield Beach, FL: Health Communications. 1996.

Canfield, Jack, Hansen, Mark Victor, Aubery, Patty, and Mitchell, Nancy, RN. *Chicken Soup for the Surviving Soul: 101 Stories of Courage and Inspiration from Those Who Have Survived Cancer*. Deerfield Beach, FL: Health Communications. 1996.

Campbell, Joseph. *The Hero with a Thousand Faces*. Princeton, NJ: Bollingen. 2004.

Carlson, Richard, PhD. *Don't Sweat the Small Stuff ... and It's All Small Stuff: Simple Ways to Stop the Little Things from Taking over Your Life*. New York: Hyperion. 1997.

Carlson, Richard, and Shield, Benjamin. *Handbook for the Soul*. Boston: Little, Brown. 1996.

Chilton Pearce, Joseph. *The Biology of Transcendence: A Blueprint of the Human Spirit*. South Paris, ME: Park Street Press. 2002.

Chodron, Pema. *When Things Fall Apart: Heart Advice for Difficult Times*. Boston: Shambhala. 2005.

Chopra, Deepak, MD. *Ageless Body, Timeless Mind: The Quantum Alternative to Growing Old*. New York: Harmony Books. 1993.

Chopra, Deepak, MD. *Quantum Healing: Exploring the Frontiers of Mind/Body Medicine*. New York: Bantam Books. 1990.

Chopra, Deepak, MD. *Unconditional Life: Mastering the Forces That Shape Personal Reality*. New York: Bantam Books. 1991.

Clifford, Christine. *Not Now ... I'm Having a No Hair Day: Humor & Healing for People with Cancer*. Duluth, MN: Pfeifer-Hamilton Publishers. 1996.

Cousins, Norman. *Anatomy of an Illness as Perceived by the Patient*. New York: W. W. Norton. 2005.

Cousins, Norman. *Head First: The Biology of Hope*. New York: E. P. Dutton. 1990.

Cunningham, Alastair J., PhD. *The Healing Journey, Overcoming the Crisis of Cancer*. Toronto: Key Porter Books. 1992.

Dass, Ram. *Be Here Now*. New York: Crown Publishers. 1971

Dass, Ram (compiler). *Miracle of Love. Stories About Neem Karoli Baba*. Santa Fe, NM: Hanuman Foundation. 1995.

Ellenberger, Henri F. *The Discovery of the Unconscious*. New York: Basic Books. 1981.

Gawain, Shakti, with King, Laurel. *Living in the Light: A Guide to Personal and Planetary Transformation*. San Rafael, CA: New World Library. 1998.

Gaynor, Mitchell, MD. *Healing Essence: A Cancer Doctor's Practical Program for Hope and Recovery*. New York: Kodansha America. 1995.

Gaynor, Mitchell, MD. *Sounds of Healing: A Physician Reveals the Therapeutic Power of Sound, Voice, and Music.* New York: Broadway Books. 1999.

Gordon, James S., MD. *Manifesto for a New Medicine.* Reading, MA: Addison-Wesley. 1997.

Grof, Stanislov, MD. *The Adventure of Self-Discovery.* Albany: State University of New York Press. 1988.

Grof, Stanislov, MD. *Beyond the Brain: Birth, Death, and Transcendence in Psychotherapy.* Albany: State University of New York Press. 1986.

Grof, Stanislov, MD. *Psychology of the Future: Lessons from Modern Consciousness Research.* Albany: State University of New York Press. 2000.

Hanh, Thich Nhat. *The Heart of the Buddha's Teaching: Transforming Suffering into Peace, Joy, and Liberation.* New York: Broadway Books. 1999.

Havorson-Boyd, Glenna, and Hunter, Lisa K. *Dancing in Limbo: Making Sense of Life After Cancer.* San Francisco: Jossey-Bass. 1995.

Hayward, Susan. *A Guide for the Advanced Soul: A Book of Insight.* Boston, MA: Little, Brown. 1995.

Jung, Carl, MD. *Memories, Dreams, Reflections.* New York: Vintage. 1989.

Jung, Carl, MD. *Modern Man in Search of Soul.* New York: Taylor & Francis. 2001.

Katie, Byron. *Loving What Is.* New York: Three Rivers Press. 2003.

Kornfield, Jack, PhD. *After the Ecstasy, the Laundry.* New York: Bantam Books. 2001.

Levine, Stephen, and Levine, Ondrea. *Embracing the Beloved: Relationship as a Path of Awakening.* New York: Doubleday. 1996.

Maslow, Abraham. *The Farther Reaches of Human Nature.* New York: Penguin Books. 1993.

Millman, Dan. *Sacred Journey of the Peaceful Warrior.* Tiburon, CA: H. J. Kramer/New World Library. 2004

Moore, Thomas. *Care of the Soul: A Guide for Cultivating Depth and Sacredness in Everyday Life.* New York: HarperCollins Publishers. 1992.

Naparstek, Belleruth. *Your Sixth Sense: Activating Your Psychic Potential.* New York: HarperCollins Publishers. 1997.

Pert, Candace B., PhD. *Molecules of Emotion: Why You Feel the Way You Feel.* New York: Scribner. 1997.

Radner, Gilda. *It's Always Something.* New York: Avon. 1995.

Remen, Rachel Naomi, MD. *Kitchen Table Wisdom: Stories That Heal.* New York: Riverhead Books. 1997.

Remen, Rachel Naomi, MD. *My Grandfather's Blessings: Stories of Strength, Refuge, and Belonging.* New York: Riverhead Books. 2001.

Rodegast, Pat. *Emmanuel's Book: A Manual for Living Comfortably in the Cosmos. 3 Volumes.* New York: Bantam Books. 1985.

Ryder, Brent G. *The Alpha Book on Cancer and Living.* Alameda, CA: The Alpha Institute. 1993.

Schulz, Mona Lisa, MD, PhD. *Awakening Intuition: Using Your Mind-Body Network for Insight and Healing.* New York: Harmony Books. 1998.

Siegel, Bernie, MD. *Love, Medicine, and Miracles: Lessons Learned About Self-Healing from a Surgeon's Experience with Exceptional Patients.* New York: HarperCollins Publishers. 1986.

Simon, David, MD. *The Wisdom of Healing: A Natural Mind-Body Program for Optimal Wellness.* New York: Harmony Books. 1997.

Simonton, O. Carl, MD. *Getting Well Again.* New York: Bantam Books. 1992.

Tolle, Eckhart. *The Power of Now: A Guide to Spiritual Enlightenment.* Novato, CA: New World Library. 2000.

Topf, Linda Noble, MA. *You Are Not Your Illness: Seven Principles for Meeting the Challenge.* New York: Simon & Schuster. 1995.

Trivieri, Larry. *Health on the Edge: Visionary Views of Healing in the New Millennium.* New York: Jeremy P. Tarcher. 2003.

Vaughn, Frances, PhD. *Shadows of the Sacred: Seeing Through Spiritual Illusions.* Backinprint.com. 2005.

Vaughan, Frances, PhD, and Walsh, Roger, MD, PhD. *A Gift of Peace: Selections from a Course in Miracles.* Los Angeles: Jeremy P. Tarcher. 1992.

Walsh, Roger, MD, PhD, and Vaughan, Frances, PhD (editors). *Paths Beyond Ego: The Transpersonal Vision.* New York: G. P. Putnam's Sons. 1993.

Warner, Gale, Kreger, David, and Siegel, Bernie S., MD. *Dancing at the Edge of Life: A Memoir.* New York: Hyperion. 1998.

Walsch, Neale Donald. *Conversations with God: An Uncommon Dialogue. 3 volumes.* New York: G. P. Putnam's Sons. 1998.

Weil, Andrew MD. *Health and Healing.* Boston: Houghton Mifflin. 1998.

Weil, Andrew, MD. *Healthy Aging: A Lifelong Guide to Your Physical and Spiritual Well-Being.* New York: Alfred A. Knopf. 2005.

Weil, Andrew, MD. *Spontaneous Healing: How to Discover and Enhance Your Body's Natural Ability to Maintain and Heal Itself.* New York: Alfred A. Knopf. 1995.

Welwood, John, PhD. *Toward a Psychology of Awakening: Buddhism, Psychotherapy, and the Path of Personal and Spiritual Transformation.* Boston: Shambhala. 2002.

Wilber, Ken. *Grace and Grit: Spirituality and Healing in the Life and Death of Treya Killam Wilber.* Boston: Shambhala. 1993.

Wilber, Ken. *The Marriage of Sense and Soul. Integrating Science and Religion.* New York: Broadway Books. 1999.

Wilber, Ken. *No Boundary: Eastern and Western Approaches to Personal Growth.* Boston: Shambhala. 2001.

Wilber, Ken. *The Spectrum of Consciousness.* 2nd edition. Wheaton, IL: Quest Books. 1993.

AUDIO PROGRAMS

The following audio programs provide wonderful guidance for deep relaxation, visualization, guided imagery, and self-healing for patients and families.

1. *Anxiety-Free*. Paraliminal. Paul R. Scheele. Learning Strategies Corporation. Minnetoka, MN. 2005.
2. *Cancer as a Turning Point: From Surviving to Thriving.* Jeanne Achterberg, PhD, et al. Sounds True. Louisville, CO. 2004.
3. *Contacting Your Inner Healer: A Guided Imagery Relaxation Tape with Action Plan.* Neil F. Neimark, MD. R. E. P. Technologies. Irvine, CA. 2002.
4. *Creative Visualization Meditations*. Shakti Gawain. New World Library. San Rafael, CA. 2002.
5. *Deep Relaxation*. Paraliminal. Paul R. Scheele. Learning Strategies Corporation. Minnetoka, MN. 2005.
6. *The Ease of Being: Guided Meditations for Centering and Healing*. Mary Maddux and Richard Maddux. Heart of Healing. Sonoma, CA. 2002.
7. *Effective Meditations for Health and Healing*. Meditation Contemporary. Effective Learning Systems. Bonita Springs, FL. 1995.
8. *Effective Meditations for Stress Relief. Contemporary Meditation Series.* Deirdre Griswold. Effective Learning Systems. Port Richmond, CA. 1995.
9. *Healing Journey*. Marci Archambeault. The Quest. Leominster, MA. 1996.
10. *Health Journeys: A Meditation to Help You with Chemotherapy*. Belleruth Naparstek. Time Warner AudioBooks. Los Angeles. 1991.
11. *Health Journeys: A Meditation to Help You with Radiation Therapy*. Belleruth Naparstek. Time Warner AudioBooks. Los Angeles. 1999.
12. *Health Journeys: For People with Cancer*. Belleruth Naparstek. Time Warner AudioBooks. Los Angeles. 2001.
13. *Health Journeys: For People with Depression*. Belleruth Naparstek. Time Warner AudioBooks. Los Angeles. 2000.
14. *Health Journeys: For People Experiencing Grief*. Belleruth Naparstek. Time Warner AudioBooks. Los Angeles. 1993.
15. *Health Journeys: For People Experiencing Stress*. Belleruth Naparstek. Time Warner AudioBooks. Los Angeles. 2000.
16. *Health Journeys: For People Managing Pain*. Belleruth Naparstek. Time Warner AudioBooks. Los Angeles. 2001.
17. *How to Meditate*. Lawrence LeShan. Audio Renaissance. New York. 2004.
18. *The Inner Art of Meditation*. Jack Kornfield. Sounds True. Louisville, CO. 2004.
19. *Meditation for Beginners*. Jack Kornfield. Sounds True. Louisville, CO. 2004.
20. *The Miracle of Mindfulness: A Manual on Meditation*. Abridged Audio Cassettes: Thich Nhat Hanh. Harper Audio. Carlsbad, CA. 1995.

21. *Peaceful Body, Quiet Mind: A Healing Program of Curative Images, Positive Affir-mations, and Serene Music.* Harriett Sanders. New Harbinger Publishers. Oakland, CA. 1995.

22. *Perfect Health.* Paraliminal. Paul R. Scheele. Learning Strategies Corporation. Minnetoka, MN. 2005.

23. *Self-Healing: Creating Your Health.* Louise L. Hay. Hay House Audio. Carlsbad, CA. 2004.

24. *Self Healing with Guided Imagery: How to Use the Power of Your Mind to Heal Your Body.* Andrew Weil, MD, and Martin L. Rossman, MD. Sounds True. Louisville, CO: 2004.

25. *The Soul of Healing Meditations.* Deepak Chopra. Rasa Music. New York. 2001.

26. *10-Minute Supercharger.* Paraliminal. Paul R. Scheele. Learning Strategies Corporation. Minnetoka, MN. 2005.

MUSIC

The following CDs offer warm, soothing music to facilitate rest, relaxation, meditation, healing, and the experience of joy and inner peace.

1. *Celtic Spirit: Narada Collection Series.* Celtic Legacy/Narada Media. 1996.

2. *Chant: The Benedictine Monks of Santo Domingo de Silos.* Angel. 1994.

3. *Cristofori's Dream.* David Lanz. Narada. 1999.

4. *In the Enchanted Garden.* Kevin Kern. Real Music. 1996.

5. *Following the Circle.* Dik Darnell. Variena Music. 1994.

6. *Graceful Passages: A Companion for Living and Dying.* Gary Malkin and Michael Stillwater. Wisdom of the World. 2001.

7. *Inner Voices.* R. Carlos Nakai. Canyon Records. 1999.

8. *The Magic of Healing Music, Kapha: Invigorating.* Bruce BecVar and Brian BecVar. Gus Swigert Management. 1998.

9. *The Magic of Healing Music, Pitta: Calming.* Bruce BecVar and Brian BecVar. Gus Swigert Management. 1998.

10. *The Magic of Healing Music, Vata: Relaxing.* Bruce BecVar and Brian BecVar. Gus Swigert Management. 1998.

11. *Music as Medicine.* Nawang Khechong and R. Carlos Nakai. Gemini Sun Records. 2005.

12. *O'cean: Flute Music with Humpback Whale Sounds.* Larkin. Narada. 1985.

13. *Praises for the World.* Jennifer Berezan. Edge of Wonder. 2002.

14. *Reiki: Hands of Light.* Deuter. New Earth Records. 2002.

15. *Returning.* Jennifer Berezan. Edge of Wonder. 2001.

16. *The Silent Path.* Robert Haig Coxon. RHC Productions. 1996.

APPENDIX 2

CANCER SUPPORT ORGANIZATIONS

American Brain Tumor Association
2720 River Road
Des Plaines, IL 60018
(800) 886-2282
www.abta.org

American Cancer Society National Headquarters
1599 Clifton Road, N.E.
Atlanta, GA 30329
(800) 227-2345
www.cancer.org

American Pain Society
4700 West Lake Avenue
Glenview, IL 60025
(847) 375-4715
www.ampainsoc.org

American Society of Clinical Oncology
1900 Duke Street, Suite 200
Alexandria, VA 22314
(703) 299-0150
www.asco.org

American Urological Association Foundation
1000 Corporate Boulevard
Linthicum, MD 21090
(800) 828-7866
www.auanet.org

Brain Tumor Society
124 Watertown Street, Suite 3H
Watertown, MA 02472
(800) 770-8287
www.tbts.org

Caitlin Raymond International (Bone Marrow) Registry
University of Massachusetts Medical Center
55 Lake Avenue North
Worcester, MA 01655
(800) 726-2824
www.crir.org

Cancer Care, Inc.
275 Seventh Avenue
New York, NY 10001
(800) 813-4673
www.cancercare.org

Cancervive
11636 Chayote Street
Los Angeles, CA 90049
(310) 203-9232
www.cancervive.org

Candlelighters Childhood Cancer Foundation
3910 Warner Street
Kensington, MD 20895
(800) 366-2223
www.candlelighters.org

CANHELP
P.O. Box 103
Port Gamble, WA 98364
(800) 565-1732
www.canhelp.com

Children's Hospice International
901 North Pitt Street, Suite 230
Alexandria, VA 22314
(800) 242-4453
www.chionline.org

Commonweal
Cancer Help Program
P.O. Box 316
Bolinas, CA 94924
(415) 868-0970
www.commonweal.org

Corporate Angel Network
Westchester County Airport
One Loop Road
White Plains, NY 10604
(914) 328-1313
www.corpangelnetwork.org

Gilda Radner Familial Ovarian Cancer Registry
Roswell Park Cancer Institute
Elm and Carlton Streets
Buffalo, NY 14263
(800) 682-7426
www.ovariancancer.com

Hospice Education Institute
3 Unity Square
Machiasport, ME 04655
(800) 331-1620
www.hospiceworld.org

International Myeloma Foundation
12650 Riverside Drive, Suite 206
North Hollywood, CA 91607
(800) 452-2873
www.myeloma.org

Leukemia and Lymphoma Society
1311 Mamaroneck Avenue, Suite 310
White Plains, NY 10605
(800) 955-4572
www.leukemia-lymphoma.org

Lymphoma Foundation of America
814 North Garfield Street
Arlington, VA 22201
(703) 875-9800
www.lymphomahelp.org

Lymphoma Research Foundation of America
111 Broadway, 19th Floor
New York, NY 10006
(800) 235-6848
www.lymphoma.org

Make-a-Wish Foundation of America
3550 North Central Avenue, Suite 300
Phoenix, AZ 85012
(800) 722-9474
www.wish.org

National Alliance of Breast Cancer Organizations
9 East 37th Street, 10th Floor
New York, NY 10016
(212) 719-0154
www.nabco.org

National Breast Cancer Coalition
1101 17th Street, NW, Suite 1300
Washington, DC 20036
(800) 622-2838
www.natlbcc.org

National Cancer Institute
Building 31, Room 10A19
9000 Rockville Pike
Bethesda, MD 20892
(800) 422-6237
www.cancer.gov

National Center for Complementary and Alternative Medicine
NCCAM Clearinghouse
P.O. Box 7923
Gaithersburg, MD 20898
(888) 644-6226
www.nccam.nih.gov

National Coalition for Cancer Survivorship
1010 Wayne Avenue, Suite 770
Silver Spring, MD 20910
(301) 650-9127
www.cansearch.org

National Family Caregivers Association
10400 Connecticut Avenue, Suite 500
Kensington, MD 20895
(800) 896-3650
www.thefamilycaregiver.org

National Hospice and Palliative Care Organization
1700 Diagonal Road, Suite 625
Alexandria, VA 22314
(800) 658-8898
www.nhpco.org

National Leukemia Research Association
585 Stewart Avenue, Suite 18
Garden City, NY 11530
(516) 222-1944
www.childrensleukemia.org

National Lymphedema Network
1611 Telegraph Avenue, Suite 1111
Oakland, CA 94612
(800) 541-3259
www.lymphnet.org

National Ovarian Cancer Coalition
500 Spanish River Boulevard, Suite 8
Boca Raton, FL 33431
(888) 682-7426
www.ovarian.org

National Patient Air Transport Helpline
4620 Haygood Road, Suite 1
Virginia Beach, VA 23455
(800) 296-1217
www.patienttravel.org

Prostate Cancer Foundation
1250 Fourth Street, Suite 360
Santa Monica, CA 90401
(800) 757-2873
www.prostatecancerfoundation.org

Ronald McDonald House Charities
1 Kroc Drive
Oak Brook, IL 60523
(630) 623-7048
www.rmhc.org

Skin Cancer Foundation
245 Fifth Avenue, Suite 1403
New York, NY 10016
(800) 754-6490
www.skincancer.org

Smith Farm Center for the Healing Arts
1632 U Street, NW
Washington, DC 20009
(202) 483-8600
www.smithfarm.com

Susan G. Komen Breast Cancer Foundation
5005 LBJ Freeway, Suite 250
Dallas, TX 75244
(800) 462-9273
www.komen.org

United Ostomy Associations of America
19772 MacArthur Boulevard, Suite 200
Irvine, CA 92612
(800) 826-0826
www.uoaa.org

US TOO International
5003 Fairview Avenue
Downers Grove, IL 60515
(800) 808-7866
www.ustoo.org

Visiting Nurse Association of America
99 Summer Street, Suite 1700
Boston, MA 02110
(888) 866-8773
www.vnaa.org

Wellness Community National Headquarters
2716 Ocean Park Boulevard, Suite 1040
Santa Monica, CA 90405
(310) 314-2555
www.twc-wla.org

Y-ME National Breast Cancer Organization
212 West Van Buren Street, Suite 1000
Chicago, IL 60607
(312) 986-8338
www.y-me.org

APPENDIX 3

CANCER INFORMATION RESOURCES ON THE INTERNET

The World Wide Web is an extraordinary source of information about cancer, cancer treatment, health, and wellness for patients, family members, caregivers, and friends. Here is a list of some of the best Web sites that may be of assistance to you.

GENERAL CANCER INFORMATION SITES

American Cancer Society
  www.cancer.org
American Society of Clinical Oncology
  www.asco.org
Association of Cancer Online Resources
  www.acor.org
Association of Community Cancer Centers
  www.accc-cancer.org
Cancer Guide: Steve Dunn's Cancer Guide
  www.cancerguide.org
Cancer Research Institute
  www.cancerresearch.org
CancerWEB
  http://cancerweb.ncl.ac.uk
Caring4Cancer
  www.caring4cancer.com
Centers for Disease Control (CDC): Cancer Prevention and Control
  www.cdc.gov/cancer

National Cancer Institute Cancer Information Service
    http://cis.nci.nih.gov
National Society of Genetic Counselors
    www.nsgc.org
OncoLink: The University of Pennsylvania Cancer Center Resource
    www.oncolink.upenn.edu

SITES FOR SPECIFIC TYPES OF CANCER

BREAST CANCER

National Action Plan on Breast Cancer
    www.womenshealth.gov/napbc
National Breast Cancer Coalition
    www.stopbreastcancer.org
Susan G. Komen Breast Cancer Foundation
    www.komen.org
Y-ME National Breast Cancer Organization
    www.y-me.org

COLORECTAL CANCER

Colon Cancer Alliance
    www.ccalliance.org
Colorectal Cancer (CDC Cancer Prevention and Control)
    www.cdc.gov/colorectalcancer
Colorectal Cancer Network
    www.colorectal-cancer.net

LEUKEMIA/LYMPHOMA

Leukemia & Lymphoma Society of America
    www.leukemia.org
Lymphoma.com
    www.lymphoma.com
Lymphoma Foundation of America
    www.lymphomahelp.org
Lymphoma Research Foundation of America, Inc.
    www.lymphoma.org

LUNG CANCER

Lung Cancer Alliance
  www.lungcanceralliance.org
Lung Cancer Awareness Campaign
  www.lungcancer.org
Lung Cancer Online
  www.lungcanceronline.org

MYELODYSPLASTIC SYNDROMES

Aplastic Anemia and MDS International Foundation
  www.aamds.org
Myelodysplastic Syndromes (MDS) Foundation
  www.mds-foundation.org

MYELOMA

International Myeloma Foundation
  www.myeloma.org
Multiple Myeloma Research Foundation
  www.multiplemyeloma.org

OVARIAN CANCER

Gilda Radner Familial Ovarian Cancer Registry
  www.ovariancancer.com
National Ovarian Cancer Coalition
  www.ovarian.org
Ovarian Cancer (CDC Cancer Prevention and Control)
  www.cdc.gov/cancer/ovarian

PROSTATE CANCER

National Prostate Cancer Coalition
  www.fightprostatecancer.org
Prostate Cancer Foundation
  www.prostatecancerfoundation.org

Prostate Cancer Research Institute
    www.prostate-cancer.org
US TOO International: Prostate Cancer Education and Support
    www.ustoo.org

MISCELLANEOUS

American Brain Tumor Association
    www.abta.org
National Bone Marrow Transplant Link
    www.nbmtlink.org
Caitlin Raymond International Bone Marrow Registry
    www.crir.org
National Brain Tumor Foundation
    www.braintumor.org
National Cervical Cancer Coalition
    www.nccc-online.org
National Childhood Cancer Foundation
    www.curesearch.org
Pancreatic Cancer Research Center
    www.path.jhu.edu/pancreas
Thyroid Cancer Survivors' Association
    www.thyca.org

COMPLEMENTARY AND ALTERNATIVE MEDICINE SITES

Alternative Medicine
    www.alternativemedicine.com
The Cancer Project
    www.cancerproject.org
Healthweb: Alternative Medicine
    www.healthweb.org/alternative
National Center for Complementary and Alternative Medicine
    http://nccam.nih.gov
M. D. Anderson Cancer Center Complementary/Integrative
    Medicine Education Resources
    www.mdanderson.org/departments/CIMER
WholeHealthMD
    www.wholehealthmd.com

GENERAL HEALTH SITES

Health Network
    www.ahni.com
HealthWorld Online
    www.healthy.net
Office of Men's Health (OMH) Resource Center
    www.menshealthoffice.info
Office on Women's Health (OWH)
    www.womenshealth.gov/owh
WebMD Health
    www.webmd.com

SUPPORT SITES FOR PEOPLE LIVING WITH CANCER

Cancer Care, Inc.
    www.cancercare.org
Cancer Survivorship
    www.cdc.gov/cancer/survivorship
CANSearch: National Coalition for Cancer Survivorship
    www.cansearch.org
Commonweal
    www.commonweal.org
Corporate Angel Network
    www.corpangelnetwork.org
InterNet Resources for Cancer
    www.cancerindex.org/clinks1.htm
Living Beyond Breast Cancer
    www.lbbc.org
National Coalition for Cancer Survivorship
    www.canceradvocacy.org
National Organizations Offering Cancer Services
    www.cancer.gov/cancertopics/factsheet/support/organizations
National Patient Air Transport Helpline
    www.patienttravel.org
People Living with Cancer
    www.plwc.org
Smith Farm Center for the Healing Arts
    www.smithfarm.com
The Wellness Community
    www.thewellnesscommunity.org

APPENDIX 4

NCI-DESIGNATED
COMPREHENSIVE CANCER CENTERS

The following have been designated "comprehensive cancer centers" by the National Cancer Institute.

ALABAMA

University of Alabama at Birmingham
Comprehensive Cancer Center
1824 Sixth Avenue South
Birmingham, AL 35293
(205) 975-8222
www.ccc.uab.edu

ARIZONA

University of Arizona Cancer Center
1515 North Campbell Avenue
Tucson, AZ 85724
(520) 626-2900
www.azcc.arizona.edu

CALIFORNIA

Chao Family Comprehensive Cancer Center
University of California at Irvine
101 The City Drive, Building 23, Route 81
Orange, CA 92868
(714) 456-8200
www.ucihs.uci.edu/cancer

City of Hope National Medical Center and Beckman Research Institute
1500 East Duarte Road
Duarte, CA 91010
(626) 256-4673
www.cityofhope.org

Comprehensive Cancer Center and Cancer Research Institute
University of California at San Francisco
2340 Sutter Street, Box 0128
San Francisco, CA 94115
(415) 353-9888
www.cc.ucsf.edu

Jonsson Comprehensive Cancer Center
University of California at Los Angeles
10833 Le Conte Avenue
Los Angeles, CA 90095
(310) 825-5268
www.cancer.mednet.ucla.edu

Norris Comprehensive Cancer Center
University of Southern California
1441 Eastlake Avenue
Los Angeles, CA 90033
(323) 865-3000
http://ccnt.hsc.usc.edu

Rebecca and John Moores Cancer Center
University of California at San Diego
3855 Health Sciences Drive
La Jolla, CA 92093
(858) 534-7600
www.cancer.ucsd.edu

COLORADO

University of Colorado Cancer Center
1665 North Ursula Street
Aurora, CO 80045
(720) 848-0300
www.uccc.info

CONNECTICUT

Yale Cancer Center
Yale University School of Medicine
333 Cedar Street, Box 208028
New Haven, CT 06520
(203) 785-4095
www.info.med.yale.edu/ycc

DISTRICT OF COLUMBIA

Lombardi Cancer Research Center
Georgetown University Medical Center
3800 Reservoir Road, N.W.
Washington, DC 20057
(202) 444-4000
http://lombardi.georgetown.edu

FLORIDA

H. Lee Moffitt Cancer Center and Research Institute
12902 Magnolia Drive
Tampa, FL 33612
(813) 972-4673
www.moffitt.usf.edu

ILLINOIS

Robert H. Lurie Comprehensive Cancer Center
Northwestern University
676 N. St. Clair Street, Suite 1200
Chicago, IL 60611
(312) 695-0990
www.cancer.northwestern.edu

IOWA

Holden Comprehensive Cancer Center
University of Iowa
200 Hawkins Drive
Iowa City, IA 52242
(319) 356-4200
www.uihealthcare.com/depts/cancercenter

MARYLAND

The Sidney Kimmel Comprehensive Cancer Center
Johns Hopkins University
401 North Broadway
Baltimore, MD 21231
(410) 955-8964
www.hopkinskimmelcancercenter.org

MASSACHUSETTS

Dana-Farber Cancer Institute
44 Binney Street
Boston, MA 02115
(617) 632-3000
www.dfhcc.harvard.edu

MICHIGAN

Barbara Ann Karmanos Cancer Institute
Wayne State University
4100 John R.
Detroit, MI 48201
(800) 527-6266
www.karmanos.org

Comprehensive Cancer Center
University of Michigan
1500 East Medical Center Drive
Ann Arbor, MI 48109
(800) 865-1125
www.cancer.med.umich.edu

MINNESOTA

Mayo Clinic Cancer Center
200 First Street, S.W.
Rochester, MN 55905
(507) 284-9589
http://mayoresearch.mayo.edu/mayo/research/cancercenter

University of Minnesota Cancer Center
Box 806, 420 Delaware Street, S.E.
Minneapolis, MN 55455
(612) 624-8484
www.cancer.umn.edu

NEW HAMPSHIRE

Norris Cotton Cancer Center
Dartmouth-Hitchcock Medical Center
One Medical Center Drive
Lebanon, NH 03756
(603) 650-6600
www.cancer.dartmouth.edu

NEW JERSEY

The Cancer Institute of New Jersey
Robert Wood Johnson University Hospital
195 Little Albany Street
New Brunswick, NJ 08903
(732) 235-2465
www.cinj.org

NEW YORK

Herbert Irving Comprehensive Cancer Center
College of Physicians & Surgeons
Columbia University
161 Fort Washington Avenue
New York, NY 10032
(212) 305-9237
www.ccc.columbia.edu

Memorial Sloan-Kettering Cancer Center
1275 York Avenue
New York, NY 10021
(212) 639-2000
www.mskcc.org

Roswell Park Cancer Institute
Elm and Carlton Streets
Buffalo, NY 14263
(800) 767-9355
www.roswellpark.org

NORTH CAROLINA

Comprehensive Cancer Center
Wake Forest University Baptist Medical Center
Medical Center Boulevard
Winston-Salem, NC 27157
(336) 713-5440
www.wfubmc.edu/cancer

Duke Comprehensive Cancer Center
Duke University Medical Center
Box 3843
Durham, NC 27710
(919) 684-3377
www.cancer.duke.edu

UNC Lineberger Comprehensive Cancer Center
University of North Carolina Chapel Hill
102 West Drive
Chapel Hill, NC 27599
(919) 966-3036
http://cancer.med.unc.edu

OHIO

Comprehensive Cancer Center
Arthur G. James Cancer Hospital &
Richard J. Solove Research Institute
Ohio State University
300 West 10th Avenue
Columbus, OH 43210
(614) 293-3300
www.osuccc.osu.edu

Ireland Cancer Center
Case Western Reserve University
11100 Euclid Avenue
Cleveland, OH 44106
(216) 844-5432
http://cancer.case.edu

PENNSYLVANIA

Abramson Cancer Center
University of Pennsylvania
3400 Spruce Street
Philadelphia, PA 19104
(215) 662-7900
www.penncancer.org

Fox Chase Cancer Center
333 Cottman Avenue
Philadelphia, PA 19111
(215) 728-6900
www.fccc.edu

University of Pittsburgh Cancer Institute
5150 Centre Avenue, Suite 500
Pittsburgh, PA 15232
(412) 647-2811
www.upci.upmc.edu

TENNESSEE

Vanderbilt-Ingram Cancer Center
Vanderbilt University
777 Preston Research Building
Nashville, TN 37232
(615) 322-6053
www.vicc.org

TEXAS

M.D. Anderson Cancer Center
University of Texas
1515 Holcombe Boulevard, Box 91
Houston, TX 77030
(713) 792-2121
www.mdanderson.org

VERMONT

Vermont Cancer Center
University of Vermont
210 Colchester Avenue
Burlington, VT 05405
(802) 656-4414
www.vermontcancer.org

WASHINGTON

Fred Hutchinson Cancer Research Center
P.O. Box 19024
1100 Fairview Avenue North
Seattle, WA 98109
(206) 288-1024
www.fhcrc.org

WISCONSIN

Comprehensive Cancer Center
University of Wisconsin
600 Highland Avenue
Madison, WI 53792
(608) 265-1700
www.cancer.wisc.edu

ABOUT THE AUTHOR

JEREMY R. GEFFEN, MD, FACP, is a board-certified medical oncologist, a pioneer in the field of integrative medicine and oncology, and the founder of Geffen Visions International, Inc. (www.geffenvisions.com). In 1994 he founded the Geffen Cancer Center and Research Institute (GCCRI) in Vero Beach, Florida, which he directed until 2003. GCCRI was one of the first cancer centers in the United States explicitly designed to provide leading-edge, integrative care for patients and their loved ones.

Dr. Geffen is a summa cum laude graduate of Columbia University and received his MD degree with honors from New York University School of Medicine. He completed residency training in internal medicine at the University of California at San Diego Medical Center and fellowship training in hematology and oncology at the University of California at San Francisco Medical Center. He is a Fellow in the American College of Physicians and has testified before the United States Congress as an expert witness on integrative medicine and oncology.

Dr. Geffen has also traveled extensively and has more than thirty years of experience exploring the great spiritual and healing traditions of the East, including Ayurveda, Tibetan medicine, yoga, meditation, and other approaches to self-awareness. He lectures widely and offers seminars and retreats on the Seven Levels of Healing; the multidimensional aspects of health and wellness; and the interface among science, medicine, and spirituality. He also advises individuals and organizations on integrative programs for medicine and healing.